AF884701

JUNG AND THE EPIC OF TRANSFORMATION

Vol. 1

Wolfram von Eschenbach's "Parzival" and the Grail as Transformation

By Paul Bishop

CHIRON PUBLICATIONS • ASHEVILLE, NORTH CAROLINA

© 2024 by Chiron Publications. All rights reserved. No part of this publication may be reproduced, stored in a retrieval system, or transmitted, in any form by any means, electronic, mechanical, photocopying, recording, or otherwise, without the prior written permission of the publisher, Chiron Publications, P.O. Box 19690, Asheville, N.C. 28815-1690.

www.ChironPublications.com

Interior and cover design by Danijela Mijailovic
Printed primarily in the United States of America.

ISBN 978-1-68503-225-8 paperback
ISBN 978-1-68503-226-5 hardcover
ISBN 978-1-68503-227-2 electronic
ISBN 978-1-68503-228-9 limited edition paperback
ISBN 978-1-68503-497-9 limited edition hardcover

Library of Congress Cataloging-in-Publication Data

Names: Bishop, Paul, 1967- author.
Title: Jung and the epic of transformation / by Paul Bishop.
Description: Asheville, North Carolina : Chiron Publications, 2024- | Includes bibliographical references. | Contents: v. 1. Wolfram von Eschenbach's "Parzival" and the grail as transformation | Summary: "What have the Middle Ages got to do with us? For Jung, it seems, quite a lot; after all, he tells us: "I must catch up with a piece of the Middle Ages - within myself," adding: "We have only finished the Middle Ages - of others." In Wolfram von Eschenbach's "Parzival" and the Grail as Transformation, Paul Bishop considers the significance for Jung of a masterpiece of medieval German literature, and a major work in the tradition of the legendary Holy Grail. Wolfram's Parzival epic depicts a three-fold quest: for the hero's identity, for vröude ("joy"), and for the mysterious Grail. In the course of this quest, Parzival himself is transformed from a fool into the lord of the Grail, and the power of the Grail brings about a collective transformation as well. This is the first volume in a series of books, examining key texts in German literature and thought that were, in Jung's own estimation or by scholarly consent, highly influential on his thinking. The project of Jung and the Epic of Transformation consists of four titles, sequentially arranged to explore great works from a Jungian perspective and in turn to highlight their importance for interpreting The Red Book"-- Provided by publisher.
Identifiers: LCCN 2024023460 | ISBN 9781685032258 (paperback) | ISBN 9781685032265 (hardcover) | ISBN 9781685032272 (ebook)
Subjects: LCSH: German literature--History and criticism. | Jung, C. G. (Carl Gustav), 1875-1961. | Psychology and literature. | Wolfram, von Eschenbach, active 12th century. Parzival. | Goethe, Johann Wolfgang von, 1749-1832. Faust. | Nietzsche, Friedrich Wilhelm, 1844-1900. Also sprach Zarathustra. | Jung, C. G. (Carl Gustav), 1875-1961. Liber novus. | LCGFT: Literary criticism.
Classification: LCC PT143.P83 B57 2024 | DDC 830.9/002--dc23/eng/20240531 LC record available at https://lccn.loc.gov/202402346

Contents

List of Abbreviations

BB = C.G. Jung, *The Black Books, 1913-1932: Notebooks of Transformation*, ed. Sonu Shamdasani, trans. Martin Liebscher, John Peck, and Sonu Shamdasani, 7 vols. (New York and London: Norton, 2020).

CW = C.G. Jung, *Collected Works*, ed. Sir Herbert Read, Michael Fordham, Gerhard Adler, and William McGuire, 20 vols. (London: Routledge & Kegan Paul, 1953-1983). Cited in the text with volume number and paragraph reference.

DKV = Wolfram von Eschenbach, *Parzival*, ed. Eberhard Nellmann, trans. Dieter Kühn, 2 vols. (Frankfurt am Main: Deutscher Klassiker Verlag, 2006).

ETG = *Erinnerungen, Träume, Gedanken von C.G. Jung*, ed. Aniela Jaffé (Olten und Freiburg im Breisgau: Walter-Verlag, 1990).

H = *The Holy Bible, according to the Douay and Rheimish Version* [1859], ed. George Leo Haydock (Duarte, CA: Catholic Treasures, 2006).

MDR = *Memories, Dreams, Reflections of C.G. Jung*, ed. Aniela Jaffé, trans. Richard and Clara Winston (London: Routledge & Kegan Paul, 1963).

NJB = *The New Jerusalem Bible*, general ed. Henry Wansbrough (London: Darton, Longman & Todd, 1985).

PU = C.G. Jung, *Psychology of the Unconscious: A Study of the Transformations and Symbolisms of the Libido: A Contribution to the History of the Evolution of Thought*, trans. Beatrice M. Hinkle (London: Moffat, Yard, and Co., 1916) (cited with paragraph references as reprinted [London: Routledge, 1991]).

RB = C.G. Jung, *The Red Book: Liber Novus* [Reader's Edition], ed. Sonu Shamdasani, trans. Mark Kyburz, John Peck, and Sonu Shamdasani (New York and London: Norton, 2012).

SNZ = C.G. Jung, *Nietzsche's "Zarathustra": Notes of the Seminar given in 1935-1939*, ed. James L. Jarrett, 2 vols (London: Routledge, 1989).

Grail Studies
(in chronological order)

David Nutt, *Studies on the Legend of the Holy Grail: With Especial Reference to the Hypothesis of its Celtic Origin* (London: David Nutt, 1888).

Sebastian Evans, *In Quest of the Holy Grail* (London: Dent, 1898).

Arthur E. Waite, *The Hidden Church of the Holy Graal: Its Legends and Symbolism Considered in Their Affinity with Certain Mysteries of Initiation and Other Traces of a Secret Tradition in Christian Times* (London: Rebman, 1909).

Julius Evola, *The Mystery of the Grail: Initiation and Magic in the Quest for the Spirit* [1934; 1937], trans. Guido Stucco (New York: Simon & Schuster, 2018).

Emma Jung and Marie-Louise von Franz, *The Grail Legend* [1960], trans. Andrea Dykes [1970] (Boston; London; Sigo Press; Coventure, 1986).

Roger Sherman Loomis, *The Grail: From Celtic Myth to Christian Symbolism* (Cardiff and New York: University of Wales Press and Columbia University Press, 1963).

D.D.R. Owen, *The Evolution of the Grail Legend* (London: Oliver & Boyd, 1968).

John Matthews, *The Grail: Quest for the Eternal* (London: Thames & Hudson, 1981).

Richard Barber, *The Holy Grail: Imagination and Belief* (London: Allen Lane, 2004).

Giles Morgan, *The Holy Grail* (Harpenden: Pocket Essentials, 2005).

Juliette Wood, *Eternal Chalice: The Enduring Legend of the Holy Grail* (London: Tauris, 2008).

John Michael Greer, *The Ceremony of the Grail: Ancient Mysteries, Gnostic Heresies, and the Lost Rituals of Freemasonry* (Woodbury, MN: Llewellyn Publications, 2022).

Parzival/Parsifal Studies
(in chronological order)

Edwin H. Zeydel and Bayard Quincy Morgan (eds), *The "Parzival" of Wolfram von Eschenbach: Translated into English Verse with Introduction, Notes, Connecting Summaries* (Chapel Hill, NC: University of North Carolina Press, 1951).

Heinz Rupp (ed.), *Wolfram von Eschenbach* [*Wege der Forschung*, vol. 57] (Darmstadt: Wissenschaftliche Buchgesellschaft, 1966).

Wolfram von Eschenbach, *Parzival*, trans. A.T. Hatto (Harmondsworth: Penguin, 1980).

Wolfram von Eschenbach, *Parzival: Mittelhochdeutscher Text nach der Ausgabe von Karl Lachmann – Übersetzung und Nachwort von Wolfgang Spiewok* (Stuttgart: Reclam, 1981).

D.H. Green, *The Art of Recognition in Wolfram's "Parzival"* (Cambridge: Cambridge University Press, 1982).

Robert A. Johnson, *He: Understanding Masculine Psychology, Based on the Legend of Parsifal and His Search for the Grail, Using Jungian Psychological Concepts* [1974] (New York: Harper & Row, 1986).

Will Hasty (ed.), *A Companion to Wolfgang's "Parzival"* (Rochester, NY, and Woodbridge: Camden House, 1999).

Wolfram von Eschenbach, *Parzival: Studienausgabe, 2. Auflage: Mittelhochdeutscher Text nach der sechsten Ausgabe von Karl Lachmann – Übersetzung von Peter Knecht – Mit Einführungen zum Text der Lachmannschen Ausgabe und in Probleme der „Parzival"-Interpretation von Bernd Schirok* (Berlin and New York: de Gruyter, 2003).

Wolfram von Eschenbach, *Parzival: With "Titurel" and the Love-Lyrics*, trans. Cyril Edwards, and with an essay on the Munich *Parzival* illustrations by Julia Walworth (Cambridge: D.S. Brewer, 2004).

William Kinderman and Katherine R. Syer (eds), *A Companion to Wagner's "Parsifal"* (Rochester, NY, and Woodbridge: Camden House, 2005).

G. Ronald Murphy, SJ, *Gemstone of Paradise: The Holy Grail in Wolfram's "Parzival"* (Oxford and New York: Oxford University Press, 2006).

Joachim Heinzle (ed.), *Wolfram von Eschenbach: Ein Handbuch*, 2 vols in 1 [vol. 1, *Autor Werk, Wirkung*; vol. 2, *Figuren-Lexikon, Beschreibendes Verzeichnis der Handschriften, Bibliographien, Register, Abbildungen*] (Berlin and Boston: de Gruyter, 2011).

Online resource: *MediaeWiki, das Mediävistik-Wiki*, especially http://mediaewiki.de/wiki/Kategorie:Parzival

Editions cited

Wolfram von Eschenbach, *Parzival: A Knightly Epic*, trans. Jessie L. Weston [1894], 2 vols. (New York: Stechert, 1912).

Johann Wolfgang Goethe, *Faust: Parts I and II*, trans. Albert G. Latham (London; New York: Dent; Dutton, 1908).

Friedrich Nietzsche, *Thus Spake Zarathustra: A Book for All and None* [*Complete Works of Friedrich Nietzsche*, ed. Oskar Levy, vol. 4], trans. Thomas Common (Edinburgh and London: Foulis, 1909).

Acknowledgements

I should like to thank colleagues at Chiron Publications, especially Len Cruz and Steve Buser, for their interest in this project at an early stage and for their support in turning it into a reality; many thanks to Jennifer Fitzgerald for her invaluable contribution to managing the project.

I am extremely grateful to the Academic Sub-Committee of the IAAP for its financial support for this project, without which it would have not been possible to bring it to publication. And I should like to thank Joe Cambray for his advice and support, for which I am likewise extremely grateful.

Over the years I have incurred a number of debts to innumerable colleagues in *Germanistik* and Jung Studies alike, especially Roger Stephenson; Jim Walker (at Camden House); and students and colleagues in the School of Modern Languages and Cultures (SMLC) at the University of Glasgow; as well as Alan Cardew; Terence Dawson; Leslie Gardner; Phil Goss; Lucy Huskinson; Peter Kingsley; Christiana Ludwig; Martin Liebscher; Roderick Main; Catriona Miller; Susan Rowland; Andrew Samuels (and other colleagues at the Department of Psychosocial and Psychoanalytic Studies, formerly the Centre for Psychoanalytic Studies, at the University of Essex); Sonu Shamdasani; and Murray Stein (whose invitations to contribute to the Zurich Lecture Series and to *Jung's Red Book for Our Time* have repeatedly encouraged me to focus on various aspects of Jung's relation to German culture). And an invitation in 2022 from the Training Committee of the AJA (Association of Jungian Analysts) speak about the Grail Myth in relation to Jungian thinking about the transcendent function and spirituality for the JATQP (Jungian Analytic Training for Qualified Psychotherapists) program helped focus my thoughts at a crucial stage in the writing of this book.

Above all, I am grateful as always for support from Helen, not to mention Ruben.

Preface

This project consists of a series of four books examining key texts in German literature and thought that were, in Jung's own estimation or by scholarly consent, highly influential on his thinking. The works in question are Wolfram von Eschenbach's *Parzival*, Goethe's *Faust*, and Nietzsche's *Zarathustra* — all of which can be seen as notable works in a tradition of epic that culminates in Jung's *Red Book* or *Liber Novus*. These four titles are sequentially arranged to explore great works from a Jungian perspective and in turn to highlight their importance for interpreting *The Red Book*.

In part, my motivation for working on such a proposal has been the experience of lockdown during the COVID-19 pandemic and the sense that there is an appetite for returning anew to foundational texts in the Western tradition; in part, it has been because these works, while often referred to, are actually very little known beyond their titles, and so the series will aim to reawaken interest in these works and to frame *The Red Book* within a tradition I would describe as "the epic of transformation." And in part, because it seems to me that one of the achievements of Jung in *The Red Book* is to enable us to look back with fresh eyes on the sources of the Western tradition.

After all, some of Jung's key tenets were discovered (if the transcriptions of his vision in his *Red Book* are to be believed) against the backdrop of the outbreak of World War I and, in a remarkable and unexpected way, the global coronavirus pandemic that began in March 2020, the Black Lives Matter protests that took place in the summer of 2020, the outbreak of the Russo-

Ukrainian War on 24 February 2022 with the distant, yet possible, threat of nuclear war, and the Israel-Hamas conflict that began in October 2023 — all serve as a call to focus on what really matters. In the words of Angelus Silesius (c. 1624-1677), *Mensch werde wesentlich!* — "Eternal essence be! The world will fall away, / The accidental perish, essence alone will stay."[1] It is the devout wish of the present author that this series of books will encourage the reader to discover (or return to) the original works by Wolfram, Goethe, and Nietzsche, as well as to gain a new depth of appreciation for what Jung has achieved in his *Red Book*.

This first book in the series is devoted to Wolfram von Eschenbach's *Parzival*, the great medieval romance written in Middle High German which centers on one of the heroes of Arthurian legend, Perceval (as he is called in English; known as *Perceval* in French, *Parzival* in Middle High German, and *Parsifal* in modern German) and his quest for the Holy Grail. It is an unresolved question, but it is nevertheless worth asking: What *is* the Grail?

The Grail and Arthurian legend

In the Canon of the Mass according to the rites before the Second Vatican Council, the priest narrates the first offering and institution of the unbloody sacrifice by Jesus Christ at the Last Supper with his apostles in the Cenacle. After the words of consecration and the elevation of the Host, the priest places it on the corporal and adores it, before uncovering the chalice and taking it in both hands, and he then says: *Hic est enim calix sanguinis mei* ("For this is the Chalice of My Blood") … The chalice … the blood … On some accounts of the Arthurian legend of the quest for the Holy Grail, this *is* the Grail — the cup used by Jesus at the Last Supper (and, by extension, the

---

[1] Angelus Silesius, *The Cherubinic Wanderer*, trans. Maria Shrady, ed. Josef Schmidt (New York and Mahwah: Paulist Press, 1986), p. 58.

cup in which his blood was caught as it dripped from his wounds on the Cross).

In other accounts, however, the Grail is a stone; in yet another, such as *Peredur son of Efrawg* (one of the Three Welsh Romances associated with the *Mabinogion*), it is a platter which contains a kinsman's severed head, swimming in blood. Together with another artifact of the Crucifixion, the spear which the Roman centurion used to pierce the side of Christ,[2] the Grail is said to have been brought to England by Joseph of Arimathea, the rich man and disciple of Jesus to whose tomb the body of Jesus was taken for burial after his death on the Cross. Those entrusted with the custody of the Grail were descendants of Joseph and known as the Grail keepers.

In the story of the mysterious Grail, different sources mix and mingle: biblical allusion, the Arthurian cycle, Celtic myth.[3]

---

[2] The identification of the Grail legend with the lance of Longinus, the Last Supper, and the Crucifixion is explored at length by the great German scholar Konrad Burdach (1859-1936), in his last work, *Der Graal* (1938; reprinted 1974). For further discussion of the Holy Spear (otherwise known as the Holy Lance, the Lance of Longinus — after the name of the Roman centurion — or the Spear of Destiny), identified by Richard Wagner in his *Parsifal* with the bleeding spear in the Grail Castle and the spear that has wounded the Fisher King, see Franz Kirchweger (ed.), *Die Heilige Lanze in Wien: Insignie – Reliquie – Schicksalsspeer* (Vienna: Kunsthistorisches Museum, 2005); for an anthroposophical approach, emphasizing its occult significance and political implications, see Trevor Ravenscroft (1921-1989), *The Spear of Destiny: The Occult Power Behind the Spear Which Pierced the Side of Christ* [1973] (Boston, MA; York Beach, ME: Weiser Books, 1982); and, with a critique of Ravenscroft, see Alec Maclellan, *The Secret of the Spear: The Mystery of the Spear of Longinus* (London: Souvenir Press, 2004).

[3] As Henry and Renée Kahane put it in their entry on the Grail, the Grail legend has four components:

- Christian legend
- Celtic folkore
- the *Isis Book* (in the *Metamorphoses* of Apuleius, book 1, which describes the initiation into the Mysteries of Isis)
- the *Corpus Hermeticum*

(see *Encyclopedia of Religion*, general ed. Mircea Eliade (New York and London: Macmillan, 1987), vol. 6, pp. 89-94). Alternatively it has been suggested that, rather than from Celtic mythology, the core of the Arthurian and Holy Grail traditions

(Correspondingly, a study of modern [and postmodern] adaptations of the Grail legend has argued that there are three parallel trends in Grail scholarship and in how the legend has been appropriated by differing worldviews: (i) controversy over its Christian or pagan origins, (ii) attempts at secularization by way of humanism, and finally (iii) esoteric mysticism.)[4] On the Arthurian side, a key source was Geoffrey of Monmouth (c. 1095-c. 1155), a cleric from Wales (as his name suggests) and the author of a chronicle, the *History of the Kings of Britain* (*Historia Regum Britanniae*), which founded the body of literary and legendary material known as the "Matter of Britain" — as opposed, that is, to the "Matter of France," focusing on the legends of Charlemagne, and the "Matter of Rome," centered on Greek and Roman mythology, notably such military heroes as Alexander the Great and Julius Caesar, as well as the stories of the Trojan War and the adventures of Aeneas, including the founding of Rome. In the *Brut* (or the *Roman du Brut*) (c. 1155), the Norman poet Robert Wace (c. 1110- after 1174) produced a poetic version in octosyllabic couplets of Geoffrey's *Historia*. Dedicated to Eleanor, queen of Henry II, its half (or one-quarter) historical, half (or three-quarters) fictional account of the *Geste des Bretons* (or "Deeds of the Britons"), as Wace himself referred to it, related how Britain had been founded by Brutus of Troy, a legendary great-grandson of the Trojan hero Aeneas, before going on to narrate the story of King

derives rather from the folklore of the peoples of ancient Scythia (or what are now the South Russian and Ukrainian steppes); for further discussion, see C. Scott Littleton and Linda A. Malcor, *From Scythia to Camelot: A Radical Reassessment of the Legends of King Arthur, the Knights of the Round Table, and the Holy Grail* [1994] (New York and Abingdon: Routledge, 2000).

[4] See John B. Marino, *The Grail Legend in Modern Literature* (Cambridge: D.S. Brewer, 2004). The notion of the "esoteric" (even the word itself!) is controversial, but it can be defined as "that organism which consists of various teachings about the supersensory powers and effects hidden in the world and their relation to what is sensorily-physically perceptible," as Michael Frensch describes it in his historical sourcebook of esotericism; see *Lust an der Erkenntnis: Esoterik: Von der Antike bis zur Gegenwart: Ein Lesebuch*, ed. Michael Frensch (Munich and Zurich: Piper, 1991), p. 15.

Leir of Britain, the Roman conquest, the arrival of Christianity, the end of Roman rule and the Anglo-Saxon settlement, concluding on the reign of king Cadwallader (Cadwaladr ap Cadwallon) in the seventh century. Wace foregrounded the figures of King Arthur and Merlin, giving them sufficient prominence to launch the legends of the Round Table — and the French tradition of Arthurian romances, notably Chrétien de Troyes (see below).

In turn, in the late 12th and early 13th century, the English priest and poet Layamon tried to do in Middle English what Wace had done in Norman-French verse. Drawing mainly on Wace, but also on Bede's *Ecclesiastical History of the English People* and Geoffrey's *Historia Regum Britanniae*, Layamon's verse in his *Brut* uses alliteration, but also syllabic strictness, rhyme, and assonance, and he expands Wace's account of the life and deeds of King Arthur. Layamon introduced the idea that, after his last great battle, Arthur was carried away to the Isle of Avalon to recover from his wounds — awaiting his return: "And afterwards I will return to my kingdom and dwell among the Britons with great joy."[5] Between them, Geoffrey of Monmouth, Wace, and Layamon may be said to have invented the legends of King Arthur.[6]

Over time, the Arthurian legend became predominant and entered high culture: To this tradition belong the 15th-century Middle English prose reworking of the legend by Sir Thomas Malory (c. 1415-1471), *Le Morte d'Arthur* (1485), which became

[5] Wace and Layamon, *Arthurian Chronicles*, trans. Eugene Mason (London and Melbourne: Dent, 1962), p. 264. (Note that this edition translates only the Arthurian section of both works.) For further discussion, see F.H.M. Le Saux, *A Companion to Wace* (Cambridge: D.S. Brewer, 2005).

[6] For further discussion, see Leah Tether and Johnny McFadyen, with Keith Busby and Ad Putter (eds), *Handbook of Arthurian Romance: King Arthur's Court in Medieval European Literature* (Berlin and Boston: de Gruyter, 2017); Roberta L. Krueger (ed.), *The Cambridge Companion to Medieval Romance* (Cambridge and New York: Cambridge University Press, 2000); and Alan Lupack, *The Oxford Guide to Arthurian Literature and Legend* (Oxford and New York: Oxford University Press, 2005).

the definitive account of King Arthur's life and death and the associated Grail quest for later writers;[7] the revival of the Arthurian tales by Edmund Spenser (1552-1599) in his epic allegorical poem *The Faerie Queene* (1590; 1596);[8] and the cycle of 12 narrative poems about the Arthur's love for Guinevere, and the rise and fall of his kingdom, the *Idylls of the King* (written 1833-1874, published 1859-1885) by Alfred, Lord Tennyson (1809-1892), in which Sir Percivale recalls the moment when he saw the Grail:

> And in the blast there smote along the hall
> A beam of light seven times more clear than day:
> And down the long beam stole the Holy Grail
> All over covered with a luminous cloud,
> And none might see who bare it, and it past.
> But every knight beheld his fellow's face
> As in a glory, and all the knights arose,
> And staring each at other like dumb men
> Stood, till I found a voice and sware a vow.[9]

(Framed by a "Dedication" [to the Prince Consort] and an epilogue "To the Queen," and by two idylls, "The Coming of Arthur" and "The Passing of Arthur," the remaining 10 idylls are titled "Gareth and Lynette," "The Marriage of Geraint," "Geraint and Enid," "Balin and Balan," "Merlin and Vivien," "Lancelot and Elaine," "The Holy Grail," "Pelleas and Ettarre," "The Last Tournament," and "Guinevere." At one point, Sir Percivale expresses the

---

[7] For further discussion, see Elizabeth Archibald and A.S.G. Edwards (eds), *A Companion to Malory* (Cambridge: D.S. Brewer, 1996).

[8] For further discussion, see Andrew Hadfield (ed.), *The Cambridge Companion to Spenser* (Cambridge: Cambridge University Press, 2001).

[9] *Tennyson: A Selected Edition*, ed. Christopher Ricks (Harlow: Longman, 1989, p. 880. For further discussion, see F.B. Pinion, *A Tennyson Companion: Life and Works* (Basingstoke: Macmillan Press, 1984), pp. 172-194; and Laurence W. Mazzeno, *Alfred Tennyson: A Companion* (Jefferson, NC: McFarland & Company, 2020).

frustration of all those who quest for — or write books about — the Grail, when he says, "Lo, if I find the Holy Grail itself / And touch it, it will crumble into dust" [889].)

In the 19th century, the legend of the Grail exercised a huge attraction on the influential group of artists known as the Pre-Raphaelites: Dante Gabriel Rossetti (1828-1882), John Everett Millais (1829-1896), and William Holman Hunt (1827-1910). Rossetti, for instance, painted in 1855 a watercolor, "Arthur's Tomb," based on the description of the final meeting of Guinevere and Lancelot in Book 21 in Malory's *Morte d'Arthur*, and produced a number of wood engravings on Arthurian themes for a new edition of Tennyson's poems. Malory's *Morte d'Arthur* was also admired by the artist and designer William Morris (1834-1896) as well as by the painter Edward Burne-Jones (1833-1898), who produced a series of tapestries called "The Quest of the Holy Grail" (1891-1894). Meanwhile in Germany, Richard Wagner repeatedly turned to Arthurian legends (and, in his *Ring* cycle, Scandinavian and Germany mythology) for the subject matter of his operas: *Tannhäuser* (1845), *Lohengrin* (1850), *Tristan und Isolde* (1865), and his final opera, *Parsifal* (1882). (Wagner is said to have visited Rennes-le-Château in France because of its connections with the chalice around 1865; even less likely is the story that Wagner traveled to Nanteos Mansion, near Aberystwyth in North Wales, because of the Nanteos Cup, a medieval wooden bowl said to have been fashioned from a piece of the True Cross and attributed — but only from the 19th century onward — with supernatural healing properties.) In his poem *The Vision of Sir Launfal* (1848), the American Romantic poet James Russell Lowell (1819-1891), associated with the New England fireside poets, described the Grail as something attainable in a mystic vision: whereas, in Tennyson, the discoverer of the Grail is Sir Galahad, in the case of this work it is Sir Launfal:

"My golden spurs now bring to me,
 And bring to me my richest mail,
For to-morrow I go over land and sea
 In search of the Holy Grail;
Shall never a bed for me be spread,
Nor shall a pillow be under my head,
Till I begin my vow to keep;
Here on the rushes will I sleep,
And perchance there may come a vision true
Ere day create the world anew."
 Slowly Sir Launfal's eyes grew dim,
 Slumber fell like a cloud on him,
And into his soul the vision flew.[10]

At the same time, the idea emerged that the Grail legend contained a secret occult lore, passed down through the generation in parallel to the Church: Proponents of this idea included G.R.S. Mead (1863-1933), the founder of the Quest Society.[11]

In the anthroposophical tradition associated with Rudolf Steiner (1861-1925), Walter Johannes Stein (1891-1857) developed an account which identifies historical people and events in the Grail epic and, in particular, offers a reading of Wolfram von Eschenbach's *Parzival* as an esoteric document with a secret message, containing instructions on an inner path of human development.[12] "Thus

[10] James Russell Lowell, *The Vision of Sir Launfal* (Cambridge, MA: George Nichols, 1848).

[11] See Massimo Introvigne, "Grail Traditions in Western Esotericism," in Wouter J. Hanegraaff et al. (eds), *Dictionary of Gnosis & Western Esotericism* (Leiden and Boston: Brill, 2006), pp. 416-418.

[12] See W.J. Stein, *The Ninth Century and the Holy Grail* [1928], trans. Irene Groves, revised John M. Wood (Forest Row: Temple Lodge Publishing, 2009). For Steiner's own approach to the Grail, see Rudolf Steiner, *The Holy Grail: The Quest for the Renewal of the Mysteries: Selections from the Work of Rudolf Steiner*, trans. revised by Christian von Arnim (Forest Row: Sophia Books, 2001); *The Mysteries of the Holy Grail: From Arthur and Parzival to Modern Initiation*, ed. and trans. Matthew Barton

the history of the Grail," Stein maintained, "is the History of the wisdom descending from above downwards, the wisdom which was to become the vessel of love, and which became so the more, as it took its way from East to West" (80). Unhappily (and not entirely unconnected to these esoteric readings), the story of the Grail also became caught up with the Nazi interest in the occult.[13]

Inspired by the Neo-Catharism of the French mystic and historian Antonin Gadal (1877-1962) and the French magistrate and anthroposophist Déodat Roché (1877-1978), who proposed that the Grail was associated with the medieval Catharist movement of the 12th to 14th centuries, the German SS Officer and Ariosophist Otto Rahn (1904-1939) visited southern France in search of the actual Grail, in the belief that a medieval heretical sect, the Cathars — also known as the Albigensians — had hidden it there. In *Crusade Against the Grail* (1933), Rahn identified Munsalväsche in Wolfram's *Parzival* with the Cathar stronghold of Montségur (the site of the last stand against the "Albigensian crusade" launched by Pope Innocent III in 1209 that continued for decades until 1243), thus taking Wolfram's work at face value as historically valid fact.[14] In *Lucifer's Courtiers* (1937), he developed this hypothesis, suggesting that the Cathars had been Aryans, who had venerated the Grail as a symbol of Lucifer. And an even more esoteric reading of the Grail legend can be found in *In the Light of Truth: The Grail*

(Forest Row: Rudolf Steiner Press, 2010); and (based on lectures given in 1913 in Berlin) *The Mysteries of Initiation: From Isis to the Holy Grail* [*Collected Works*, vol. 144] (Forest Row: Rudolf Steiner Press, 2021). For a recent approach to *Parzival* on anthroposophical principles, see Heinz Mosmann, *Der "Parzival" Wolframs von Eschenbach: Erkenntnis und imaginative Gestaltung des Gralsmysteriums* (Stuttgart: Verlag Freies Geistesleben, 2020).

[13] Nicholas Goodrick-Clarke, *Black Sun: Aryan Cults, Esoteric Nazism, and the Politics of Identity* (New York and London: New York University Press, 2003).

[14] See Otto Rahn, *Kreuzzug gegen den Gral: Die Geschichte der Albingenser* [1933] (Engerda: Arun, 2000). For a biography of Rahn (who is said once to have remarked, "My ancestors are witches and I am a heretic"), see Hans-Jürgen Lange, *Otto Rahn und die Suche nach dem Graal* (Engerda: Arun, 1999).

Message (*Im Lichte der Wahrheit: Neue Graalsbotschaft*), published in 1926 (and in an expanded edition in 1931) by Oskar Ernst Bernhardt (1875-1941) under the pen name Abd-ru-shin (or "Son of Light" in Persian). Consisting of 91 lectures (to which a further 59 were added), this work (and Bernhardt's self-identification as the Messiah) inspired the Grail Movement, originating in Germany in the 1940s (and still internationally active today).[15]

In some respects, the 20th century was a free-for-all as far as interpretations of the Grail legend was concerned, as the case of Jessie L. Weston's study *From Ritual to Romance* (1920) shows. This work, along with Sir James Frazer's *The Golden Bough* (2 vols., 1890; 3 vols., 1900; and 12 vols., 1906-1915), was hugely influential on a poetic masterpiece and a key work in Modernism, *The Waste Land* (1922). Time and again, T.S. Eliot has recourse to motifs from the Grail story: the Fisher King, "fishing in the dull canal / On a winter evening round behind the gashouse"; a questing knight's journey through a desert landscape undertaken to the ruined Grail chapel, after which a flash of lightning brings life-renewing rains; and the remaining self-doubt of the Fisher King, who asks himself, "Fishing, with the arid plain behind me / Shall I at least put my lands in order?" In the case of the historical drama film *Perceval le Gallois* (1978) written and directed by Éric Rohmer (1920-2010) and the opera film *Parsifal* (1982) directed by Hans-Jürgen Syberberg (in which the Grail itself is represented by Wagner's Bayreuth Theatre), as well as the epic fantasy trilogy *The Lord of the Rings* by J.R.R. Tolkien (1892-1973) and the popular retellings of the Arthurian legends by T.H. White (1906-1964), to say nothing of the 1960 Broadway musical *Camelot* and the British comedy film *Monty Python and the Holy Grail* (1975), the Grail became something of a modern (or even postmodern) obsession.

[15] See Introvigne, "Grail Traditions in Western Esotericism," in Hanegraaaff et al. (eds), *Dictionary of Gnosis & Western Esotericism*, pp. 436-438.

Seven further examples confirm the pattern of a remarkable revival of interest during the 20th century in the Grail legend. First, in his encyclopedic compendium of esoteric doctrines (Masonic, Hermetic, Kabbalistic, and Rosicrucian) published as *The Secret Teachings of All Ages* (1928), the Canadian esoteric philosopher Manly P. Hall (1901-1990) placed the Grail legend along with the Arthurian tales and alchemical symbolism in the context of his view of so-called Mystic Christianity. Like the *Schethiyâ* (i.e., the divine sapphire on which the Tables of the Law were traced), the *lapis exilis* (or the crown jewel of the archangel Lucifer) is said to have fallen from heaven. During the conflict between, on the one hand, Lucifer and his legions of rebellious spirits and, on the other, Michael and the angelic hosts, the *lapis exilis* was struck from Lucifer's coronet by the flaming sword of Michael — and (in Hall's dramatic words) "the green stone fell through all the celestial rings into the dark and immeasurable Abyss," and the Holy Grail is said to have been fashioned from this "radiant gem."[16] Around this account Hall constellated a number of mystical mythologems:

- as custodian of the Grail and the spear of Longinus, Joseph of Arimathea carried them to a distant country, finally placed, according to some accounts, in Glastonbury Abbey in England, according to others in a castle on Mount Salvat in Spain (309)
- the Knights of the Holy Grail belonged to a powerful organization of Christian mystics, "perpetuating the Ancient Wisdom under the rituals and sacraments of the oracular Cup" (309)
- the quest for the Grail is "the eternal search for truth," and identifiable (in Albert G. Mackey's account of the history of

[16] Manly P. Hall, *The Secret Teachings of All Ages* [Reader's Edition] (New York: Tarcher/Penguin, 2003), pp. 308-309.

Freemasonry) with the legend of the Lost Word sought by the brethren of the Craft (309)

- the story of the Grail is an "elaboration of the early pagan Nature myth" that has become "engrafted upon the cult of Christianity," and accordingly the Grail is "a type of the ark or vessel in which the life of the world is preserved," signifying the body of the Great Mother, i.e., Nature (309)
- its green colour relates the Grail to:
    - Venus and the mystery of generation
    - Islamic faith, whose sacred color is green and whose Sabbath is Friday, the day of Venus
- thus, the Grail is a symbol of the lower (or irrational) world *and* the bodily nature of humankind → as receptacles for the living essences of superior worlds
- to the Christian, it symbolizes the heart in which "continually swirls the living water of eternal life"
- thus, the search for the Holy Grail is "the search for the real Self which, when found, is the consummation of the *magnum opus*" (309).

In the Arthurian cycle itself, Hall highlighted the "strange and mysterious figure" of Merlin — a figure of great significance for Jung (as we shall see in in Volume 4, Chapter 3). And as well as suggesting that many of the legends about Charlemagne became associated with Arthur, Hall argued that Arthur's personality represented a form of the "ever-current cosmic myth":

- as the prince of Britain, Arthur → the sun
- Arthur's knights → the zodiac
- his flashing sword → the sun's ray with which he fights and vanquishes the dragons of darkness
- the Round Table → the universe
- the *Siege Perilous* → the throne of the perfect man (590).

At the same time, in its "terrestrial sense" the figure of Arthur was the "Grand Master" of a "secret Christian-Masonic brotherhood of philosophic mystics who termed themselves *Knights*" (590), and while adding that the medieval Rosicrucians were "undoubtedly in possession of the true secret of the Arthurian Cycle and the Grail legend," Hall noted that, although it is the "most obvious of all keys to the *Christos* mystery," the Grail legend has "received the least consideration" (591).[17]

Second, in *Le Roi du monde* (1927) René Guénon (1886-1951), an exponent of the Traditionalist or Perennialist School, dedicated a chapter to the Grail. (This work took as its starting point the notion introduced by Ferdynand Antoni Ossendowski (1876-1945) in his *Beasts, Men and Gods* (1922) of the "king of thc world," a mysterious figure who is said to direct the spiritual development of humankind from Agartha, a legendary subterranean country.)[18] In its fifth chapter, Guénon rehearses those accounts that relate how the Grail chalice was fashioned by angels from an emerald that had dropped from Lucifer's forehead at the time of his fall (recalling the "urna," or Hindu frontal jewel, depicting the place of the third eye of Shiva) and that it had been entrusted to Adam in the terrestrial Paradise but lost when he was banished from Eden (26). On this account, the loss of the Grail (or of one of its symbolic equivalents) "signifies the loss of tradition with all that this conveys"; or, more precisely, that "the tradition is hidden rather than lost, or [...] that it can be lost only to lesser spiritual centres that have ceased to maintain a direct contact with the supreme centre" (27). After discussing the nature of this terrestrial Paradise, the Round Table, and the location of Mont Salvat, Guénon returned to the Grail itself, saying that "it is

[17] In 1949, Hall dedicated the first of his series of volumes, *The Adepts in the Western Esoteric Tradition*, to the "Orders of the Quest," distinguishing three main divisions in the "European descent of the Mysteries": first, the Orders of the Quest, dedicated to the "restoration of the secret sciences through search and discovery"; second, the Orders of the Great Work; and third, the Orders of Universal Reformation (Manly Palmer Hall, *The Adepts in the Western Esoteric Tradition: Orders of the Quest* (Los Angeles, CA: Philosophical Research Society, 1949), p. 7).

[18] René Guénon, *Le Roi du monde* (Paris: Charles Bosse, 1927). Cited here from *The Lord of the World*, trans. Carolyn Shaffer and Olga de Nottbeck, rev. Anthony Cheke and Anthony Blake (Ellingstring: Coombe Springs Press, 1983).

easy to see that its primary significance is basically the same as that which the sacred vase has everywhere it is found; which, especially in the East, was the sacrificial vessel which originally contained the Vedic Soma or Mazdean Haoma, the 'draught of immortality,' that bestows upon or restores to the drinker who receives it with the due rites his 'sense of eternity'" (29).[19]

Third, in his *Revolt Against the Modern World* (1934), Julius Evola (1898-1974) included an appendix titled "Mystery of the Grail." Three years later he expanded this appendix into a full-length book, published in Bari, Italy, by Laterza Publishers, whose list included works by Jung, Freud, and Richard Wilhelm. In this work, Evola proposed, as part of his "suprahistorical" analysis of medieval chivalry and sacred regality, the following three theses (as summarized by H.T. Hansen):

- the Grail was not a Christian mystery, but a Hyperborean mystery (i.e., a product of an ancient Nordic culture, since disappeared)
- the legend of the Grail is concerned with the mystery of initiation
- the Grail itself is a symbolic expression of the ambition of the Ghibellines (one of two factions, this one supporting the Holy Roman Emperor, and the other — the Guelphs — supporting the Pope) to reunite the Western world on a transcendental, spiritual basis as a new Holy Empire.[20]

---

[19] For further discussion of how, in the Grail, Guénon found "an answer" to the effects of modernity which he both described and deplored, see Simon Wilson, "René Guénon and the Heart of the Grail," *Temenos Academy Review*, 18 (2015), 146-167 (p. 146): "The Grail was perhaps *the* quintessential symbol for Guénon, containing all the meanings of the heart, of Eden and of the transcendent Centre. Our predicament, adrift as we are in the quantified and chaotic modern world, can be summed up in terms of the loss or withdrawal of the Grail. […] [T]he Grail's rediscovery promises the end of the dispersal and confusion of the modern world and a return to the paradise of light and love and vision at the heart of the world: it can also take us beyond that paradise" (p. 153).

[20] Julius Evola, *The Mystery of the Grail: Initiation and Magic in the Quest of the Spirit*, trans. by Guido Stucco (Rochester, VT: Inner Traditions, 1997), p. vii; cf.

(Evola's statement of the so-called "Traditional method" stands, mutatis mutandis, for many esoteric approaches to the Grail: "The order of things that I [...] deal with [...] is that in which all materials having a 'historical' and 'scientific' value are the ones that matter the least; conversely, all the mythical, legendary, and epic elements denied historical truth and demonstrative value acquire here a superior validity and become the source for a more real and certain knowledge," he wrote, adding: "From the perspective of 'science' what matters in a myth is whatever historical elements maybe extracted from it. From the perspective that I adopt, what matters in history are all the mythological elements it has to offer.")[21]

Fourth, in a lecture given in 1938 at the K.R. Cama Oriental Institute titled "The Legend of the Holy Grail," the Indian economist and scholar of ancient Iranian mythology Jahangir Cooverji Coyajee (1875-1936) argued that parallels between the Grail legends and aspects of Iranian epic tradition suggested that the Celts had come into contact with the cult of Mithras and its mysteries, so that "it is to Mithraism that we must turn, with confidence, to find the source of important contributions to the Grail Legend."[22] On this account, the notion of the Holy Grail can be identified with the Khvarenah, an Avestan word for the Zoroastrian concept of "divine" or "royal

pp. 23-24. In this way, Evola rephrases the definition of mythology offered by the Roman historian Sallust in *On the Gods and the World*, §4, "Now these things never happened, but always are. And Mind sees all things at once, but Reason (or Speech) expresses some first and others after. Thus, as the myth is in accord with the Cosmos, we for that reason keep a festival imitating the Cosmos, for how could we attain higher order?" (see Appendix, "Translation of the Treatise by Sallustius, 'On the Gods and the World,'" in Gilbert Murray, *Five Stages of Greek Religion* [³1955] (Mineola, NY: Dover, 2002), pp. 191-211 [p. 195]. Based on a course of lectures originally given in 1912 as *Four Stages of Greek Religion* (and revised as *Five Stages* in 1925), this work by Gilbert Murray (1866-1957) sought to defend the Olympian deities against the chthonic spirits championed by Jane Ellen Harrison (1850-1928).

[21] Julius Evola, *Revolt Against the Modern World* [*Rivolta contra il mondo moderno*, 1934], trans. Guido Stucco (Rochester, VT: Inner Traditions, 1995), p. xxxiv.

[22] J.C. Coyajee, *Studies in Shāhnāmeh* (Bombay: Taraporevala, 1939), pp. 37-126 (p. 40; cf. pp. 80-91).

glory" — a kind of divine mystical energy bestowed on kings or rulers. (Like the Khvarenah, the Grail can take various forms, but is typically associated with a dazzling radiance.)[23] Coyajee compared the Grail and the "royal glory" in five respects: (1) the nature of the Grail and the "glory," including their respective relation to the element of water; (2) the varied forms assumed by each of them (in the case of the Grail, as a stone, as a cup, and its association with the lance); (3) the character of the quest for each of them; (4) the problem of the identity of the "Fisher King," a solution to which lies in the relation between the family of the keepers of the Grail and the heroes of the quest in the *Shāhnāmeh*; and (5) the heroes of the quest and their exploits in the Grail Castle and elsewhere, including the "great fool tale" of Perceval (or Parzival) and the figure of Kai Khusrau and the hypothesis of the "Aryan expulsion and return formula," the "vengeance quest," and the theme of the quest in the Indo-Aryan texts and in the *Avesta*.

(Without citing Jung, Coyajee's work echoes his in significant respects: the attention paid to Aryan mythology, the emphasis on Mithraism, and the notion of the phenomenon of *mana*. Like Jung, Coyajee moves with ease across world mythology and in this case across the ritual theory or the Adonis theory, i.e., the hypothesis proposed by Jessie L. Weston that the basic idea of the Grail legend can be understood as an initiation into the cult of Adonis; the mysteries of Eleusis and of Samothrace; and the so-called folklore theory, i.e., the hypothesis that folklore was saturated with Mithraic conceptions in those lands where the legends of Arthur and of the Holy Grail also flourished.) On Coyajee's account, "both Iranian and Indian myths might be used to throw light on the legend of the Grail" and "the idea prevailing in ancient Irān and India on the subject were very similar"; nor should this be wondered at,

[23] For further discussion, see Jeanine Miller, "Holy Vessel, Holy Grail," *The Theosophist*, October 1989, 18-24.

since "the ancient and central mass of Aryan tradition [...] lies behind, and [...] imparts [...] remarkable similarity to the Iranian traditions," i.e., as found in the *Shāhnāmeh* as well as the *Mihir Yasht* and the *Zamyād Yasht* in the *Avesta*) as well as "the allied Indian myths" — and beyond, to Arthurian legend (126).

Fifth, in 1965 Henry R. Kahane (1902-1992) and Renée Kahane (1907-2002), Romance philologists and linguists at the University of Illinois working in collaboration with Angelina R. Pietrangeli (1907-1984), a professor of Spanish and Italian, published a study in which they argued that important elements in Wolfram's *Parzival*, including the word "grail" itself, derived from the corpus of writings attributed to the legendary Hellenistic figure Hermes Trismegistus.[24] Building on the work of the historian of religion Arthur D. Nock (1902-1963) and of the French Dominican friar and Neoplatonist scholar André-Jean Festugière (1898-1982), the Kahanes examined the features common to both Hermeticism and *Parzival* to support their claim that Wolfram worked basic concepts and characters from the *Corpus Hermeticum* into his adaptation of Chrétien's *Perceval*, discussed the historical problems involved in the transmission of a Greek text written in the second or third century in Egypt to Wolfram in the 12th century in Germany, and considered the techniques used by Wolfram in his artistic conversion of this material. On their account, for instance, the *kratēr* of Hermeticism as found in the *Corpus*

[24] Henry and Renée Kahane with Angelina Pietrangeli, *The Krater and the Grail: Hermetic Sources of the "Parzival"* (Urbana, IL: University of Illinois Press, 1965). See also their study *Magic and Gnosticism in the "Chanson de Roland"* (Oakland, CA: University of California Press, 1959). Elsewhere the Kahanes point to correspondences between the "Isis Book" of Apuleius's *Metamorphoses* (book 1, §9-§11 and §22-§23) and Chrétien's account of the Grail procession, especially details of the prelude of the Isis procession or the Anteludia; and between the Latin *Asclepius*, ascribed to Hermes Trismegistus, notably its sanctuary setting with the presence of four men; the use of the Hermetic term *malitia* (or "evil") for *agnosia* or what Chrétien calls *mal*; the motif of the wasteland in the form of an apocalyptic vision of Egypt; and conclusion of the conversion with a "pure meal."

Hermeticum (discourse 4, §4), is the same as Wolfram's *grâl*, both conceptually (as the symbol around which a select ethico-religious brotherhood gathers) and linguistically.[25]

Sixth, during the last 14 years of his life the Grail came to occupy an increasingly prominent place in the work of the theologian and Iranologist Henry Corbin (1903-1978), sometimes associated with the Traditionalist School.[26] Corbin — also a close associate of Jung —[27] viewed the Grail as representing something like the Western equivalent of the esoteric tradition of Shīʿite Islam in Iran. For Corbin, the mere coincidence in medieval France of Arthurian legend and narratives of Christ's Passion is insufficient to explain the emergence of the Grail; rather, borrowing an idea from the Persian Sufi mystic, Shihab al-Din al-Suhrawardi (1154–1191), Corbin describes the event of the encounter of these two narrative traditions as taking place in the invisible or imaginal realm of the *Malakūt* — as a spiritual event that "happens" outside social, literary, or intellectual history.[28] In this sense, the Grail belongs to the category of "spiritual facts [*faits spirituels*] constituting the history of the soul which, always in the present, breaks the irreversibility of time" and is "not simply a conjecture which results

[25] Kahane, *The Krater and the Grail*, pp. 14-15; cf. Henry and Renée Kahane, "Wolframs Gral und Wolframs Kyot," *Zeitschrift für deutsches Altertum und deutsche Literatur*, 89 (1958-1959), 191-213 (pp. 192-194). On this account, the source transmitted by Kyot to Wolfram was the *Corpus Hermeticum* attributed to Hermes Trismegistus, who appears in the mystagogic figure of Trevrizent and even in his name (*treble escient* = *Trevrizent*).

[26] See John Carey, "Henry Corbin and the Secret of the Grail," *Temenos Academy Review*, 14 (2011), 159-178 (p. 159).

[27] For further discussion, see Peter Kingsley, *Catafalque: Carl Jung and the End of Humanity*, 2 vols (London: Catafalque Press, 2018), vol. 1, pp. 363-400; vol. 2, pp. 723-771; and Henry Corbin, *Jung, Buddhism, and the Incarnation of Sophia: Unpublished Writings from the Philosopher of the Soul*, ed. Michel Cazenave (Rochester, VT: Inner Traditions, 2019).

[28] Henry Corbin, *En Islam iranien: Aspects spirituels et philosophiques*, vol. 2, *Sohrwardî et les Platoniciens de Perse* (Paris: Gallimard, 1971), pp. 166-167; cited in Carey, "Henry Corbin and the Secret of the Grail," p. 165.

from reconstituting the fading material traces of a vanished past."[29] In a long essay titled "De l'épopée héroïque à l'épopée mystique" (first delivered as an Eranos lecture in 1966), Corbin argued that "heroic" epic became "mystical" epic, "oriented" toward the spiritual dimension; as examples, he elsewhere cited *The Shepherd of Hermas*, the *Roman de la rose*, the *Chymical Wedding of Christian Rosenkreutz*, and Wagner's *Ring* cycle.[30] As the "mystical epic in the West" par excellence, the cycle of the Grail took its place alongside these works as "initiatic tales," which required reading "with new eyes, with those eyes which have long been shut in the philosophy and civilization of the West, and which our 'oriental' theosophers have kept open to the *mundus imaginalis*."[31]

Noting the way in which the Grail romances involve a hidden succession of Grail keepers outside the ecclesiastical structures of Roman Catholicism, Corbin detected — influenced by Arthur E. Waite (1857-1942) and *The Hidden Church of the Holy Graal* (1909) — the concealed presence of a subterranean Church (one paying homage to John the Apostle, not to Peter), analogous to the Shīʿite doctrine of the hidden Imām. Thus "Where is the Imām?" and "Where is the Grail?" amount to the same question, since hiddenness is a quintessential characteristic of the Grail: "Whether one says that Parsifal conveys the Holy Grail into the Orient, or that it is conveyed by Galahad to Sarras[[32]] whence it is taken up into Heaven, the event signified [...] is the same; for 'Orient' and 'Sarras' are, like Hûrqâlya, places of the 'eighth climate,' invisible to the senses of those who have not been 'baptized in the *kratēr*,'" he argues, adding: "This transfer is the tranfiguration of the mystic,

[29] Corbin, *En Islam iranien*, vol. 2, p. 155; translated in Carey, p. 166.
[30] Carey, "Henry Corbin and the Secret of the Grail," p. 167. (For a similar constellation of works on the part of Jung, see CW 15 §141, where he lists examples of the "visionary" mode of artistic creation.)
[31] Corbin, *En Islam iranien*, vol. 2, p. 365; translated in Carey, pp. 167-168.
[32] In *The Quest of the Holy Grail*, Galahad travels to the city of Sarras, beholds the mysteries within the Grail, and dies, while the Grail itself is taken up into heaven.

anticipating his personal eschatology."[33] Tellingly, Corbin believed, one of the forms taken by the Khvarenah was a vessel known as the "Cup of Jamshid" (or *jām-e Jam*), also known as the "Cup which mirrors the universe" (*jām-gītī-nemā*), and identified by Corbin as — the Grail (174).

And finally, in *Johannes ist sein Name* (1993) the Austrian Catholic Traditionalist philosopher Gerd-Klaus Kaltenbrunner (1939-2011) presented a study of the mythological figure of Prester John, the legendary Christian patriarch who was said to rule East Africa or Central Asia.[34] In his opening sentence, Kaltenbrunner declared that "Prester John has never lived and is nonetheless one of the most influential figures of the Middle Ages," going on to develop a complex picture of this "suprahistorical" (or metahistorical) individual, involving not only Prester John himself, but his spiritual ancestor John the Evangelist and his disciple John the Presbyter. Positing the existence of an esoteric school of "Johannides," Kaltenbrunner was able to link Prester John to the legend of the Holy Grail, interpreting some of the Grail epics in the light of this putative Johannide philosophy and its mythological-symbolic way of thinking.

Meanwhile, the Grail was maintaining its presence within esoteric thinking. In 1975, in *Experience of the Inner Worlds*, the appropriately named ritual magician Gareth Knight (1930-2022) included a chapter on the Grail in his self-described course in "Christian Qabalistic magic."[35] In this chapter, Knight locates the quest for the Grail in the Christian Platonic tradition, identifies the period 1100 to 1300 as two significant centuries, and surveys the

[33] Corbin, *En Islam iranien*, vol. 2, p. 154; translated in Carey, p. 172.

[34] Gerd-Klaus Kaltenbrunner, *Johannes ist sein Name: Priesterkönig, Gralshüter, Traumgestalt* (Zug/Schweiz: Die Graue Edition, 1993).

[35] "The Holy Grail," in Gareth Knight, *Experience of the Inner Worlds: A Course in Christian Qabalistic Magic* (Cheltenham: Helios Book Service, 1975; Skylight Press, 2010). My thanks to James Ellis for this reference.

Crusades, the tradition of "courtly love," and the persecution of the Cathars and the Albigensians, before turning to the resurgence of the Divine Feminine (especially in the vision of Dante), the relation between the Grail and key symbols of Celtic mythology, and finally the Matter of Britain considered as a "drama of the soul." Ultimately, he argues, the search for the Grail is "not a literary, but a practical Quest" (and, in a concluding practical exercise, he invites readers to meditate on the verse, "A Chalice shall you be, a Holy Grail, / All emptied and receptive to my filling," to regard the Grail as the "receptivity of ourselves to the divine vocation that we are called to perform," and to use the Grail as "an ace of consecration and one's readiness to become aware of the Will of God in one's own life and destiny" — while realizing that "one is never alone, however lone or long the furrow one has to plough may seem" …) (98-99).

In 1983, Knight expanded this analysis into an entire book, titled *The Secret Tradition in Arthurian Legend.*[36] Drawing both on such authors as Chrétien de Troyes, Robert de Boron, and Wolfram von Eschenbach, as well as on such works as Rudolf Steiner's *Universe, Earth and Man* (based on 11 lectures delivered in Stuttgart in August 1908) and W. Scott-Elliot's *The Story of Atlantis* (1896), Knight proposed the view that the Arthurian legends in general (and the story of the quest for the Grail in particular) enshrine "a secret Mystery Tradition that stems from beyond the Western Ocean" and was "the guiding force behind the old stone circles and the ancient trackways of Western Europe" (13). While preserved in Celtic myth and legend and recast in poetic form by the troubadours and trouvères of the 12th century, this "ancient tradition" finds unique expression in Arthurian legend, inasmuch as it provides "a complete run through from the depths of our primeval spiritual yearnings to the heights of mystical experience […] from the ancient tradition

[36] Gareth Knight, *The Secret Tradition in Arthurian Legend: The Archetypal Themes, Images and Characters of the Arthurian Cycle and the Place in the Western Magical Tradition* (Wellingborough: Aquarian Press, 1983).

of the cauldron of inspiration and rebirth won from the King of the Underworld, to Galahad, the perfect medieval Christian knight, returning his soul to God after achieving the Grail Quest" (13).

In the context of Knight's division of the Arthurian Mysteries into three primary grades (the "Lesser Mysteries" of the Grade of the Powers of Arthur, the Grade of the Powers of Merlin, and the Grade of the Powers of Guenevere, beyond which lie the "Greater Mysteries" of the Quest and Achievement of the Holy Grail) (14), Percivale (i.e., Parsifal) is seen as an "archetypal figure representing all humanity" and, as such as corresponding to the "innocent Fool of the Tarot" (110).[37] As a 12th-century version of the Fool of the Tarot, Percivale is a more universal figure than another figure of the Grail Quest legend, namely Galahad, who is said to represent "the natural sequence of the ancient Atlantean dynastic pattern conceived by Merlin, his masters and the faery women" (231). In contrast to the figure of Sir Balin (a figure found in Thomas Malory's *Le Morte d'Arthur*, based on the continuation of the second book of the Post-Vulgate cycle of legend, the *Suite du Merlin*, but not present in Eschenbach's version) who, as the "knight of the two swords," represents the "split or divided spiritual will," Percivale is a "cosmic representation of the human condition" in another respect (232). For Percivale is "the pagan innocent, the natural man who, without the Fall, would have wandered around the cycle of incarnation, blundering at first, but achieving spiritual maturity through natural experience in the created universe" (232). So whereas Balin is "the pattern of man as agent of a cosmic disaster," Percivale represents "how things would and could have been without the Fall" (232). Whereas Balin's difficulties in the relationship with the mother are reflected in his beheading of the Lady of the Lake for allegedly having murdered *his* mother, in the case of Percivale, the "innocent pilgrim

[37] For further discussion, see Caitlín Matthews and John Matthews, *The Arthurian Tarot* (Wellingborough: Aquarian Press, 1990), and *Hallowquest: Tarot Magic and the Arthurian Mysteries* (Wellingborough: Aquarian, 1990).

soul," he "comes forth into manifestation forgetting his origins in the womb of the Cosmic Mother" (235).

In his chapter on the Knights on the Grail Quest, Gareth Knight describes Percivale as "a Grail winner who brings with him much that is outside the mainstream of native Arthurian tradition," noting that his tale is developed particularly by Wolfram, "whose *Parzival* is regarded by many as one of the two great peaks of mediaeval visionary poetry" — the other being Dante's *Divine Comedy* (260). Arguing that Chrétien's tale is based on "old Celtic sources, via the Breton, adapted to Norman French court tastes" and that Wolfram's both comes from the same root as well as being "infused and transformed by later esoteric teaching from the Near East" (261), Knight's interpretation tends to draw on Malory and on the Vulgate *Queste del Saint Graal* rather than on Wolfram's *Parzival* (230) — and, in the case of his discussion of Dindrane, Percivale's sister, on *The Arthurian Poems* of Charles Williams (1886-1945) (111). Ultimately, Knight highlights how, in Wolfram's *Parzival* and especially in Albrecht von Scharfenberg's *Der jüngere Titurel*, the Grail Castle is "more universal than the parallel associations of any particular place and time," even echoing "a description of a 'model universe' so familiar to students of magic from Marsilio Ficino to the present day" and how the Grail itself in this cycle "has a more cosmic and pre-Christian ambience" (264). As the human "Fool" and an "uncouth youth" who, "unaware of his own high lineage or of the very fact of knighthood," nevertheless "through his own inherent, unrealized virtue [...] find his way to knighthood and eventual achievement of the Holy Grail," Percivale differs greatly from such other questing knights as Lancelot, Gawain,[38] Bors, and Galahad, yet common to all these stories is a key principle of the Arthurian cycles — their status as "an inspiration, instruction and

[38] For further discussion, see John Matthews, *Gawain: Knight of the Goddess: Restoring an Archetype* (Wellingborough: Aquarian Press, 1990).

challenge" and as an expression of a "a living Mystery Tradition," "embody[ing] the ultimate Vision of Perfection, reinterpreteted throughout the ages for different times and seasons" (271).

Subsequently, in the 1980s, a new controversy over the Grail had emerged in the form of the book *The Holy Blood and the Holy Grail* (1982), coauthored by Michael Baigent (1948-2013), Richard Leigh (1943-2007), and Henry Lincoln (1930-2022). In 1969, during a holiday in France, Lincoln happened to come across a book called *Le Trésor Maudit de Rennes-le-Château* (or "The Accursed Treasure of Rennes-le-Château"), the paperback edition of *L'Or de Rennes, ou La Vie insolite de Bérenger Saunière, curé de Rennes-le-Château* (or "The Gold of Rennes, or The Strange Life of Bérenger Saunière, Priest of Rennes-le-Château"), written by Gérard de Sède (in collaboration with Pierre Plantard) and first published in 1967 (and as a paperback in 1968). At the center of this book was the apparently mysterious story of Bérenger Saunière, a former priest at Rennes-le-Château, and an alleged secret (in the form of hidden treasure and/or documents), and this became the basis for a series of documentaries for BBC Television in its *Chronicle* series ("The Lost Treasure of Jerusalem," broadcast in February 1972; "The Priest, the Painter and the Devil," broadcast in October 1974; and "The Shadow of the Templars," shown in November 1979).

In turn, these documentaries laid the groundwork for the central thesis of Baigent, Leigh, and Lincoln, namely, that Jesus had been married to Mary Magdalene and that their children (or their descendants) had traveled to southern France, where they had intermarried with noble families and founded the Merovingian dynasty, whose claim to the throne of France was supported by a secret society called the Priory of Sion. Thus, the Holy Grail was a symbol of the womb of Mary Magdalene — or, more precisely, of the sacred royal bloodline to which she had given birth. In short, their entire thesis is captured in a play on words: the Holy Grail (= *San Greal* = *San Graal* = *Sangréal*) is really the Royal Blood (= *Sangréal*

= *Sang Réal* = *Sang Royal*).[39] Into this semantic and argumentational vessel, a whole host of conspiracy theories and esoteric doctrines could be poured: Mary Magdalene was Jesus's wife and the bearer of the true Christian message, Leonardo da Vinci and others were in on this secret as members of the secretive Priory of Sion, the *Protocols of the Elders of Zion* reveals the Priory's master plan, etc.

Together, Baigent, Leigh, and Lincoln went on to write a sequel, *The Messianic Legacy* (1986), while Baigent and Leigh followed this up with *The Temple and the Lodge* (1989). Other writers have jumped on this band waggon: in 1993 Margaret Starbird (b. 1942) published *The Woman with the Alabaster Jar: Mary Magdalene and the Holy Grail*, repeating the hypothesis that Jesus and Mary Magdalene had been married and that Mary Magdalene *was* the Holy Grail, and adding the claim that Saint Sarah (whose name in Hebrew means "Princess"), associated with the legend of the cult at Saintes-Maries-de-la-Mer, was their daughter and the forgotten descendant of the *sang real,* or the royal bloodline, of the King of the Jews. And in 1996 the "alternative historian" Laurence Gardner (1943-2010) published *Bloodline of The Holy Grail: The Hidden Lineage of Jesus Revealed*, which quickly became a *Sunday Times* bestseller and was followed by *Genesis of the Grail Kings: The Astonishing Story of the Ancient Bloodline of Christ and the True Heritage of the Holy Grail* (1999) and by *Realm of The Ring Lords: The Ancient Legacy of the Ring and the Grail* (2003). This body of work as a whole (or, as Baigent and Leigh were to argue in a famous lawsuit, *The Holy Blood and the Holy Grail* in particular) became the inspiration in 2003 for the bestselling novel by the American novelist Dan Brown called *The Da Vinci Code*

[39] This etymology was originally proposed in the 15th century by the English chronicler John Hardying (1378-1465), and it was subsequently adopted by Malory (see Richard Barber, *The Holy Grail: Imagination and Belief* (London: Allen Lane, 2004), pp. 213-215; and Juliette Wood, *Eternal Chalice: The Enduring Legend of the Holy Grail* (London and New York: Tauris, 2008), pp. 36-37).

(and in 2006 its film adaptation). Not surprisingly, these pseudo-historical theses have provoked a number of critiques, including Damian Thompson's *Counterknowledge: How We Surrendered to Conspiracy Theories, Quack Medicine, Bogus Science and Fake History* (2008), yet the remarkable success of the Holy-Blood-Holy-Grail thesis does not just prove the validity of the remark attributed to G.K. Chesterton — namely, that "when people stop believing in God, they don't believe in nothing, they believe in everything" — but also points to the lasting, perennial fascination of the Grail *as a symbol*, that is, as a cultural-historical archetype.

Most recently, Ralph Ellis — an independent researcher into biblical and Egyptian history — has developed an account of the Grail that forms part of a wider set of remarkable claims about biblical history; tellingly, this radical reassessment of Arthurian history is published as the *fourth* (!) volume of the "King Jesus Trilogy."[40] According to Ellis:

- the history of King Arthur was modeled upon the life of Jesus
- Jesus-Arthur had 12 disciple-knights of the Round (Last Supper) Table
- the son of Jesus-Arthur was the king of Palmyra in Syria.

In short, Ellis's "radical reassessment" of Arthurian history is based on the premise that the Classical Arthur never actually existed, a claim which seeks to explain why, until the early 12th century, there is no mention of King Arthur for nearly 600 years.

On this account, the Arthurian genre was only born when the Templar Crusaders returned to Normandy from Syria and Judaea because King Arthur served as an alter ego for the biblical King Jesus of Judaea and Edessa. Although the Templar Crusaders had

[40] Ralph Ellis, *The Grail Cypher: The Secrets of Arthurian Legends Revealed* (Chester: Edfu Books, 2015; expanded 2017). The other titles in this "trilogy" are *Cleopatra to Christ* (2006), *King Jesus* (2008), and *Jesus, King of Edessa* (2012), in addition to which a fifth volume has appeared, *Mary Magdalene: Princess of Orange* (2011).

discovered in Syria a manuscript revealing the true monarchical and military life of King Jesus and his family, the heretical and consequently dangerous nature of this historical insight led to the Norman Templars confecting an alternative pseudo-history about a "British" monarch called King Arthur, effectively recording and preserving while disguising this history. On the basis of this premise, Ellis goes on to make a series of even more startling claims, including that St Peter had been a guardian of the Holy Grail, that the Grail itself had been brought to Earth by aliens (or, as Wolfram von Eschenbach called them, angels), and that Jesus-Arthur is buried at Stonehenge.

So much for its reception in the 20th century. What can be said about the origin of the Grail legend?

An overview of the main sources for the Grail legend may be presented as follows:

1. Chrétien des Troyes's *Perceval ou le Conte du Graal*, together with:
    (a) a first continuation attributed to (Pseudo-)Wauchier de Denain
    (b) a second continuation, also attributed to (Pseudo-)Wauchier
    (c) a third continuation by Manessier
    (d) a fourth continuation by Gerbert de Montreuil
2. the cycle of Robert de Boron, which includes:
    (a) *Joseph of Arimathea*
    (b) *Merlin*
    (c) *Perceval*
3. the so-called *Grand Saint Graal*, a French prose romance (early 13th century)
4. the *Perlesvaus* (edited by Charles Potvin as *Perceval le Gallois, ou le Conte du Graal*), written in prose
5. the *Queste del Saint Graal* → the penultimate part of the *Lancelot* cycle, written in prose

6. Wolfram von Eschenbach's *Parzival*, associated with
   (a) Albrecht von Scharfenberg's *Der jüngere Titurel* (or *The Younger Titurel*)
   (b) the *Sängerkrieg* (minstrel contest) or the *Wartburgkrieg* (Wartburg contest) held at Wartburg, a castle in Thuringia, in 1207
7. Sir Thomas Malory's *Le Morte d'Arthur*
8. Heinrich von dem Türlin's *Diu Crône* (or *The Crown*)

The *Urtext* (or "primordial text"), if such a thing can be said to exist, is *Perceval or the Story of the Grail* (*Perceval ou le Conte du Graal*), the last and unfinished verse romance by Chrétien de Troyes, written in Old French in the late 12th century.[41] Chrétien's patron was Marie of France, Countess of Champagne (1145-1198), and in five major poems composed in rhyming eight-syllable couplets, he brought Arthurian legend into high literary tradition. Preceding the incomplete *Perceval or the Story of the Grail* (written between 1181 and 1190), Chrétien had written four courtly epics in the 1170s: *Erec and Enide* (c. 1170), *Cligès* (c. 1176), *Yvain or the Knight of the Lion* (c. 1180) and *Lancelot or the Knight of the Cart* (c. 1180). In his final work, one notices some immediate differences between the later Grail tradition and Chrétien's understanding of the Grail: He refers to "*a* grail" (*un graal*), not *the* Grail; he does not describe it as holy; and equal significance accrues to the lance, which appears at the same time.

Despite sticking strictly to the traditional form of octosyllabic verse in rhymed couplets, Chrétien used this form with

[41] For the original Old French and a modern French translation, see Chrétien de Troyes, *Œuvres complètes*, ed. Daniel Poirion et al. (Paris: Gallimard, 1994), pp. 683-911; and for an English translation, see Chrétien de Troyes, *Arthurian Romances*, trans. D.D.R. Owen (London: Dent, 1987), pp. 374-495. For further discussion, see Rupert T. Pickens, "*Le Conte du Graal*: Chrétien's Unfinished Last Romance," in Norris J. Lacy and Joan Tasker Grimbert (eds), *A Companion to Chrétien de Troyes* (Cambridge: D.S. Brewer, 2005), pp. 169-187.

considerable sophistication: He creates a remarkable variety of rhythms, achieves a striking fluency of expression, shows himself to have been a master of dialogue, and demonstrates a richness of vocabulary.[42] Even if he describes Chrétien's technique of using existing motifs as revealing him to be "a more brilliant re-creator than creator," D.D.R. Owen recognizes that this "lack of outright inventiveness" was disguised by "a mask of new detail" (xii). Owen suggests that there is "no reason" not to take Chrétien at his word when he claims to have derived his romances from some kind of written or oral source — and, in the case of *Cligés* and the *Conte du Graal*, from a book. In no case, however, do we actually have access to a source that could have served as a prime model for any of his romances, although three texts in the collection of Welsh prose tales, the *Mabinogion*, are of particular relevance to Chrétien.[43] (The Celtic sources in the *Mabinogion* and, in particular, the tale of Culhwch and Olwen, were analyzed from a psychological perspective by the anthropologist and Jungian analyst John Layard [1891-1974] in a posthumously published study in 1975.)[44] Chrétien's originality, then, lies in part in *how* he uses his sources, and, in the case of *Cligés* and *Lancelot*, presenting stories of adulterous love in terms of one of the great Christian mysteries surrounding the Crucifixion, death, and Resurrection of Christ, including his Harrowing of Hell (xv). The challenge remains for the reader, then (in medieval times) as now, in discerning, amid these fantastic tales of adventure, what Chrétien in his prologue

[42] D.D.R. Owen, "Introduction," in Chrétien de Troyes, *Arthurian Romances*, trans. Owen, pp. ix-xviii (pp. xi-xii).
[43] The tales in question are "Gereint Son of Erbin," "The Lady of the Fountain" (or "Owein"), and "Peredur Son of Efrawg"; see *The Mabinogion*, trans. Gwyn Jones and Thomas Jones (London; New York: Dent; Dutton, 1974).
[44] John Layard, *A Celtic Quest: Sexuality and Soul in Individuation*, ed. by Anne S. Bosch (Dallas, TX: Spring Publications, 1985). For more recent discussion of Celtic analogues of the French Arthurian cycle, see John Carey, *Ireland and the Grail* [Celtic Studies Publications, 11] (Aberystwyth: Celtic Studies Publications, 2007).

to *Lancelot* defined as their *sen*, that is, their implicit meaning (including a moral one) (xv).

On the one hand, the topic of sexual relationships seems to have been at the forefront of Chrétien's mind. In *Erec*, a happy marriage leads a husband to neglect his duties as a knight, causing him to set out in search of opportunities to prove his valor — with his forbearing spouse as witness. In *Yvain*, we find the reverse situation: This time a hero abandons his bride all too soon after winning her, putting love at risk and prompting him to turn *away* from tournaments to establish his reputation as a worthy husband. In *Cligés*, two tales explore the blossoming of young love — and the conversion of extramarital passion into honorable fulfillment. In *Lancelot*, the adulterous love of a knight for his lord's wife is the central theme. And in *Perceval,* we see the development of true love, while the figure of Gawain reminds us how easy it is to be deflected by romance from the path of duty (xvi).

On the other, an even more important topic is the question of chivalry. In *Erec*, the service of society is contrasted with the private world of love. In *Yvain*, domestic approval is contrasted with the search for adventure and glory. In *Cligés*, the relationship between honor and love is explored in the context of the chivalric ethic. In *Lancelot*, love is shown to have the power to make the wise look foolish. And in the case of *Perceval*, we shall never know — because the work is incomplete — whether Perceval's tentative apprenticeship in courtly love would prove to be the beginning of his initiation into the chivalric ethic and whether Gawain would learn from the error of his romantic ways (xvi-xvii).

Yet as D.D.R. Owen suggests, ultimately these are two aspects of the same chivalric coin: In *Erec*, the purity of love is shown as leading to an ideal marriage; in *Yvain*, passion can be subordinated to marital vows; in *Lancelot*, untutored passion leads to adultery; and in the case of *Perceval*, the challenges of the relation between love and chivalry remain unresolved because the work was never completed. On Owen's account, Chrétien was "a man of intellect rather than of high emotion," inasmuch as "for him with his schoolman's training the debate held greater delights than the declaration of preconceived truths"; indeed, Owen even goes so far as to detect the possibility of an ironic dimension to Chrétien's works, suggesting that he "flaunted the high ideal, while constantly hinting that this was but a poet's dream" (xvii-xviii). In his opening *incipit* to *Perceval ou le Conte du Graal,* Chrétien claims to have used a written source, referring to a book given to him by Philip I, Count of Flanders, known as Philip of Alsace (1143-1191), and to have been commanded by Philip "to tell in rhyme the finest story ever related in a royal court" — the "story of the Grail" (ll. 63-68; trans. Owen, pp. 374-375). And he places the work in a theological framework, doing so in the prologue in two respects. First, by citing Jesus's words on the need for almsgiving in secret and the advice, "let not thy left hand know what thy right hand doth" (Matthew 6:3), and interpreting the left hand as signifying "vainglory, which stems from false hypocrisy," and the right hand as "charity, which does not boast of its good works" (ll. 39-44; trans. Owen, p. 374). And second, by quoting (as will later Wolfram) from the First Epistle of St. John, "God is charity: and he that abideth in charity, abideth in God, and God in him" (4:16) — although curiously he misattributes this quotation to St. Paul (perhaps because Paul, in his First Epistle to the Corinthians, penned his famous encomium of love [13:1-13]) (ll. 47-50; trans. Owen, p. 374).

When it makes its appearance in *Perceval*, however, the Grail is simply — well, a grail, inasmuch as it is neither a holy relic nor associated with the blood of Christ. Nevertheless, the sheer drama of the scene has something compelling about it:

> A damsel, who came with the youths
> and was fair and attractive and beautifully adorned,
> held in both hands a grail.

Once she had entered
with this grail that she held,
so great a radiance appeared
that the candles lost their brilliance […].
After her came another maiden,
holding a silver carving-dish.
The grail, which proceeded ahead,
was of pure refined gold.
And this grail was set with
many kinds of precious stones,
the richest and most costly
in sea or earth:
those stones in the grail
certainly surpassed all others. […]
The young man [i.e., Perceval] saw them pass,
but did not dare ask
who was served from the grail,
for he kept continually in his heart
the words of that wise gentleman [i.e., Gornemant].

(ll. 3220-3228 and 3230-3239 and 3243-3247; trans. Owen, p. 417)

On this occasion in the castle of the wounded Fisher King,[45] the grail is not described as a cup but rather as a kind of dish or platter, nor is it associated with blood, but its miraculous properties become clearer in a later episode when the hermit (who turns out to be Perceval's uncle) explains the relationship between the Fisher King and the Grail:

[45] The Fisher King (*roi pêcheur*) is sometimes called the Rich Fisher (*riche pêcheur*), a semantic ambiguity which opens up vast interpretative possibilities, given Jung's interest (notably in *Aion*) in the fish as a symbol of Christ on the basis of the first-century acrostic, Ἰησοῦς Χρῖστός Θεοῦ Υἱός Σωτήρ (*Iēsoûs Khrīstós, Theoû Huiós, Sōtḗr*, i.e., "Jesus Christ, God's Son, Savior").

And the rich Fisher King, believe me, is
the son of that king who has himself
served from the grail.
But don't imagine he has
pike, lamprey or salmon:
he's served with a single conscrated wafer
brought to him in that grail —
that supports his life in full vigour,
so holy a thing is the grail
[*Tant sainte chose est li Graax*].

(ll. 6417-6425; trans. Owen, p. 459)

Here the Grail is imagined as a dish large enough to contain a fish, yet its mysterious power lies in the fact that it contains just a single Communion wafer (*oiste*), which is sufficient to sustain the Fisher King's crippled father (and has done so, the hermit adds, for 12 years). We are certainly far removed from a later continuation of the *Perceval* romance which talks in another context of a hundred boars' heads being served on grails (*graaus*)![46] For Chrétien died before having completed the work, which breaks off abruptly after line 9234, in the midst of a subplot about how Gawain liberates a castle whose inhabitants include his long-lost mother (Morgause), his grandmother (Ygerne), and his sister (Clarissant). Subsequently, in a series of texts known as the *Four Continuations*, to which two prologues known as the *Elucidation* and *Bliocadran* should be added, various writers tried to complete what Chrétien had left unfinished.[47]

---

[46] *Continuations of the Old French Perceval*, ed. William Roach (Philadelphia: University of Pennsylvania Press, 1949), vol. 1, *The first Continuation, Redaction of mss. TVD*, p. 262. Cf. *Sir Gawain and the Lady of Lys*, trans. Jessie L. Weston [Arthurian Romances Unrepresented in Malory's "Morte d'Arthur," no. 7] (London: David Nutt, 1907), p. 29.

[47] For an English translation, see *The Complete Story of the Grail: Chrétien de Troyes' "Perceval" and its Continuations*, trans. Nigel Bryant (Cambridge: D.S. Brewer, 2015). For further discussion, see Annie Combes, "The Continuations of the

In the *First Continuation*, formerly attributed to Wauchier de Denain, the figure of Gawain moves to the fore.[48] In one episode, he sees the Grail and, accompanying it, a lance; and he tries to mend a broken sword (107-109). The account of the procession of the Grail is reminiscent of Chrétien's, but on the second occasion when he sees the Grail again (and learns that the bleeding lance is the one that Longinus, the Roman soldier, had plunged into the side of Christ on the cross), there is a far greater emphasis on its physical power:

> And then, coming through a door, Sir Gawain saw the wondrous grail, which promptly served the bread, placing it swiftly before all the knights. Then it performed the butler's duty, serving the wine in great goblets of fine gold, setting them on every table for lords and retainers alike. Without more ado it served the next course to each table in great silver bowls. Sir Gawain gaped in astonishment as the grail served them so, with no other servant to be seen — he was utterly amazed: he could hardly bring himself to eat. [...] It was a long and leisurely meal, and all the while the grail served them with perfect, brisk and wondrous ease. (216)

By contrast, it is in the trilogy of prose romances attributed to Robert de Boron around 1180 or 1190 that other contours of the Grail legend as we customarily think of it emerge.

Conte du Graal," in Lancy and Grimbert (eds), *A Companion to Chrétien de Troyes*, pp. 191-201.

[48] In the Middle English tradition, Gawain is at the center of the 14th-century alliterative poem *Sir Gawain and the Green Knight*, thought to be written by the same author who wrote *Pearl*, *Cleanness*, and *Patience*. For further discussion, see Derek Brewer and Jonathan Gibson (eds), *A Companion to the Gawain-Poet* (Cambridge: D.S. Brewer, 1997).

It is Boron, for instance, who identifies the chalice of the Last Supper with the one obtained by Joseph of Arimathea from Pilate and used to collect Christ's blood after his removal from the Cross. (In his account Boron seems to have drawn on the apocryphal Gospel of Nicodemus.) During his imprisonment by the Jewish authorities, Joseph survives by contemplating the Grail. Twelve years later, he is set free by the emperor Vespasian, and leaves Palestine, creating a prototype of the Round Table by founding a society of adepts who are united by sitting around a table. (One of the seats is to remain vacant, as a reminder of Judas Iscariot, and reserved for a descendant of Joseph's brother-in-law, Bron. In later Arthurian legend, this seat becomes the Siege Perilous, a seat at the Round Table kept vacant by Merlin for the successful knight in the quest for the Grail.)

As commanded by God, Joseph passes the Grail to his brother-in-law Bron, who is called the "rich Fisher King." Together with his wife (and Joseph's sister), Enigeus, Bron has 12 sons, the last of whom, Alain, remains celibate and receives instruction from his uncle Joseph. Alain is sent into the West, and God tells Joseph that "just as the world is and always will be moving towards night, so must Bron and his people move towards the setting sun — into the West": "As soon as the Fisher King has the vessel and grace bestowed upon him, he must journey westward, wherever his heart leads him. And where he comes to rest, there he must await the coming of the son's son" — who will in turn becomes the guardian of the Grail (42-43). In Boron's *Joseph of Arimathea*, his *Merlin*, and his *Perceval*, the biblical associations, the Arthurian associations, and the link to the figure of Merlin all become clearer.[49] (This trilogy is known as the Little or Lesser Grail Cycle, to distinguish it from the Lancelot-Grail or Vulgate Cycle; see below).

[49] For an English translation, see *Merlin and the Grail: Joseph of Arimathea, Merlin, Perceval*, trans. Nigel Bryant (Cambridge: D.S. Brewer, 2001).

Dating to the first decade of the 13th century, another romance in Old French known as the *Perlesvaus* or *Li Hauz Livres du Graal* (*The High Book of the Grail*) represents another attempt at a continuation of Chrétien's unfinished work.[50] It differs from other versions by purporting to be a translation of a supposed Latin source found in Avalon and attributed to someone called Josephus (presumably the Jewish historian, Flavius Josephus [c. 37-c. 100]) in an attempt to lend their work authenticity: "The Latin text from which this story was set down in the vernacular was found in the Isle of Avalon, in a holy abbey which stands at the edge of the Lands of Adventure; there lie King Arthur and the queen, by the testimony of the worthy monks who dwell there, and who have the whole story, true from the beginning to the end."[51] Whereas in Chrétien's *Perceval ou le Conte du Graal* the Grail is depicted as something rich and splendid, and associated in some strange way with the Mass, and in Wauchier's *Continuation* as something preeminently physical (dishing out food and drink aplenty), in the *Perlesvaus,* the Grail seems hardly material at all and more like some sort of mystic aura. At one point (in Branch 6, §19-§20), viewing the Grail seems to plunge Gawain into a kind of catatonic state:

> Suddenly two maidens appeared from a chapel: in her hands one was carrying the Holy Grail [...] Sir Gawain gazed at the Grail and thought he saw therein a chalice, which at that time was a rare sight indeed [or: albeit

[50] See *Le Haut Livre du Graal: Perlesvaus*, ed. William A. Nitze and T. Atkinson Jenkins, 2 vols (Chicago, IL: University of Chicago Press, 1932-1937; reprinted New York: Phaeton Press, 1972). For an English translation, see *The High Book of the Grail: A Translation of the Thirteenth-Century Romance of Perlesvaus*, trans. Nigel Bryant (Cambridge: D.S. Brewer, 2007).

[51] *The High Book of the Grail*, trans. Bryant, p. 272; cf. Nitze and Jenkins (eds), *Perlesvaus*, vol. 2, pp. 176-179; and Benn Ramm, "Locating Narrative Authority in *Perlesvaus: Le Haut Livre du Graal*," in *Arthurian Literature XII*, ed. Keith Busby and Roger Dalrymple (Cambridge: D.S. Brewer, 2005), pp. 1-19 (pp. 12-13).

> none there was as at this time] [...] Sir Gawain was deep in thought, so deep in joyful thought that he could think only of God. [...] Then the two maidens came out of the chapel and passed once more before Sir Gawain. And he thought he saw three angels where before he had seen but two, and in the Grail he thought he could see the figure of a child. The foremost knight cried out to Sir Gawain, but he, looking before him, saw three drops of blood drip on to the table, and was so captivated by the sight that he did not say a word. [...] Thereupon the two maidens passed once more before the table, and to Sir Gawain it seemed that there were three; and looking up it appeared to him that the Grail was floating in mid-air. And above it he saw, he thought, a crowned king nailed to a cross, and the lance was thrust in his side. Sir Gawain was filled with sorrow at the sight, and he could think of nothing save the pain that the king was suffering. Again the foremost knight cried out to him to speak, saying that if he delayed longer, the chance would be lost forever. But Sir Gawain remained gazing upwards in silence, hearing nothing that the knight had said.[52]

Aside from its emphasis — in common with Chrétien and other versions — on the importance of the Grail lineage (which can leave the reader struggling with the complex genealogies), the *Perlesvaus* is strikingly different in tone and in focus: harsher and darker than other Arthurian romances, its focus shifts from Perceval to the other knights of the Round Table and their quest for the Grail, notably Lancelot and Gawain.

---

[52] *The High Book of the Grail*, trans. Bryant, p. 68; cf. Loomis, *The Grail: From Celtic Myth to Christian Symbol*, pp. 116-117.

The length of these works varies, but taken in their entirety, they are less than the Lancelot-Grail or Vulgate Cycle of the 13th century.[53] This cycle of chivalric romances expands on the work of Chrétien and Robert de Boron by chronicling a number of episodes in the legend of Arthur, including the quest for the Grail but also the affair between Lancelot and Guinevere. The over 150 surviving manuscripts of the Cycle from the 13th, 14th, and 15th centuries can be arranged in various ways:

- *History of the Holy Grail* (*L'Estoire del Saint Graal*), relating how Joseph of Arimathea and his son, Josephus, bring the Grail over to England
- *History of Merlin* (*L'Estoire de Merlin*), or the Vulgate Merlin, consisting of
    - the Merlin Proper (or *Roman de Merlin*)
    - the *Story of Merlin* (or *Suite du Merlin*), also known as *The First Deeds of King Arthur* (*Les Premiers Faits du roi Arthur*)
- the Lancelot Trilogy (*Lancelot en prose*, *L'Estoire de Lancelot*, or the *Lancelot–Queste–Mort Artu* trilogy):
    - the Vulgate Lancelot Proper (*Lancelot propre*, or the *Roman de Lancelot* or just *Lancelot du Lac*) is inspired by and partially based on Chrétien's *Lancelot*, and constitutes half of the entire cycle.
- *The Quest for the Holy Grail* (the Vulgate *Queste del Saint Graal*), which relates how the quest for Grail is achieved by Galahad, Lancelot's son
- *The Death of King Arthur* (the Vulgate *Mort le roi Artu*)

[53] For further discussion, see Carol Dover (ed.), *A Companion to the Lancelot-Grail Cycle* (Cambridge: D.S. Brewer, 2003), and William W. Kibler (ed.), *The Lancelot-Grail Cycle: Text and Transformations* (Austin: University of Texas Press, 1994).

In the edition together with a modern French translation of the Vulgate Cycle undertaken by Daniel Poirion in three volumes for the Pléiade between 2001 and 2009, the works are arranged as follows:

- Volume 1
    - *Joseph of Arimathea* (*Joseph d'Arimathie*)
    - *Merlin* (*Merlin*)
    - *The First Deeds of King Arthur* (*Les Premiers Faits du roi Arthur* or *Suite du Merlin*)
- Volume 2
    - *The Marche de Gaule*
    - *Galehaut*
    - First Part of *The Quest of Lancelot* (*La Quête de Lancelot I*)
- Volume 3:
    - Second Part of *The Quest of Lancelot* (*La Quête de Lancelot II*)
    - *The Quest of the Holy Grail* (*La Quête du Saint Graal*)[54]
    - *The Death of King Arthur* (*La Mort du roi Arthur*) [55]

Just as this Cycle was preceded by the Lesser Cycle of Robert de Boron's *Joseph of Arimathea*, *Merlin*, and *Perceval*, so in its turn the *Lancelot-Grail* Cycle was followed, after revision in the 1230s, by the much shorter Post-Vulgate Cycle, also known as the *Roman du Graal*. Here the main figure is no longer Lancelot and the story of his affair with Guinevere, and the focus shifts instead onto the quest for

[54] *The Quest of the Holy Grail*, trans. Pauline Matarasso (Harmondsworth: Penguin, 1969).
[55] *The Death of King Arthur*, trans. James Cable (Harmondsworth: Penguin, 1971).

the Grail, while the significance of a new figure emerges — Tristan, and the story of his affair with Iseut, taking this Celtic legend that had been turned into a medieval chivalric romance (as found in the *Prose Tristan* of the 1230s or 1240s) and weaving it into the Arthurian legend. This Cycle is conventionally divided into four parts:

- the Post-Vulgate *Estoire del Saint Graal*, telling the story of Joseph of Arimathea and his son, Josephus, bringing Grail to England
- the Post-Vulgate *Estoire de Merlin*, relating the story of Merlin and the early years of Arthur, including the Post-Vulgate *Suite du Merlin* (or the Huth-*Merlin*) with its additional material about the adventures of Arthur and his Knights of the Round Table (including the incestuous birth of his treacherous illegitimate son, Mordred, and his gift of the sword Excalibur from the Lady of the Lake)
- the Post-Vulgate *Queste del Saint Graal*, describing the search for the Holy Grail, achieved only by Galahad, Percival, and Bors, while including elements from the Prose *Tristan*
- the Post-Vulgate *Mort Artu*, recounting Arthur's death at the hands of Mordred and the subsequent collapse of his kingdom.

Into the midst of this rich, vibrant tradition in Old French (as well as Middle Welsh) there bursts — in the first quarter of the 13th century — the figure of Wolfram von Eschenbach, a knight-poet writing in Middle High German. Some 20 years or so after Chrétien had abandoned his narrative, Wolfram began to write his own version of the story of the Grail.

Wolfram von Eschenbach's *Parzival*

About Wolfram himself we know very little, other than that he is said to have come from Ober-Eschenbach (or as it now calls itself, Wolframs-Eschenbach) in Franconia, bordering on northern Bavaria in the center of southern Germany — in *Parzival* Wolfram talks at one point about *wir Beier* (i.e. "we Bavarians") (§121, l. 7) — but his fame as a Minnesänger (nine songs by him survive) was such that Richard Wagner included him (along with Walter von der Vogelweide) in his opera of 1845, *Tannhäuser und der Sängerkrieg auf* [*der*] *Wartburg* ("Tannhäuser and the Minnesängers' Contest at the Wartburg"). As well as writing *Parzival*, Wolfram wrote two other works, both incomplete: the fragmentary *Titurel*, which tells the story of Schionatulander and Sigune (the two lovers in *Parzival*), and the unfinished *Willehalm*, based on an Old French *chanson de geste*, *Aliscans*, which is set at the time of the conflicts between the Christians and the Saracens (as the Muslims of Arabic origin were called by medieval Christian writers).[56]

In an excursus inserted between the second and third books and commonly referred as "Wolfram's Apology," Wolfram presents himself as someone who can write songs — of which, aside from his epics, five *Tagelieder* and four *Minnelieder* (or *Werbelieder*) have survived —[57] but ultimately less as a poet and more as a knight. Indeed, he even says of his work, *Parzival*, and of himself: "Yet he who heareth shall reckon, if he fain would account me friend, / That this is no book he readeth, for no maker of books am I!" (*swer des von mir geruoche, / dern zels ze keinem buoche. / ine kan decheinen buochstap*) (§115, ll. 25-27; vol. 1, p. 66). As Hatto translates this final line, "I haven't a letter to my name!" (69). But what does this mean? That he was illiterate (which, given the complexity of *Parzival*, seems unlikely)? That he had been given a lay education (as opposed to an ecclesiastical one)? (As Joachim Bumke notes,

[56] For further discussion, see Martin H. Jones and Timothy McFarland, *Wolfram's "Willehalm": Fifteen Essays* (Rochester, NY, and Woodbridge: Camden House, 2002).
[57] For further discussion, see Franz-Josef Holznagel, "Die Lieder," in Joachim Heinzle (ed.), *Wolfram von Eschenbach: Ein Handbuch* (Berlin and Boston: de Gruyter, 2011), pp. 83-143.

in the High Middle Ages the terms *litteratus* and *illitteratus* referred to elementary schooling, such that while an "uneducated" [*illitteratus*] person was someone who could neither read nor write, an "educated" [*litteratus*] person was someone who had learned to read and write Latin, that is, who had acquired the basic subjects of the trivium, namely: grammar and rhetoric.)[58] That he was not as learned in scholarly subjects as one of his rivals, Hartmann von Aue? (Yet in such fields as astrology and mineralogy, Wolfgang exhibits remarkable technical familiarity!) Or is it an echo of Psalm 70[71]:15, "Because I have not known learning"?[59] As we shall see, Jung himself took this claim at face value, although its intention is more likely to be polemical (or, in Hatto's words, a "tactical joke").

Nevertheless, in 1963, the great scholar of medieval and Arthurian literature and historian of the Grail legend, Roger Sherman Loomis (1887-1966), wrote about Wolfram's *Parzival* that "there breathes throughout the poem a spirit bold, realistic, generous, tender, and magnanimous. For most moderns who can either read the original German or can find a satisfactory translation [...] *Parzival* is the most satisfying medieval treatment of the legend of the Grail."[60] Wolfram's *Parzival* finds a place among the list of great works of the Middle Ages in Harold Bloom's *The Western Canon* (1994).[61] It has rightly been described by one critic as "the most popular vernacular verse narrative in medieval Germany and one of the most vibrant of the High Middle Ages."[62] The German scholar Albrecht Classen has

[58] Joachim Bumke, *Courtly Culture: Literature and Society in the High Middle Ages* [1986], trans. Thomas Dunlap (Woodstock, New York, and London: Overlook Duckworth, 2000), p. 433. Bumke adds, however, that "this terminology was not without imprecision" (p. 433). For discussion of lay education in Germany at the time, see pp. 429-433.

[59] For an overview of these alternatives, see DKV, vol. 2, pp. 516-517.

[60] Roger Sherman Loomis, *The Grail: From Celtic Myth to Christian Symbol* (Princeton, NJ: Princeton University Press, 1991), p. 222.

[61] Harold Bloom, *The Western Canon: The Books and School of the* Ages (London: Macmillan, 1995), p. 533.

[62] Will Hasty, "Introduction," in Will Hasty (ed.), *A Companion to Wolfram's "Parzival"* (Woodbridge and Rochester, NY: Camden House, 1999), pp. ix-xxx (p. ix).

suggested that *Parzival* might be "one of the most intriguing works of its time in terms of intellectual and spiritual epistemology."[63] More recently, G. Ronald Murphy has written that "[n]o literary or cultural work of the Middle Ages, with the exception of the Gothic cathedral, to which *Parzival* has more than passing kinship, surpasses this story in integrated richness, luminosity, and graciousness," adding: "Wolfram's Grail story stands on a par with the *Divine Comedy*, and with Chrétien's Arthurian romances."[64]

As a work of fiction, *Parzival* is constructed as a response to his predecessor Chrétien de Troyes. In fact, as Adrian Stevens has argued, "to read *Parzival* within the context of the rise of Arthurian romance in Germany is to see Wolfram as a reader and interpreter of Chrétien, and to view *Parzival* as enacting an intensive narrative dialogue with *Li Contes del Graal* in the process of its construction as a work of fiction."[65] Wolfram departs from Chrétien's tale in significant respects, as Murphy has also noted:

- Chrétien combines Celtic and Christian motifs, Wolfram combines:
    - Muslim and Christian ones
    - husband and wife
    - astronomy and medicine
    - the contemporary and the ancient (or the archaic)

    producing an "incredibly rich medieval humanistic Christian tapestry"

[63] Albrecht Classen, "Jewish-Christian Relations in the Middle Ages — The Exploration of Alternative Voices? The Deconstruction of a Myth or Factual History? Literary-Historical Investigations," *Amsterdamer Beiträge zur Älteren Germanistik*, 58 (2003), 123-149 (p. 137).

[64] G. Ronald Murphy, SJ, *Gemstone of Paradise: The Holy Grail in Wolfram's "Parzival"* (New York: Oxford University Press, 2006), p. 11.

[65] Adrian Stevens, "Fiction, Plot and Discourse: Wolfram's *Parzival* and its Narrative Sources," in Hasty (ed.), *A Companion to Wolfram's "Parzival"*, pp. 99-123 (p. 99). For a discussion of the different modes of narrative presentation in *Parzival*, see Neil Thomas, "Wolfram von Eschenbach: Modes of Narrative Presentation," in Hasty (ed.), *A Companion to Wolfram's "Parzival,"* pp. 124-139.

- integrates the motif of the Grail as a stone and contemporary lapidary science and interest in gems
- finds a harmony between the Crusaders' quest to free the Holy Sepulcher and the quest for the Holy Grail
- integrates astrological planetary lore with the figure of Kyot, the putative (and much disputed) source of Wolfram's narrative
- finds a new connection between the Passion of Christ and the Grail
- combines the worlds of Christian and Muslim learning. (11)

Over and above these specific elements, one might highlight the following aspects of Wolfram's treatment of the Grail legend as particularly important innovations.

First, Wolfram's narrator questions the version of the Grail story provided by Chrétien des Troyes; Chrétien, he says, got it wrong! Instead, the narrator claims to have an independent source, a figure he calls Kyot Laschantiure, alias "the Provençal," an attaché to the Knights Templar. In turn, Kyot is said to have relied on an Arabic manuscript, written by a pagan astronomer and man of science called Flegetanis, who

> had won for his wisdom fame,
> And saw many a wondrous vision, (from Israel's race he came,
> And the blood of the kings of old-time, of Solomon did he share,)
> He wrote in the days long vanished, ere we as a shield might bear
> The cross of our Holy Baptism 'gainst the craft and the wiles of Hell,
> And he was the first of earth's children the lore of the Grail to tell.
>
> (§453, ll. 24-30; vol. 1, p. 262)

Second, Wolfram expounds at length on various mystical attributes of the Grail, whose bearer as the Queen of the Grail Family — Repanse de Schoye — he describes as

> a maiden, o'er the others was she the queen,
> So fair her face that they thought them 'twas the morning's dawn, I ween!
> And they saw her clad in raiment of Pfellel of Araby,
> And she bare aloft on a cushion of verdant Achmardi
> Root and blossom of Paradise garden, that thing which men call "The Grail"
> [*den wunsch von pardîs,*
> *bêde wurzeln und rîs.*
> *daz waz ein dinc, daz hiez der Grâl*].
> (§235, ll. 15-23; vol. 1, p. 135).

Third, despite this description as the roots and branches of earthly Paradise, the Grail is said to be "a stone" (*ein stein*) — a stone that lends youthfulness and brings about rejuvenation, hence it is called (in a passage which, as we shall see, attracted the attention of Jung) the *lapsit exillis* (or, on some readings, *lapis elixis*, and thus a variant on *lapis elixir*, or the philosophers' stone in alchemy),[66] and it is by this stone that the Knights Templar live:

> [...] Then know, by a *stone* they live,
> And that stone is both pure and precious — Its name hast thou never heard?
> Men call it *Lapis Exilis* [*lapsit exillis*] — by its magic the wondrous bird,

[66] See DKV, vol. 2, pp. 679-680; and Emma Jung and Marie-Louise von Franz, *The Grail Legend* [1960], trans. Andrea Dykes (Boston: London: Sigo Press; Coventure, 1986), p. 150.

The Phœnix, becometh ashes, and yet doth such virtue flow
From the stone, that afresh it riseth renewed from the ashes glow,
And the plumes that erewhile it moulted spring forth yet more fair and bright —
[…] And this stone all men call the Grail
[*der stein ist ouch genant der grâl*].
(§469, ll. 2-13 and 28; vol. 1, p. 270)

Fourth, the Grail is like a kind of magic writing-pad, inasmuch as it records the names of those that are called to its service — yet it immediately effaces them once read, so that these names cannot be read again:

On the Grail, in a mystic writing, appeareth each chosen name,
If a man it shall be, or a maiden, whom God calls to this journey blest.
And the message no man effaceth, till all know the high behest,
But when all shall the name have read there, as it came, doth the writing go […].
(§470, ll. 23-30; vol. 1, p. 271)

(In this respect, one can detect an echo of The Revelation to John, and the third — to Pergamum — of its opening seven letters to the Churches of Asia, "To him that overcometh, I will give the hidden manna, and will give him a white stone; and in the stone a new name written, which no man knoweth but he that receiveth it" [2:17]. According to the commentary in the NJB, the manna — which had been, together with the Ark of the Covenant, hidden by Jeremiah — will thus be served as the food to those who are saved in the heavenly kingdom; the white stone — the whiteness of which alludes to triumph and joy — recalls such various ancient usages as badges of honor and tablets of discharge or admission; and the "new name" signifies the spiritual rebirth of the Christian [NJB, NT, 2033].)

And fifth, whereas Chrétien de Troyes' *Perceval ou le Conte du Graal* was dedicated to Count Philip I of Flanders, and had Marie, Countess of Champagne as a patron, and its continuation by the early 13th-century Old French romance called *Perlesvaus* or *The High Book of the Grail* (*Li Hauz Livres du Graal*) portrayed the Grail knights as the guardians of a great, sacred secret, Wolfram's *Parzival* is explicit in identifying the Knights Templar as the guardians of the Grail and its family.

To these assessments one might add that Wolfram's *Parzival* goes beyond Chrétien's narrative by moving into the foreground the motif of *transformation* — which, while core to the very legend of the Grail, becomes combined with important theological and existential themes about the nature of God and the purpose of suffering. So on the one hand, *Parzival* can be seen in the context of the tradition of Arthurian romance in general and the Grail legend in particular; on the other, it has a broader significance as a key work in the tradition that stretches out to Goethe's *Faust* and Nietzsche's *Zarathustra* as a medieval exemplar of the German epic of transformation. In this sense, one might see *Parzival* (as Winder McConnell has done) as an exemplar of what Jung, in "Psychology and Literature" (1930), termed a "visionary" work of art, that is, one based on "primordial experiences" that "rend from top to bottom the curtain upon which is painted the picture of an ordered world, and allow a glimpse into the unfathomable abyss of the unborn and of things yet to be" (CW 15 §141) — a category in which Jung included Goethe's *Faust* and Nietzsche's *Zarathustra*.[67]

[67] See Winder McConnell, "Otherworlds, Alchemy, Pythagoras, and Jung: Symbols of Transformation in *Parzival*," in Hasty (ed.), *A Companion to Wolfram's "Parzival,"* pp. 203-222 (pp. 203-204).

The structure of this study is, I hope, clear and straight-forward. By way of introduction to this series as a whole and to Wolfram's *Parzival* in particular, in Chapter 1, we consider the genre of epic and its allegorical significance, notably in relation to the theme of transformation. In Chapter 2, we examine Wolfram's epic work *Parzival* in some detail, uncovering its major themes and exploring of its motifs, notably the Grail itself and its transformative effects. And in Chapter 3, we discuss Jung's long-standing interest in the legend of the Grail, particularly as reflected in some of the dreams recounted in *Memories, Dreams, Reflections*. In Book 5 of *Parzival*, Wolfram's narrator anticipates that his audience, when it hears about the Grail, will say, "Such riches ye never on earth shall find," and he responds with calm self-assurance: "So many have said, yet I think me that folly doth rule their mind — / For the Grail was the crown of blessing, the fulness of earth's delight, / And Its Joys I right well may liken to the glories of Heaven's height!" (§238, ll. 18-24; vol. 1, p. 136). As a symbol, the Grail serves to express that transformative process Jung dubbed the process of individuation, granting us access to the fullness — superabundance, even — of the self, so that "each one has he liked him best / Might speak the word, and proffer the cup, and behold! 'twas filled / By the power of the Grail" (§239, ll. 2-5; vol. 1, p. 136). It is hoped that a sense of the fullness of interpretative possibilities to be found in Wolfram's epic will prove equally satisfying to the reader.

Chapter 1

An Introduction to Epic

In his *Poetics*, Aristotle distinguished among three broad categories of poetry: lyrical, dramatic, and epic. What *is* epic? Epic poetry, Aristotle tells us, "has been seen to resemble tragedy to this extent, that of being an imitation of serious subjects in metre," but it "differs from it, however, in that it is in one kind of verse and in narrative form; and also by its length — which is due to its action having no fixed limit of time, whereas tragedy endeavours to keep as far as possible within a single circuit of the sun, or something near that" (book 5, 1449b). "They differ also," he added, "in their constituents, some being common to both and others peculiar to tragedy — hence a judge of good and bad in tragedy is a judge of that in epic poetry also," while "all the parts of an epic are included in tragedy; but those of tragedy are not all of them to be found in the epic" (1449b).[1] (As John Peck has argued, there is an important correspondence between Aristotle's analysis of the structure of dramatic action in his *Poetics* and Jung's approach to dreams;[2] arguably, the same could be said to apply to Aristotle's analysis of epic.) In other words, already in Aristotle's time there existed a

[1] Aristotle, *Complete Works*, ed. Jonathan Barnes, 2 vols (Princeton, NJ: Princeton University Press, 1984), vol. 2, pp. 2319-2320.

[2] "The Aristotelian template for action in the *Poetics*, applied by Jung to dreams, was part of a consistently developed analogy between medical practice and tragedy, one that students of both literature and psychology have mostly forgotten" (John Peck, "Introduction," in C.G. Jung, *Dream Interpretation Ancient & Modern: Notes from the Seminar Given in 1936-1941*, ed. John Peck, Lorenz Jung, and Maria Meyer-Grass, trans. Ernst Falzeder with Tony Woolfson (Princeton, NJ, and Oxford: Princeton University Press, 2014), pp. xxi-lii [p. xxvi]).

sophisticated formal theory of epic. And, in English, our word *epic* derives via the Latin (*epicus*) from the ancient Greek noun ἔπος (*epos*) and the adjective ἐπικός (*epikos*).

The oldest epic is the *Epic of Gilgamesh* (c.2500-1300 B.C.E.), dating back to ancient Sumer and recounting the exploits of Gilgamesh, the king of Uruk. For centuries, the *Epic of Gilgamesh* was lost, until it was rediscovered in the Library of Ashurbanipal in 1849. Its translation in the early 1870s led to controversy, as its flood myth found in Tablet XI raised questions about the historicity of the account of the Flood in the Hebrew Bible (Genesis 6:5-9:17). Another ancient epic is also the longest, the *Mahābhārata*, one of the two major epics in Sanskrit (the other being the *Rāmāyaṇa*). It narrates the battle between two groups of cousins in the Kurukshetra War in over 200,000 verse lines (i.e., 100,000 ślokas or couplets), while incorporating lengthy philosophical or religious excurses. Arguably the most famous of these, the *Bhagavad Gita*, is a component that could be considered a work in its own right; not least because its dialogue between Prince Arjuna and his guide and charioteer, Krishna (an avatar of Lord Vishnu), invites an allegorical reading.

In fact, almost every language and culture has its epics: in ancient Greece, Homer's *Odyssey* and his *Iliad* or the *Argonautica* by Apollonius of Rhodes; in ancient Rome, Virgil's *Aeneid*; in ancient Norse, the *Edda*; in Anglo-Saxon, *Beowulf*; in Finnish, the *Kalevala*; in Middle High German, the *Nibelungenlied*;[3] in Old French, the *Song of Roland*; in Spanish, the *Cid*; in Italian, Dante's *Divine Comedy*; in Polish, Adam Mickiewicz's *Pan Tadeusz*; in modern English, Edmund Spenser's *The Faerie Queene* (1590-1596) and John Milton's *Paradise Lost* (1667; [2]1674). Even or

[3] For a useful overview of medieval German epic, see Kurt Herbert Halbach, "Epik des Mittelalters," in Wolfgang Stammler (ed.), *Deutsche Philologie im Aufriß*, second edn, vol. 2 (Berlin: Erich Schmidt, 1960), cols 397 and 683 (especially cols 557-581 on Wolfram von Eschenbach); and Joachim Bumke, *Wolfram von Eschenbach* (Stuttgart: Metzler, 2004).

especially in modern times, the epic tradition has continued: as *Star Wars* in the world of film and *Star Trek*, *Battlestar Galactica*, *Lost*, and many other TV examples demonstrate.

Older epics were composed in a culture before writing had been invented and were performed by a bard who used different kinds of rhetorical and metrical schemes in order to memorize these complex works of art: in Sumerian, repetition; in ancient Greek and Latin, dactylic hexameter; in Old English, Middle High German, and Norse, alliterative verse; in Italian, Spanish, and Portuguese, terza rima (a three-line stanza using an interlocking three-line scheme rhyming ABA BCB CDC DED, etc.) or ottava rima (a stanza of eight lines of iambic pentameters, consisting of a rhyme scheme three alternate rhymes and one double rhyme, i.e., ABABAB CC); and in modern English, heroic couplets or blank verse.

Literary critics have described epics in terms of a number of stylistic and structural characteristics or conventions, including an opening invocation to the Muse (one of the nine daughters of Zeus) or a statement of the work's theme; a narrative structure that begins *in media res* (that is, in the middle of things) and continues with flashbacks to earlier episodes in the story; the use of *enumeratio* or long lists, catalogs, and genealogies; and frequent epithets, or stock phrases. Yet perhaps even more important is the focus on the (usually, male) hero and his quest or cyclical journey; it is not for nothing that the American literary scholar Joseph Campbell (1904-1987) was apparently able in his bestselling work *The Hero with a Thousand Faces* (1949) to reduce *all* existing epics to the single "monomyth" (an expression borrowed from James Joyce) of the hero's journey, involving a threefold structure: an adventure, a crisis, and its resolution.[4] As Campbell described this structure: "A

[4] Recently Maria Tatar has provided a feminist corrective to Campbell's exclusive focus on the male hero; see her *The Heroine with a 1001 Faces* (New York: Liveright, 2022).

hero ventures forth from the world of common day into a region of supernatural wonder: fabulous forces are there encountered and a decisive victory is won: the hero comes back from this mysterious adventure with the power to bestow boons on his fellow man."[5]

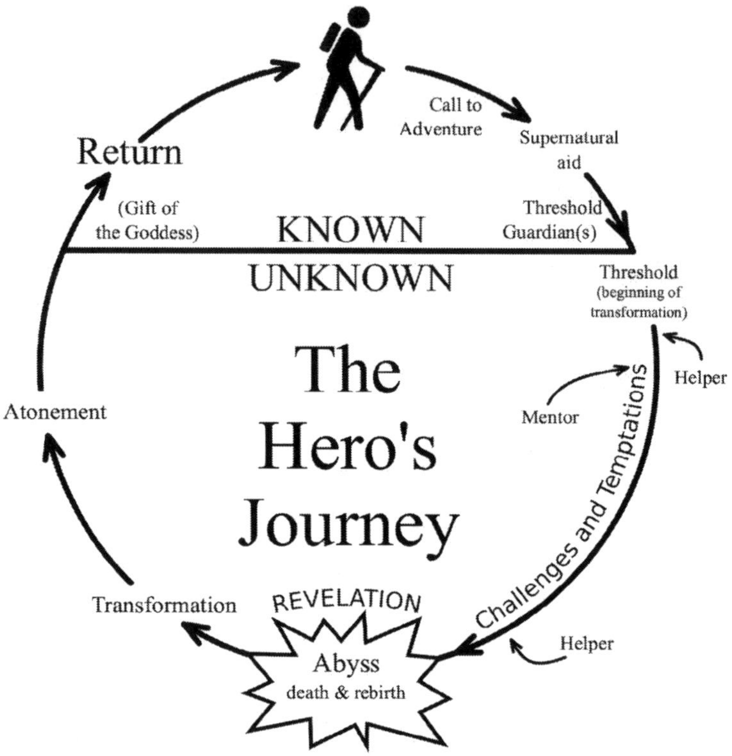

Figure 1: Diagram of the hero's journey[6]

In *The Hero with a Thousand Faces*, Campbell went on to classify no fewer than 17 stages of the monomyth, which may be collected into three phases:

[5] Joseph Campbell, *The Hero with a Thousand Faces* (Princeton, NJ: Princeton University Press, 1968), p. 30.

[6] This image outlines the basic path of the monomyth, or "Hero's Journey," and it is in the public domain. Available online https://commons.wikimedia.org/wiki/File:Heroesjourney.svg

- departure (or separation)
- initiation (subdivisible into
    - (a) descent
    - (b) initiation proper
- return

or (using the categories mentioned above):

- adventure
- crisis
- resolution.

In the final volumc, *Creative Mythology* (1968), of his four-volume study *The Masks of God* (vol. 1, *Primitive Mythology*; vol. 2, *Oriental Mythology*; vol. 3, *Occidental Mythology*), Campbell turned to a close study of the Grail legends.

In a passage from the 13th-century *La Queste del Saint Graal*, we are told (in a passage which Campbell reads as an expression of the spiritual predicament of the West) how the knights of the Round Table set off separately from the castle of King Arthur in quest of the Grail: "And now each one went the way upon which he had decided, and they set out into the forest at one point and another, there where they saw it to be thickest [*la ou il la voient plus espesse*],"[7] so that each knight would, as Campbell puts it, "experience the unknown pathless forest in his own heroic way."[8] Updating the Grail legend, Campbell adds that today, when "the walls and towers of the culture-world that then were in the building are dissolving" — and how much more true must this be in the second decade of the 21st century than at the end of the '60s of the last one — we have no choice but to set forth "from the known unto the unknown": "We today, willy-nilly, *must* enter the forest from the known to the unknown *la ou nous la voions plus espesse*:

[7] *La Queste del Saint Graal: Roman du XIIIe siècle*, ed. Albert Pauphilet (Paris: Champion, 1923), p. 26.

[8] Joseph Campbell, *The Masks of God*, vol. 4, *Creative Mythology* (New York: Viking Penguin, 1968), pp. 36-37.

and, like it or not, the pathless way is the only way now before us" (37).

Further on, Campbell identifies two "great difficulties" that confront the would-be knight errant of today, or "the questing individual who, alone, would seek beyond the tumult of the state" — which Campbell sees powerfully evoked in the chapter titled "The New Idol" in Nietzsche's *Zarathustra* (Z I 11) — "in the silences of earth and sea and the silence of his heart, the Word beyond words of the mystery of nature and his own potentiality as man" (88). The first difficulty is "breaking through and beyond the system of delusion impressed upon and built into his very nerves by the forces — at once moral and linguistic — of his youth" (88-89); and the second difficulty is — assuming one has actually been "vouchsafed an experience of one's own [...] transcending those categories written by one's people over the face of nature" and has returned to the king's court and rejoined "those others who likewise in the dark wood were vouchsafed their own experiences" — one of "establishing some kind of life, in terms not of the old 'collective faith' but of one's own" (89). (This second difficulty is addressed in the document known as "Analytical collectivity," attributed variously to Jung or to Maria Moltzer.)[9]

In *Creative Mythology*, Campbell showed himself to be alert to the roots of the Grail legend in the ancient Mediterranean mystery cults, displaying parallels with Orphic, Mithraic, Gnostic, and Manichaean traditions, as well as — in the symbolism of the rotating wheel — between the revolving castles of Celtic Arthurian stories and wheel imagery in Hindu legends. Thus, while advancing the Jungian thesis of a universal, archetypal dimension to the "mythic cycle," Campbell was also as keen as Jung had been to explore the

[9] Richard Noll, *The Aryan Christ: The Secret Life of Carl Jung* (New York: Random House, 1997), pp. 143-158; and Sonu Shamdasani, *Cult Fictions: C.G. Jung and the Founding of Analytical Psychology* (London and New York: Routledge, 1998), pp. 72 and 85-89.

individual cultures in which these myths were embedded and to trace their historical transmission through space and time.

In the wake of Campbell's work on the monomyth, this basic epic scheme has been discussed, developed, and qualified by such other critics as David Adams Leeming (1981), Phil Cousineau (1990), and Christopher Vogler (2007). Although it became popular in the 1970s, more recently Campbell's monomyth approach has subsequently become a subject of criticism for failing to pay sufficient attention to the specificities of the works to which it is applied. Indeed, this could be said to be the problem of structural approaches in general, which tend to erase history and individual subjectivity from the works they discuss. (Indeed, a case can be made that structuralism and postmodernism more generally are responsible for the erosion in the arts and humanities that has taken place at the end of the 20th and the beginning of the 21st century.)[10]

A good example of how a structural analysis can bring out the latent meanings of a work is provided by the dissertation thesis written in 1939 by Howard Nemerov (1920-1991) on Thomas Mann's novel *The Magic Mountain* (1924). Entitled *The Quester-Hero: Myth as Universal Symbol in the Works of Thomas Mann*, Nemerov argued that various mythic narratives — notably the Grail legend, but also the Upanishads, the Egyptian Book of the Dead, and the Polynesian legends of Maui — informed Mann's writing in general and *The Magic Mountain* in particular. Nemerov sent a copy of his analysis of the "quester narrative" to Mann

[10] Michel Onfray, *La Résistance au nihilisme* [*Contre-histoire de la philosophie*, vol. 12] (Paris: Grasset, 2020), pp. 61-82. For a structuralist account of structuralism, see Gilles Deleuze, "A quoi reconnaît-on le structuralisme" [1967], in François Châtelet (ed.), *Histoire de la philosophie*, vol. 8, *Le XXième siècle* (Paris: Hachette, 1972), pp. 299-335; translated by Melissa McMahon and Charles Stivale as "How do We Recognize Structuralism?" and published as an appendix to Charles Stivale, *The Two-Fold Thought of Deleuze and Guattari* (New York: Guilford Press, 1998), pp. 258-282. For a critical appraisal, see Stephen R.C. Hicks, *Explaining Postmodernism: Skepticism and Socialism from Rousseau to Foucault* (Tempe, AZ, and New Berlin/Milwaukee, WI: Scholarly Publishing).

himself, who professed to be convinced by it. Not realizing that his correspondent — later to become a famous poet — was at this time an undergraduate and not a professor, Mann welcomed his study:

> I read a manuscript by a young scholar of Harvard University, Howard Nemerov, called "The Quester Hero: Myth as Universal Symbol in the Works of Thomas Mann," and it considerably refreshed my memory and my consciousness of myself. The author places *The Magic Mountain* and its simple hero in the line of a great tradition that is not only German but universal. He classifies it as an art that he calls "The Quester Legend," which reaches very far back in tradition and folklore. *Faust* is of course the most famous German representative of the form, but behind Faust, the eternal seeker, is a group of compositions generally known as the *Sangraal* or Holy Grail romances. Their hero, be it Gawain or Galahad or Perceval, is the seeker, the quester, who ranges heaven and hell, makes terms with them, and strikes a pact with the unknown, with sickness and evil, with death and the other world, with the supernatural, the world that in *The Magic Mountain* is called "questionable." He is forever searching for the Grail — that is to say, the Highest: knowledge, wisdom, consecration, the philosophers' stone, the *aurum potabile*, the elixir of life.

Mann went so far as to apply Nemerov's approach not just to his own work but to Goethe's *Wilhelm Meister* novels and to the tradition of the *Bildungsroman*:

> The Quester of the Grail legend, at the beginning of his wanderings, is often called a fool, a great fool, a guileless

> fool. That corresponds to the naivete and simplicity of my hero. [...] Goethe's Wilhelm Meister — is he too not a guileless fool? To a great extent he is identified with his creator; but even so, he is always the object of his irony. Here we see Goethe's great novel, too, falling within the Quester category. And after all, what else is the German *Bildungsroman* (educational novel) — a classification to which both *The Magic Mountain* and *Wilhelm Meister* belong — than the sublimation and spiritualization of the novel of adventure? The seeker of the Grail, before he arrives at the Sacred Castle, has to undergo various frightful and mysterious ordeals in a wayside chapel called the Atre Périlleux. Probably these ordeals were originally rites of initiation, conditions of the permission to approach the esoteric mystery; the idea of knowledge, wisdom is always bound up with the "other world," with night and death.

For his part, Mann claimed that he had not been fully conscious of what he was doing in his novel or of the extent of the influence of this "mysterious tradition":

> In *The Magic Mountain* there is a great deal said of an alchemistic, hermetic pedagogy, of *transubstantiation*. And I, myself a guileless fool, was guided by a mysterious tradition, for it is those very words that are always used in connection with the mysteries of the Grail. Not for nothing do Freemasonry and its rites play a role in *The Magic Mountain*, for Freemasonry is the direct descendant of initiation rites. In a word, the magic mountain is a variant of the shrine of the initiatory rites, a place of adventurous investigation into the mystery of life. [...]

And Mann invited his readers to adopt Nemerov's approach, aligning himself fully —albeit probably with a degree of irony — with the tradition of the Grail legend:

> Perhaps you will read the book again from this point of view. And perhaps you will find out what the Grail is: the knowledge and the wisdom, the consecration, the highest reward, for which not only the foolish hero but the book itself is seeking. You will find it in the chapter called "Snow," where Hans Castorp, lost on the perilous heights, dreams his dream of humanity. If he does not find the Grail, yet he divines it, in his deathly dream, before he is snatched downwards from his heights into the European catastrophe. It is the idea of the human being, the conception of a future humanity that has passed through and survived the profoundest knowledge of disease and death. The Grail is a mystery, but humanity is a mystery too. For man himself is a mystery, and all humanity rests upon reverence before the mystery that is man.

(Mann made these remarks in a short essay titled "The Making of *The Magic Mountain*" first published in the *Atlantic* in January 1953 and subsequently included as an appendix to the English translation of his novel by H.T. Lowe-Porter.)[11]

Yet Campbell's work on the hero and, before it, Nemerov's work on the "quester narrative" were by no means the first to sketch a psychoanalytic-cum-structural approach to the mythical figure of the hero. In 1909, Otto Rank (1884-1939) had published *The Myth of the Birth of the Hero*, publishing a second (and greatly extended)

[11] Thomas Mann, "The Making of *The Magic Mountain*," in *The Magic Mountain*, trans. H.T. Lowe-Porter (London: Secker and Warburg, 1971), pp. 719-729 (pp. 727-729).

edition in 1922. Central to his reading of the hero-myth was his focus on the fact that "the history of the birth and of the early life of these [national heroes] came to be especially invested with fantastic features, which in different nations — even though widely separated by space and entirely independent of each other — present a baffling similarity or, in part, a literal correspondence."[12] After analyzing an entire series of case studies in heroic births (Sargon, Moses, Karna, Oedipus, Paris, Telephus, Perseus, Gilgamesh, Cyrus, Tristan, Romulus, Hercules, Jesus, Siegfried, and Lohengrin), Rank comes to the following conclusion about their underlying structure:

> The hero is the child of most distinguished parents, usually the son of a king. His origin is preceded by difficulties, such as continence, or prolonged barrenness, or secret intercourse of the parents due to external prohibition or obstacles. During or before the pregnancy, there is a prophecy, in the form of a dream or oracle, cautioning against his birth, and usually threatening danger to the father (or his representative). As a rule, he is surrendered to the water, in a box. He is then saved by animals, or by lowly people (shepherds), and is suckled by a female animal or by an humble woman. After he has grown up, he finds his distinguished parents, in a highly versatile fashion. He takes his revenge on his father, on the one hand, and is acknowledged, on the other. Finally he achieves rank and honors.[13]

In his final chapter, Rank uncovers what he calls "the narrow boundary line where the contents of innocent infantile imaginings,

[12] Otto Rank, *The Myth of the Birth of the Hero and Other Writings*, ed. Philip Freund (New York: Knopf, 1959), p. 3.
[13] Rank, *The Myth of the Birth of the Hero*, p. 65.

suppressed and unconscious neurotic fantasies, poetical myth structures, and certain forms of mental disease and crime lie close together, although far apart as to their causes and dynamic forces."[14]

Although Rank himself chose to "resist the temptation to follow one of these divergent paths that lead to altogether different realms, but which are as yet unblazed trails in the wilderness," his work on the hero legend caught the attention (as it was perhaps inevitable) of C.G. Jung, who enthusiastically embraced these trailblazing opportunities. In his turn, Jung devoted a chapter of Part Two of *Transformations and Symbols of Libido* (1911-1912) to the "unconscious origin of the hero." On his account (which we shall consider in more detail in Volume 2 in this series), an analysis of libido symbolism always leads back to the fantasy of maternal incest, and the myth of the hero is nothing other than the myth of our own suffering unconscious. The fact that heroes are nearly always wanderers is, Jung argued, "a psychologically clear symbolism," for wandering is "a representation of longing, of the ever-restless desire, which nowhere finds its object, for, unknown to itself, it seeks the lost mother" (PU §317). The hero myth is the myth of our own suffering unconscious, because it has "an unquenchable longing for all the deepest sources of our own being" — for "the body of the mother, and through it for the communion with infinite life in the countless forms of existence" (PU §317). Precisely at this point in his study, Jung turns to Goethe's *Faust*, quoting *in extenso* from the Mothers Scene of Part Two and describing it as "the words of the Master who has divined the deepest roots of Faustian longings" (PU §317).

Campbell's model is, like those psychoanalytic models of Rank, Jung, and others, essentially structural in its approach, and others have arrived at similar conclusions, albeit by different routes. In 1972, for instance, the German medievalist Hugo Kuhn

[14] Rank, *The Myth of the Birth of the Hero*, p. 96.

(1909-1978) suggested that such great medieval epics as Chrétien de Troyes's *Erec*, *Yvain*, and *Perceval*, Hartmann von Aue's *Erec* and *Iwein*, and Wolfram von Eschenbach's *Parzival* were underpinned by "a general myth and fairy tale scheme," that he described as "*descensus — ascensus*, the return of a god, of a *heros*, or a fairy tale hero from death, from the Other World, from animal metamorphosis, etc."; accordingly, he designated this category of epic as *Descencusmärchen*.[15] Subsequently, this model and its associated concept of *katabasis* was applied more systematically to Wolfram's *Parzival* in 1978 by the Kansas-based Germanist Ernst S. Dick (1929-2014). He suggested that the "organizing principle" of Parzival's progress as Grail hero, from "entering the world as a fool to his ascent to the grail kingdom," is "the journey to the Other World" — and more specifically, *katabasis* as the descent to the underworld.[16]

Following the work of Richard Ganschinietz or Wolfgang Fauch,[17] Dick argued that the *katabasis* was an integral part of the epic tradition and that the descent of the hero of Homer's *Odyssey* (Book 11) and Virgil's *Aeneid* (Book 6) were imitated throughout the

[15] Hugo Kuhn, *Tristan, Nibelungenlied, Artusstruktur* [*Bayerische Akademie der Wissenschaften, Philosophisch-historische Klasse, Sitzungsberichte*, vol. 5] (Munich: Verlag der Bayerischen Akademie der Wissenschaften, 1973), p. 16.

[16] Ernst S. Dick, "*Katabasis* and the Grail Epic: Wolfram von Eschenbach's *Parzival*," *Res publica litterarum: Studies in the Classical Tradition*, vol. 1 (1978), 57-87 (pp. 57-58).

[17] Richard Ganschinietz, "Katabasis," in Pauly-Wissowa, *Realencyclopädie der classischen Altertumswissenschaft*, 85 vols (Stuttgart: Metzler, 1890-1980), vol. 10, cols 2359-2449; and Wolfgang Fauch, "Katabasis," in K. Ziegler and W. Sontheimer (eds), *Der kleine Pauly: Lexikon der Antike*, 5 vols. (Stuttgart: Metzler, 1964-1975), vol. 3, pp. 152-153. For further discussion, see Albrecht Dieterich, *Nékyia: Beiträge zur Erklärung der neuentdeckten Petrusapokalypse* (Leipzig: Teubner, 1893, ^{2}1913); Josef Kroll, *Beiträge zum Descensus ad Inferos* (Königsberg: Hartung, 1922); Josef Kroll, *Gott und Hölle: Der Mythos vom Descensuskampfe* (Leipzig and Berlin: Teubner, 1932) (reprinted 1963); and Pierre Bonnechère and Gabriela Cursaru, "Katábasis," *Cahiers des études anciennes*, 53 (2016), 7-14, as well as Raymond J. Clark, *Catabasis: Vergil and the Wisdom Tradition* (Amsterdam: Grüner, 1979); and Clifford Weber, "The Allegory of the Golden Bough," *Vergilius*, vol. 41 (1995), 3-34.

entire Classical period, thus influencing the literature of the Middle Ages right up to Dante's *Divine Comedy*. In Arthurian epic (i.e., the romances about the legendary British leader, King Arthur, and the knights of his Round Table), the motif of the hero's quest takes the specific form of the quest for the Holy Grail. This quest is pursued in a sequence of journeys, turning the hero into a *homo viator* (or "itinerant man") outside society whose epic progress is marked by his "stational path" (*Stationenweg*) through his cycle of adventures.[18] In the case of Parzival, his journeys borrow an elaborate pattern of motifs from a repertoire of traditional Otherworld journeys (as analyzed by Stith Thompson), enacting an epic progression based on the conceptual scheme of descent and ascent.[19]

On this Classical model of the journeys of Odysseus and Aeneas that inspired so many other epic wanderings, the *katabasis* marks the end of the hero's adventures, and in the case of Wolfram's *Parzival,* the central event revolves around the sacred Grail. Parzival's initiation into the secrets of the Grail takes place in the symbolically significant setting of Trevrizent's cave,[20] where Parzival acquires a new ethical orientation and insight into the spiritual mysteries of the Grail: "And to Parzival the mystery of the Grail should he now reveal" (§452, ll. 29-30; vol. 1, p. 261).[21] True, unlike Odysseus and Aeneas, Parzival does not meet his father in his *nekyia* to the underworld. But the mysterious reliquary, a casket

[18] Dick, "*Katabasis* and the Grail Epic," p. 58. For the term *Stationenweg*, see Walter Haug, "Die Symbolstruktur des höfischen Epos und ihre Auflösung bei Wolfram von Eschenbach," *Deutsche Vierteljahrsschrift für Literaturwissenschaft und Geistesgeschichte*, vol. 45 (1971), 668-705 (p. 668); and for the term *homo viator*, see Gabriel Marcel, *Homo Viator: Introduction to a Metaphysic of Hope* [1945], trans. Emma Craufurd (Chicago: Regnery, 1951).

[19] Dick, "*Katabasis* and the Grail Epic," p. 60. See Stith Thompson, *Motif-Index of Folk-Literature*, revised edn, 6 vols. (Bloomington, IN: Indiana University Press, 1955-1958), Part F, "Marvels," F0-F199, "Otherworld Journeys," in vol. 3, pp. 7-37.

[20] On the significance of the cave, see Ernst Benz, "Die heilige Höhle in der alten Christenheit und in der östlich-orthodoxen Kirche," *Eranos-Jahrbuch 1953*, vol. 22 (1954), 365-432.

[21] See note on citation style in Chapter 2.

made from precious green stone, which stands on Trevrizent's altar and had been given to him by Parzival's father, Gahmuret (cf. §498, ll. 7-12), "projects Wolfram's favorite dimension of family relationships into Parzival's cave experience."[22] And the theme of the ancestors is, as we shall see, important in one way or another to the works under consideration here. Goethe's Faust, for instance, recalls the figure of his father, a "man of honor though unsung" (*ein dunkler Ehrenmann*) (l. 1034), and embraces the principle, "What you received but as your father's heir, / Make it your own to gain possession of it!" (ll. 682-683); Nietzsche's Zarathustra issues the prophetic cry, "Not only the rationality of millenniums — also their madness, breaketh out in us. Dangerous is it to be an heir" (Z I 22 §2) while looking forward to becoming himself an ancestor to his future descendants, the "new nobles" that he hopes will arise (Z III 12 §11-§12); and in Jung's *Red Book*, the ancestors are present in the form of the dead with whom Jung enters into dialogue and whose memory he learns to respect, calling on us to "turn to the dead, listen to their lament and accept them with love" (RB, 344-345). Equally, other epic motifs recur throughout these works: Goethe's Faust realizes the true nature of Mephistopheles in his address, full of bitter regret, to the "sublime spirit" (*erhabner Geist*) in the scene "Forest and Cave"; Zarathustra goes up into the mountains to his cave from which he descends at the beginning of the Prologue and to which he periodically returns before his final descent from the cave, "glowing like the sun," in the final chapter of Part 4; and in "Descent into Hell in the Future," Jung imagines himself "stand[ing] up to [his] ankles in a dark cave," from which he crawls through "a narrow crack in the rock [to] reach an inner cave whose bottom is covered with black water [...] full of the frightful noise of shrieking voices" (RB, 147). And there are other shared motifs as well:

[22] Dick, "*Katabasis* and the Grail Epic," pp. 83-84.

- the motif of the pathless wilderness (Faust's journey through "the small world, then the great" (*die kleine Welt und die große*) (l. 2051), Zarathustra's wandering in Part 4 through the mountains to which he had retired at the outset of Part 1, Jung's journey into the desert)
- the Otherworld motif of death (Faust's journey into the afterlife at the end of Part 2, Zarathustra's dream of the *Bergburg des Todes*, the figures of the dead who "cried out in chorus, 'We have come back from Jerusalem where we found not what we sought'" [MDR, 216; cf. RB, 507-508].)
- the centrality of the symbol (in *Parzival*, the Grail; in *Faust*, the insight that "all that is transitory is but a likeness" (*alles Vergängliche ist nur ein Gleichnis*) (ll. 12105-12105); in *Zarathustra*, the importance of speaking "in likenesses" (*in Gleichnissen*); while in *The Red Book*, the symbol is everywhere).

Subsequently, Winder McConnell has placed Wolfram's *Parzival* in the category of those works C.G. Jung described as "visionary," i.e., based on "primordial experiences" that "rend from top to bottom the curtain upon which is painted the picture of an ordered world, and allow a glimpse into the unfathomable abyss of the unborn and things yet to be,"[23] and argued that the otherworldly, alchemical, and Pythagorean symbols in *Parzival* reveal how "the entry into or sojourn of the hero in the physical otherworld corresponds to a psychic transformation of great significance for his process of individuation."[24]

---

[23] Jung, "Psychology and Literature" (1930), in C.G. Jung, *The Spirit in Man, Art, and Literature* [*Collected Works of C.G. Jung*, vol. 15], trans. R.F.C. Hull (London: Routledge & Kegan Paul, 1966), §133-§162 (§141).

[24] Winder McConnell, "Otherworlds, Alchemy, Pythagoras, and Jung: Symbols of Transformation in *Parzival*," in Hasty (ed.), *A Companion to Wolfram's "Parzival,"* pp. 203-222 (p. 204).

Jung's division in "Psychology and Literature" (1930; 1950) of art into two categories, the "visionary" (see above) and the "psychological" (drawn from our conscious experience of "crucial experiences, powerful emotions, suffering, passion, the stuff of human fate in general" [CW 15 §139]) can be situated within a long tradition of aesthetics in which the nature of the epic was, in line with Aristotle, distinguished from that of other forms (the lyric, the dramatic, etc.). And within the German tradition, epic itself as genre was extensively theorized. A whole book could be written on this topic; to give a sense of the debate, however, we shall consider contributions to the discussion from Goethe, Schiller, and Hegel.

Goethe/Schiller, On Epic and Dramatic Poetry (1797)

1797 was the year that Friedrich Schiller (1759-1805) described to Johann Wolfgang Goethe (1749-1832) in a letter of 22 September 1797 as their "year of the ballads" (*Balladenjahr*), referring to their intensive epistolary collaboration on the topic of the ballad and their composition of such ballads as "The Sorcerer's Apprentice" (*Der Zauberlehrling*) by Goethe or "The Ring of Polycrates" (*Der Ring des Polykrates*) by Schiller. And it was also the year in which they jointly wrote an essay titled "On Epic and Dramatic Poetry," subsequently published in 1827 in the journal *Über Kunst und Altertum* (VI, 1), edited by Goethe. At that time, Schiller was working on his *Wallenstein* trilogy, while Goethe was working on a plan (never carried out) to treat in dramatic form the story of Nausicaa (in Book 6 of Homer's *Odyssey*) and writing an epic in hexameters against a contemporary bourgeois setting, *Hermann und Dorothea.* In fact, Goethe's reading of Homer and the Greek tragedians led him to focus, from April 1797 onward, on the question of the difference between the epic and the drama in his exchanges with Schiller, to draft the essay "On Epic and Dramatic Poetry," and to send it to Schiller for his comments on 23 December 1797 (as a kind of genre-theoretical festive gift, as it were).

Goethe and Schiller argue that epic and dramatic poets have much in common:

- subject to universal laws
  - law of unity
  - law of development
- treat similar subjects
- can use all kinds of themes.

Yet there is one great essential difference:

- the epic poet presents the event as completely past
- the dramatic poet presents the event as completely present.

For Goethe and Schiller, the subjects of the epic and the tragedy have much in common, as they are:

- purely human
- important
- full of pathos
- stand at a level of culture where self-activity is left to its own resources
- operate not morally, politically, or mechanically but rather personally.

However, the presentation of these characteristics is significantly different:

- the epic presents
  - personally limited activity
  - individuals working outside themselves
  - battles, journeys, every sort of undertaking → requires sensual breadth
- the tragedy presents
  - personally limited suffering
  - inwardly directed individuals
  - actions → need only little space

In terms of the kind of themes available to epic and tragedy in their different ways, Goethe and Schiller identified five:

1) progressive ones → advance the plot (especially in drama)
2) regressive ones → remove the plot from its goal (epic makes almost exclusive use of these)
3) impeding ones → delay action or prolong progress (used by both epic and drama)
4) reflexive ones → through which what has happened before the epoch of the poem is drawn on
5) anticipative ones → anticipate what will happen after the epoch of the poem

→ both reflexive and anticipative themes are required by the epic and the dramatic poet alike in order to make poem complete.

Correspondingly, Goethe and Schiller identified the following worlds that are "brought to view" as common to both:

1) the physical
   a) the nearest:
   drama → located in one place
   epic → moves more freely in a larger locale
   b) the more remote world:
   epic → brings this world nearer through images
   drama → makes more sparing use of these images
2) the moral:
   common to both and represented most happily in its physiological and pathological simplicity
3) the world of chimeras, presentiments, appearances, accidents, and fates
   allowed to both if brought into proximity to the sensual (and especially difficult for modern poets)

In terms of presentational technique, Goethe and Schiller distinguished between the rhapsodist (as the exponent of epic) and the mimic actor (as the exponent of drama) as follows:

the rhapsodist

- surrounded by a quietly hearkening circle
- presents what is completely past
- appears as a wise individual who, in quiet self-possession, surveys what has taken place
- tries to quiet the listeners so that they will listen protractedly and gladly
- distributes listeners' interest evenly
- because not in a position to counterbalance an overly lively impression refers backward and forward, and wanders at will
- is followed everywhere because he is exclusively concerned with the imaginative power → generates images for itself, irrespective of what kind
- should not appear as a "higher being" in the poem but read as if from behind a curtain, so one can abstract from all sense of personality and hears only the voice of the muse.

the mimic actor:

- surrounded by impatiently onlooking and listening circle
- represents himself or herself as a definite individual
- wants the spectators to identify exclusively with themselves and their closest surroundings
- wants the spectators to sympathize with their sufferings of soul and body, share predicaments, and forget themselves
- will work in stages but dares much livelier actions, because with sensuous presence, even a stronger impression can be destroyed by a weaker one
- wants the spectators to remain in a state of constant sensuous exertion, not to elevate themselves to reflection and passionately to follow
- wants the spectators' imagination to be completely reduced to silence, and for even what is narrated to be brought, as it were, graphically before their eyes.

Their discussion about the nature of the epic and the role of the rhapsodist provides a framework within which one could approach numerous ancient works with fresh eyes! Yet Schiller's collaboration with Goethe on the topic of epic and dramatic poetry was by no means his first excursion into issues of literary genre.

In his groundbreaking essay titled *On Naïve and Sentimental Poetry* (1795-1796), Schiller had distinguished between the poet who "*is* nature" and the poet who "*seeks* it," the former defining the category of the naïve and the latter the category of the sentimental (200).[25] Consequently, the naïve poet writes in a way that is direct and descriptive, while the sentimental poet writes in a way that is more self-reflective.[26] For Schiller, nearly all classical Greek poets fall into the category of the naïve, while Euripides is an example of the sentimental, but there were examples much closer to home: Goethe exemplifying the naïve, while an example of the sentimental was — Schiller himself.

In turn, sentimental poetry subdivided into three categories: satire, the elegy (to be precise, the elegiac in dramatic or epic forms), and the idyll. In different ways, these genres all stood in relationship to the ideal: either reflecting the inadequacy of reality vis-à-vis the ideal (satire) or mourning the loss of the ideal (the elegy), or celebrating the ideal (the idyll) — the idyll also being a category of the epic, exemplified in the form of the bucolic by Theocritus. Even the idyll, however, can offer only a kind of foretaste or a "preliminary appearance" (*Vorschein*) of the ideal, because as a category of sentimental poetry, it shares its essence that "nature is set off against art and the ideal against the actual."

[25] Friedrich Schiller, *Essays*, ed. Walter Hinderer and Daniel O. Dahlstrom (New York: Continuum, 2005), pp. 179-260.

[26] Daniel Dahlstrom, "Play and Irony: Schiller and Schlegel on the Liberating Prospects of Aesthetics," in Thomas Nenon (ed.), *Kant, Kantianism, and Idealism: The Origins of Continental Philosophy* [The History of Continental Philosophy, vol. 1] (Chicago: University of Chicago Press, 2010), pp. 107-129 (esp. pp. 118-119).

Thus, in its depiction of "the actual world with its limitations, civilization with its artificiality" (*die Wirklichkeit mit ihren Schranken, die Kultur mit ihrer Künstelei*), the idyll would still reproduce, rather than overcome, the gap between the ideal and reality; in short, even in the idyll, "the language bears the spirit of the time [*den Geist der Zeit*] in itself and experiences the influence of art" (212).[27] (Examples of idylls in the German tradition include the *Idylls* (*Idyllen*), 2 volumes (1756-1772), of Salomon Gessner (1730-1788), *Luise: Ein ländliches Gedicht in drei Idyllen* (1795) of Johann Heinrich Voß (1751-1826), and Goethe's great bourgeois idyll, *Hermann und Dorothea* [1797].)

In this essay by Schiller, Homer serves as the great touchstone of naïveté: He, like all ancient Greeks (and only the ancient Greeks), was "at one with himself and happy in the feeling of his humanity," as opposed to us moderns, who are "at variance with ourselves and unhappy in our experiences of humanity." This difference between the ancient and the modern is clearly expounded by Schiller when he says:

> The feeling spoken of here is thus not something that the ancients had. It is rather the same as the sort of feeling we *have for the ancients.* They felt naturally, while we feel the natural. Undoubtedly, what filled Homer's soul, as he had his divine swineherd entertain Ulysses, was a completely different feeling from what moved the soul of the young Werther when he read this song following an evening in some irritating company. Our feeling for nature is like the sick person's feeling for health. (195)

[27] Cf. William Mainland's comment on this footnote in Friedrich Schiller, *Über naïve und sentimentalische Dichtung*, ed. William F. Mainland (Oxford: Blackwell, 1957), pp. 117-118.

Underpinning this analysis is a model of history that shows humankind undergoing a process of transformation: from the state of NATURE, via the world of CULTURE, to the final stage of the IDEAL. This sort of triadic pattern can also be found in the thought of Georg Friedrich Wilhelm Hegel (1770-1831) expressed in the three stages of the dialectic as thesis, antithesis, and synthesis.

In his lectures on aesthetics, given at Heidelberg in 1818 and in Berlin in 1820/21, 1823, 1826, and 1828/29 (and subsequently published, on the basis of a — now lost — manuscript by Hegel and a series of lecture transcripts, in two volumes by Heinrich Gustav Hotho (one of Hegel's students) in 1835 (and again in 1842), Hegel identified the three basic forms of poetry as epic, lyric, and dramatic poetry.[28] In the version of these lectures given in the summer of 1826 (and compiled by Friedrich Carl Hermann and Victor von Kehler),[29] Hegel claimed that epic poetry depicts free individuals — and hence the freedom of *Geist* itself — as they are found in a world of determining circumstances and events. Or as Hegel himself put it, "in the epic individuals act and feel; but [their] actions are not independent, events [*Begebenheiten*] have their right," and consequently the epic presents "a play between actions and events" (208). To be an individual in an epic is to be an individual in a situational context and hence caught up in a larger historical event: For instance, the protagonists in Homer's *Iliad* are all involved in one way or another in the Trojan War. Their actions are determined not only by their individual will, but also by the circumstances in which they find themselves; indeed, their actions only make sense in the context of the situation in which they find

[28] G.W.F. Hegel, *Aesthetics: Lectures on Fine Art*, trans. T.M. Knox, 2 vols (Oxford: Clarendon Press, 1975).

[29] G.W.F. Hegel, *Philosophie der Kunst oder Ästhetik: Nach Hegel. Im Sommer 1826: Mitschrift. Friedrich Carl Hermann – Victor von Kehler*, ed. Annemarie Gethmann-Siefert et al. (Munich: Fink, 2004). See Stephen Houlgate, "Hegel's Aesthetics," in *Stanford Encyclopedia of Philosophy*, online https://plato.stanford.edu/entries/hegel-aesthetics/ .

themselves. Hence, epic poetry depicts the essentially *worldly* character of human freedom — and its inevitable limitations.

Thus, in Hegel's view, Alexander the Great would not have been a good subject for epic poetry, "however much he considered Achilles fortunate to have had a Homer as someone to represent him," for "the entire age does not have the character of the epic, and his world was his army": and, as *his* creation under *his* control, it did not enjoy "the same independence from him as did the Greek commanders, who were freer" (213). (Hegel's strictures overlook the existence of the 16,000-verse, 12th-century Old French romance, the *Roman d'Alexandre*, which depicts various episodes in the life of Alexander the Great. A Franco-Provençal version of the *Roman d'Alexandre* served as a model for the Early High German *Alexanderlied* by Pfaffe Lamprecht, the first German epic composed on a French model, even if it is described today as of "little poetic value."[30] But then again, the fact that it is described as a "romance" (*roman*) perhaps also makes Hegel's point that the work is a different kind of work from an epic.)

Examples of works considered by Hegel to be great epic poems are Homer's *Odyssey*, Dante's *Divina Commedia*, and the medieval Castilian epic *The Poem of the Cid*. For Hegel, however, the epic poem *par excellence* would appear to be Homer's *Iliad*, given his tendency to base most of what he says about the epic on his reading of that work.[31] Even if the existence of Homer was disputed, Hegel remarked, "his heroes live" (*Homer gesteht man nicht mehr Existenz zu; aber seine Helden leben*).[32]

At the heart of the epic, Hegel argues, lies a tension in the epic between the way it "recounts what is and what happens and

[30] See the entry on the "Alexanderlied" in Henry and Mary Garland, *The Oxford Companion to German Literature*, 2nd edn. (Oxford and New York: Oxford University Press, 1986), p. 17.

[31] Hegel, *Philosophie der Kunst oder Ästhetik*, pp. 207-208 and 217.

[32] Hegel, *Philosophie der Kunst oder Ästhetik*, p. 218.

therefore has objectivity for its content and form" and the fact that, "since it is the happening of an *action* which passes in front of us, it is precisely the individuals and their deeds and sufferings who really emerge" (1066). Consequently, Hegel believes, "only individuals, *be they men or gods*, can really act, and the more vitally they have to be interwoven with what is going on, all the more fully will they be justified in attracting the main interest" (1066-1067; my emphasis). In the works discussed in this series of books, the main figures (Parzival, Faust, Zarathustra, and Jung) are all men (i.e., human beings), yet the presence (or absence) of the god(s) forms a central part of the unfolding action of the epics in which they play the main role. In each case, there is a sense that what is at stake transcends the individual character: in the case of Parzival, the medieval mind; in the case of Faust, the outlook of the Renaissance (and the Enlightenment, and Romanticism …); in the case of Zarathustra, the predicament of modernity; and in the case of Jung, our own postmodern (or post-postmodern) condition.

From the above discussion, it is clear that what Hegel excludes from the epic he acknowledges as being true of the subject of lyric poetry. Here the subject does not undertake huge labors, voyages or adventures; instead, the subject expresses (in the forms of hymns, odes, songs) the inner feelings and ideas of the self. Sometimes this is done directly; sometimes the vehicle chosen is a rose, a glass of wine, or the beloved. Hence, Hegel's unbounded praise for Goethe's *West-östlicher Divan* (as well as Anacreon) as exemplifying how "this carefree freedom, this expansion of the heart and satisfaction of mind gives the loveliest charm of spiritual freedom and poetry" (1145). By contrast, Hegel takes to task Friedrich Gottlieb Klopstock (1724-1803) — whose *Selmar and Selma* (1771) he describes as "a miserable and tedious contest between lovers which, not without many tears, sadness, empty longing, and futile melancholy feelings, turns on the idle and lifeless speculation as to whether Selmar or Selma is to be the first to die" (1154) — for wanting to create a new "popular mythology" or "poetic mythology."[33]

In the version of his lectures as published by Hotho, Hegel seeks to clarify his claim that the basis of the epic world is "a national undertaking in which the entirety of a national spirit could be strongly marked in the earliest freshness of its heroic situations" by explaining that "on this foundation a *particular* aim must rise, the realization of which, being most intimately interwoven with the life of the whole nation, brings into view every aspect of the national character, faith, and action" (1063). *Parzival*, *Faust*, *Zarathustra*, Jung's *Red Book* — each in its own way could be said to explore the character of German culture, and to be interwoven with the life of its German-speaking readers. And each reflects what Hegel describes as the "especially remarkable" position of Dante's *Divine Comedy*: if, in the *Divine Comedy*, the epic poet himself is "the one individual to whose wanderings through Hell, Purgatory, and Paradise each and every incident is linked so that he can recount the productions of his imagination as his own experiences and therefore acquires the right [...] of interweaving his own feelings and reflections with the objective side of his work" (1066), how much more true is this of the works considered here, and their presentation of a figures wandering through the medieval forest (in the case of Parzival), through "the small world and then the large" (in the case of Faust), up and down mountains and across seas and islands (in the case of Zarathustra), and through the dream landscape of a collective imaginary (in the case of Jung).

After all, in the opening lines of *Transformations and Symbols of the Libido*, Jung notes the centrality in Freudian psychoanalysis of the Oedipus complex and compares "the impression made by this simple reference" to the Greek myth with "that wholly peculiar feeling which arises in us if, for example, in

[33] Hegel, *Aesthetics: Lectures on Fine Art*, trans. Knox, vol. 2, p. 1154-1155; Hegel, *Philosophie der Kunst oder Ästhetik*, p. 218.

the noise and tumult of a modern street we should come across an ancient relic," such as a Corinthian capital in a walled-in column or the fragment of an inscription: "Just a moment ago we were given over to the noisy ephemeral life of the present, when something very far away and strange appears to us, which turns our attention to things of another order; a glimpse away from the incoherent multiplicity of the present to a higher coherence in history. [...] While we are still engaged with the confusing impressions of the variability of the individual soul, suddenly there is opened a revelation of the simple greatness of the Oedipus tragedy — that never extinguished light of the Greek theatre" (PU §1). And in a footnote at the end of chapter 2, Jung cites the view of the great Swiss historian Jacob Burckhardt (1818-1897) to the effect that "every Greek of the classical era carried in himself a fragment of the Oedipus, just as every German carries a fragment of Faust."[34] Seen in this light, not just Faust but Parzival, Zarathustra, and the Jung figure in *The Red Book* are fully the equivalent of Homer's heroic figures: Achilles in the *Iliad* or Odysseus in the *Odyssey*; or, for that matter, the Cid.

Although Hegel places great emphasis on the *national* aspect of epic, he also argues that "what rules in epic" — "though not, as is commonly supposed," he adds, "in drama" — "is fate" (*das Schicksal*) (1070). For Hegel, the difference between the

[34] In a footnote, Jung invites us to consider Burckhardt's letter to Albert Brenner of 11 November 1855: "I have absolutely nothing stored away for the special interpretation of Faust. You are well provided with commentaries of all sorts. Hark! let us at once take the whole foolish pack back to the reading-room from whence they have come. What you are destined to find in Faust, that you will find by intuition. Faust is nothing else than pure and legitimate myth, a great primitive conception, so to speak, in which everyone can divine in his own way his own nature and destiny. Allow me to make a comparison: What would the ancient Greeks have said had a commentator interposed himself between them and the Oedipus legend? There was a chord of the Oedipus legend in every Greek which longed to be touched directly and respond in its own way. And thus it is with the German nation and Faust" (PU §56; see Hans Brenner-Eglinger, "Briefe Jakob Burckhardts an Albert Brenner," *Basler Jahrbuch 1901*, 87-110 [p. 92]).

drama and the epic resides in this point: Whereas, in the former, a character "creates his fate *himself*," in the latter a character "has his fate made for him" (1070). Parzival, Faust, Zarathustra, and Jung himself: All find themselves caught up in a process of transformation that is larger than themselves, and their goal — or, if one prefers, their *Schicksal* — is not the perfecting of the ego, but the constellation of the self. (In Stoic terms, one is transforming the exterior constraint of *fate* into the interior freedom of *destiny*.)[35] Or in Hegel's words, they exemplify the epic as a genre which begins with works that show "the dark working of a power which is not itself specifically individualized as *this* power in its divine dominion or presented poetically in its activity" (1071) and ends with works that display "the complete interweaving of all human fates and natural occurrences with the decree, will, and action of a world of manifold gods as we find it in, for example, the great Indian epics, in Homer, Virgil, etc." (1072). Here, too, Klopstock is his target: Compared with such figures as Abbadona, the repentant devil in *The Messiah* (see Canto 2, ll. 627-850) and such abstract ideas as the resurrection, "the blood-drinking phantoms in Homer, their return to the life of memory and speech, have infinitely more poetic truth and reality" (1076).

Now in Book 11 of the *Odyssey*, Odysseus makes a libation to the dead in order to enable them to speak; and, commenting on this episode, Walter Burkert noted that "the dead drink the pourings and indeed the blood — they are invited to come to the banquet, to the satiation with blood; as the libations seep into the earth, so the dead will send good things up above."[36] As we know from Goethe's *Faust*, blood is "a very special juice" (*Blut ist ein ganz besonderer Saft*) (l. 1740); in "Of Reading and Writing," Nietzsche's *Zarathustra* tells us, "Of all writings I love only that which is written with blood" (Z

[35] Bertrand Vergely, *Pascal ou l'expérience de l'infini* (Paris: Milan, 2007), p. 17.
[36] Burkert, *Greek Religion*, trans. John Raffan (Oxford: Blackwell, 1985), pp. 194-195.

I 7); and in "Nox Quarta" in *The Red Book*, Jung asks, "What is this crazy desire craving satisfaction? Whose mad cries are these? Who among the dead suffers thus? Come here and drink blood so that you can speak" (RB, 367). Indeed, in *Transformations and Symbols of the Libido*, Jung echoed this Homeric episode and used it in a metaphorical sense when, in a footnote, he wrote about Miss Frank Miller that, "like Odysseus," he had "tried to let this phantom drink only enough blood to enable it to speak, and in so doing betray some of the secrets of the inner life" (PU §57, fn.).

Mock-epic

For all the high-minded and eminently serious discussions of the epic found in Goethe, Schiller, and Hegel, it should not be overlooked how in the 17th century a tradition of so-called mock-heroic, mock-epic or heroi-comic writing had arisen. As the name suggests, these works satirize, parody, or in some other way mock the classical figure of the hero. Although the mock-epic style became popular in 17th-century Italy and in the post-Restoration and Augustan periods in Great Britain (i.e., the "restoration" of the Stuart monarchy in England, Scotland, and Ireland in 1660 when King Charles II returned from his exile in Europe, and the period of the reigns of Queen Anne, King George I, and George II in the first half of the 18th century until the 1740s, thus named after the *Epistle to Augustus* addressed by Alexander Pope (1688-1744) to George II, associating his reign with the corresponding period in Roman history after the end of the reign of Julius Caesar), it was not new. Already at the time of Alexander the Great, a parody of the *Iliad* ascribed by the Romans to Homer called the *Batrachomyomachia* (or *Battle of the Frogs and Mice*) was circulating. (Plutarch ascribed the work to Pigres of Halicarnassus, others to Lucian, but the author remains unknown.) Famous examples of mock-epic include *Hudibras* (1662-1674) by Samuel Butler (1613-1680); Pope's *Rape of the Lock* (1712-1714) and *The Dunciad* (1728-1743); and various works by Jonathan Swift (1667-1745), notably *A Tale of a Tub* (1704), *An Argument Against Abolishing Christianity* (1712), *Gulliver's Travels* (1726), and *A Modest Proposal* (1729).

It would, however, be incorrect to think of the mock epic as a purely English affair, and its European dimensions have been explored in detail by Ritchie Robertson.[37] In addition to Pope's *The Dunciad* (1728; ^{2}1729; ^{2}1743) and Byron's *Don Juan* (1819-1824), he considers such famous examples as Voltaire's *La Pucelle d'Orléans* (1752), Goethe's *Hermann und Dorothea*, and Heinrich Heine's *Atta Troll* (written 1841, pub. 1847) together with some less well-known examples as Joseph Franz Ratschky's *Melchior Striegel* (1793) and Évariste de Parny's *La Guerre des Dieux* (1799). Robertson highlights the pivotal role in establishing the mock-epic tradition played by Ludovico Ariosto (1474-1533) and his romance epic *Orlando Furioso* (1516), satirizing the chivalric tradition in its account of the battles between Charlemagne, Orlando (i.e., Roland), and the Franks against the Saracens. (Inasmuch as the work presents itself as a continuation of the unfinished romance *Orlando Innamorato* (or *Orlando in Love*), published posthumously in 1494 by Matteo Maria Boiardo (1440-1494), it highlights the need for literary works to be seen within the terms of the tradition of which they form a part — as is the case with the four works studied in this and subsequent volumes.) While the intentions of its close relative, mock-heroic poetry, are essentially parodic, Robertson argues, the mock epic is also parodic but more complex, involving:

- intertextual allusion
- narratorial irony
- a noncensorious, broadly sympathetic, and sometimes libertine presentation of sexual relations
- a range of satirical devices.

[37] Ritchie Robertson, *Mock-Epic Poetry from Pope to Heine* (New York: Oxford University Press, 2009).

Within the works studied in this series, too, we shall come across passages that are ironic or satirical in nature. Mock epic achieved three things: First, it offered a reaction and a response to the decline of serious epic against a context of rapid political and social change; and second, it contributed to the so-called *querelle des anciens et des modernes*, an artistic and intellectual debate that took place, initially within the Academie française, between two camps: one, led by Nicolas Boileau (1684-1711), that argued that great art has its roots in antiquity; and another, led by Charles Perrault (1628-1703), that argued for the validity of modern aesthetic criteria. (Of course, those criteria looked modern to *them*; to us, they look almost as ancient as the criteria they were replacing, confirming Pascal's thesis — see below — that, once upon a time, even the *anciens* were *modernes* to themselves.) The *querelle* questioned the literary and artistic authority of the epics of Homer and Virgil, but even as it did so, it helped entrench that authority; for if Homer and Virgil had been so unimportant, it would not have been worth questioning their authority. And so, third, mock epic succeeded — ironically enough — in preserving the tradition of epic poetry and bringing it into the modern period (whenever that might be said to have begun).

As Peter Morgan has emphasized, in England such middle-class writers as Samuel Butler and Alexander Pope used the mock-epic as a satirical political weapon. While in Germany from the 1740s until the 1780s, the works of Moritz August von Thümmel (1738-1817), Friedrich Wilhelm Zachariä (1726-1777), and Christoph Martin Wieland (1733- 1813) focused on the disparities one could observe among social, literary, and intellectual life, the mock-epic was less openly political. Rather, it served the function of a means of self-irony of the nobility (as in the case of Thümmel's *Wilhelmine, oder der vermählte Pedant* [1764]) and/or the intelligentsia (as in the case of Wieland or Zachariä, notably his *Der Renommiste: Ein komisches Heldengedicht* [1744]). The mock-epic culminated in verse form in Wieland's *Oberon* (written in 1778-1780, published in 1780, and revised for the final time in 1796); named after the mythological king of the fairies and based on the medieval French epic romance *Huon de Bordeaux*, the work was used as the basis for Carl Maria von Weber's opera *Oberon* in 1826. (Its opening lines, "Saddle up the hippogryph one more time, ye Muses, / For a ride into the old, romantic land!" [*Noch einmal sattelt mir den Hippogryphen, ihr Musen, / Zum Ritt ins alte romantische Land!*], capture its playful, humorous tone, as well as anticipating the fascination with magic and with the fairy tale associated with Romanticism.) In the 1790s, the mock-epic was transformed by Johann Paul Friedrich Richter (1763-1825), known as Jean Paul, into the prose idyll.[38]

The persistence of the epic tradition under the form of the mock-epic reminds us of something essentially ambiguous about our concept of modernity as it applies to literary texts (as well as to other works). As the French philosopher and commentator Bertrand Vergely has suggested, there are two false pictures one can have about modernity: The first is to diabolize modernity; the second to is to declare it sacred.[39] On this account, those who diabolize modernity respond to the tensions of the present moment by creating a nostalgia for a past which they idealize, and in so doing forget that there has never been innovation without tension, and that in the past there were the same tensions as there are for us today. By contrast, those who declare modernity sacred respond to the successes and triumphs of the present by idealizing the present, and in so doing forget that great things were achieved in the past, without which the innovations of today would never have seen the light of day. In other words, modernity is a much more complex phenomenon than it is usually understood to be.

[38] Peter Morgan, *The Critical Idyll: Traditional Values and the French Revolution in Goethe's "Hermann und Dorothea"* (Columbia, SC: Camden House, 1990), pp. 20-21.

[39] Bertrand Vergely, *Boulevard des philosophes: De la Renaissance à aujourd'hui* (Paris: Milan, 2005), pp. 119-122.

For what we have to grasp, as Vergely insists, is that modernity began a long time before modernity. In this sense, the first moderns were really the ancients, and this is an argument we find in Pascal and his *Préface sur le traité du Vide*: "Those whom we call ancient were really new in all things, and properly constituted the infancy of humankind; and as we have joined to their knowledge the experience of the centuries which have followed them, it is in ourselves that we should find this antiquity that we revere in others." [40] (This passage recalls the famous expression about "dwarfs standing on the shoulders of giants," attributed to Bernard of Chartres by John of Salisbury.) Pascal's point here is that the past is not something that is finished and over with the arrival of the modern world, but rather that it persists among us in thousands of different ways. (C.G. Jung is someone who also makes this point: i.e., the ancients are not outside of us, in the past, but are still among us, today; this is the dimension that Jung refers to as *the archaic*.[41] As he once memorably put it, "we should never think we are living in modern times — we are living three or four hundred years behind our times, our feeling life is not up to date. [...] You step into a streetcar in Zurich and there is a Neanderthal man sitting right opposite you, his psychological level of humanity."[42] In a sense, Jung's position is an eminently logical one; after all, as Dilthey argued, "the present never *is*; what we experience as present always contains the memory of what has just been present").[43]

[40] Pascal, *Œuvres complètes*, ed. Louis Lafuma (Paris: Seuil, 1963), pp. 231-232.
[41] See Jung's essay "Archaic Man" (1931); CW 10, §104-§147. For an exploration and a defence of the notion of the archaic, see Paul Bishop (ed.), *The Archaic: The Past in the Present* (London and New York: Routledge, 2012).
[42] C.G. Jung, *Visions: Notes of the Seminar given in 1930-1934*, ed. Claire Douglas, 2 vols (London: Routledge, 1998), vol. 1, pp. 59-60.
[43] Wilhelm Dilthey, *The Formation of the Historical World in the Human Sciences* [*Selected Works*, vol. 3], ed. Rudolf A. Makkreel and Frithjof Rodi (Princeton, NJ, and Oxford: Princeton University Press, 2002), p. 216.

For there to be mock-epic, there has to be true epic, and in the case of German literature (as we have seen), there was — including the *Hildebrandslied* (9th century), the *Nibelungenlied* (12th century), and Wolfram von Eschenbach's *Parzival* (in Middle High German). Sometimes these works drew on and reworked classical material, as in the case of the *Eneas*, written by a Norman cleric between 1150 and 1160, and the *Eneide* (1170-1185), written in German by the Flemish poet Heinrich von Veldeke; sometimes they drew on Germanic or Scandinavian sources, as in the case of the *Nibelungenlied*, the heroic lays of the Poetic Edda, and the *Völsunga saga*. In fact, the epic became crucial in founding and developing a tradition of German literature (as opposed to, on the one hand, the classical inheritance of Greece and Rome, and, on the other, to the "national" literatures of France and England).

In this study, we propose to discuss four epic works: Wolfram von Eschenbach's *Parzival*, Goethe's *Faust*, Nietzsche's *Thus Spoke Zarathustra*, and — as the latest newcomer to this tradition, so to speak, and as its most recent exponent — *The Red Book* of C.G. Jung. Is, however, this tradition a purely literary tradition, or is there another dimension to (German) epic as well? In other words, are we talking in these works (to use the terms of the Swiss classicist Maria Laura Gemelli Marciano) about "literary concepts" or "attitudes," or are we talking about "hard inner experience?"[44] Or is this itself a false binary?

Epic as Psychology

In their mania for categorizing and classifying different types of epic, literary critics tend to overlook the experiential dimension

[44] Peter Kingsley, *Catafalque: Carl Jung and the End of Humanity*, 2 vols (London: Catafalque Press, 2018), vol. 2, pp. 493-494, n. 52; citing M. Laura Gemelli Marciano et al, *Parmenide: suoni, immagini, esperienza* (Sankt Augustin: Academia Verlag, 2013), pp. 231-233 and 280.

of literature — as well as its philosophical importance. As Luc Ferry has argued, there is a clear line of connection from Homer to Plato, and it is no exaggeration to describe epic as the birthplace of philosophy.[45] For although, at first glance, the use of the dialogue form can make Plato's philosophy look easy, behind this surface simplicity lies a complex philosophical architecture.

The background to Plato's epoch, i.e., Greece of the fifth century B.C.E., is the so-called "Greek miracle" — the birth of Western philosophy. Intellectual life in Athens in the fifth century and then the fourth century B.C.E. was characterized by numerous philosophical schools, not just Plato and his Academy: There were the Lyceum (here Aristotle taught), the Cynic school, the Atomist school (Leucippus and Democritus), the Sophist school (Protagoras, Gorgias), the Garden of Epicurus, and the *Stoa* (the arcades after which the Stoic philosophers were named). The question is: Why did this "miracle" take place?

The first key to understanding this so-called Greek miracle lies in the name of *philosophia* itself, i.e., the "love of wisdom" (from *philo* = "to love" and *sophia* = "wisdom"). In this context, love acquires the meaning of a search or a quest: and, in the case of Socrates, this love of wisdom is not merely a search but an attempt to embody and practice it. How does philosophical discourse, i.e., the quest for wisdom, relate to such other types of discourse as the great religions or the great mythologies, especially Greek mythology? Ferry suggests that it does so in relation to "moral" as well as to "spiritual" values (and he insists on the distinction between these two). For the distinction between moral and spiritual values can help us to understand what philosophy can add to religions and mythologies that is new, and how it can lead to a *spiritualité laïque*, i.e., the search for good life without reference to

[45] See Luc Ferry, *De Homère à Platon: La naissance de la philosophie* (Paris: Flammarion, 2012); revised in *Sagesses d'hier et d'aujourd'hui* (Paris: Flammarion, 2014), pp. 9-52.

God or faith. For fundamentally, philosophy is a search for the good life without recourse to faith or to god(s).

Whereas the essence of morality involves a respect for others combined with good wishes for their well-being, many other matters — e.g., love, death, the stages of life, or grief for loss of a loved one — involve *values*, but not moral ones. Rather, these matters involve "spiritual" values (or, as Hegel puts it in the Preface to the *Phenomenology of Spirit* in a passage that has been read as alluding to the rites of the Orphic Mysteries in ancient Greece, to the Crucifixion and Resurrection of Christ, or to the dismemberment and rebirth of Dionysos Zagreus), it is a question of *das Leben des Geistes* (or "the life of the spirit").[46] Not all definitions of the good life involve a reference to God or to faith, whereas all great philosophies or kinds of *spiritualités laïques* involve acceptance of human condition, i.e., human "finitude."

The second key to understanding the "Greek miracle" lies in the way that, instead of formulating the great themes of Greek mythology in the literary form of myth, it expresses themes of mythology in a rational or conceptual (i.e., "secularized") way. To be sure, numerous myths can be found in Plato, such as the *Gorgias* myth (523a-527a), the myth of the androgyne (*Symposium*, 189d-193d), the *Phaedo* myth of the afterlife (107c-115a), the myth of Er (*Republic*, 614a-621d), the myth of the winged soul (*Phaedrus*, 246a-249d), the myth of Theuth (*Phaedrus*, 274c-275e), the cosmological myth of the *Statesman* (268-274e), the Atlantis

[46] "But the life of mind is not one that shuns death, and keeps clear of destruction; it endures death and in death maintains its being. It only wins to its truth when it finds itself utterly torn asunder" (*Aber nicht das Leben, das sich vor dem Tode scheut und von der Verwüstung rein bewahrt, sondern das ihn erträgt und in ihm sich erhält, ist das Leben des Geistes. Er gewinnt seine Wahrheit nur, indem er in der absoluten Zerrissenheit sich selbst findet*) (G.W.F. Hegel, *Preface and Introduction to the Phenomenology of Mind*, ed. Lawrence S. Stepelevich (New York and London: Macmillan, 1990), p. 88; cf. Hegel, *Texts and Commentary: Hegel's Preface to His System in a New Translation*, ed. and trans. Walter Kaufmann (Notre Dame, IN: University of Notre Dame Press, 1977), p. 51).

myth (*Timaeus*, 21e-26d, *Critias*), and the *Laws* myth (903b-905b). Some of these myths are traditional — such as the story of Gyges (*Republic*, 359d-360b), the myth of Phaethon (*Timaeus* 22c7) or the myth of the Amazons (*Laws* 804e4) — some traditional but modified — such as the myth of the noble lie in the *Republic* (414b-415d), which combines the Cadmeian myth of autochthony and the Hesiodic myth of ages — and some that are unique to Plato — such as the myth of Er and the myth of Atlantis. Of the tales that one tells children, Socrates says in the *Republic* that "surely they are, as a whole, false, though there are true things in them too" (377a),[47] and the same is true of the Platonic myths.[48] Yet Plato's philosophy, like Greek philosophy in general, can be seen to translate great themes of mythology into a rational vocabulary, using lay arguments without reference to personifications of the divine.

Ferry reminds us that Plato was writing in the wake of Homer's *Odyssey*, the first great text written in Greek from the eighth century B.C.E. It was a work that Plato knew by heart and to which he makes repeated reference, and Aristotle — Plato's greatest disciple — taught this work to Alexander the Great. Ferry notes that Greek philosophers knew their mythology extraordinarily well: After all, it formed part of the common culture of their time and, beneath its literary appearance, it was full of the most profound metaphysical ideas. On this account, philosophy consisted of a rational, secular presentation of some of the great themes of mythology, especially Homer's immense and magnificent epic, the *Odyssey*. Thus, the *Odyssey* — a work which recalls the name

[47] Plato, *The Republic*, ed. and trans. Allan Bloom (New York: Basic Books, 1991), p. 54.

[48] For further discussion, see J.A. Stewart (trans.), *The Myths of Plato*, London: Macmillan, 1905; Ludwig Edelstein, "The Function of the Myth in Plato's Philosophy," *Journal of the History of Ideas*, vol. 10, no. 4 (Oct. 1949), 463-481; and Josef Pieper, *The Platonic Myths*, trans. Dan Farrelly (South Bend, IN: St. Augustine's Press, 2011).

of its central, questing character, i.e., Odysseus — constitutes the matrix of all Greek philosophy, and even the history of philosophy in general. (It was not for nothing that, for example, in the middle of the 20th century, Theodor W. Adorno and Max Horkheimer turned to Homer's *Odyssey* for corroboration at key points in their argument in their great philosophical response to Fascism, *Dialectic of Enlightenment* [1947].)

Homer's epic charts the path from chaos to harmony; from war — i.e., the Trojan War — to the return of Odysseus to his native city of which he is king — i.e., Ithaca. The beginning of this story is marked by the most massive chaos and misfortune imaginable: the terribly cruel and bloody conflict that is the Trojan War. (Some of the suffering described in certain passages of the *Odyssey* and even more the *Iliad* is so atrocious that we cannot, Ferry notes, easily read these descriptions today.) From this point of departure involving war, conflict, disharmony, discord, and hatred, the *Odyssey* relates how Odysseus tries throughout his long journey to rediscover harmony, peace, and love. These he finally finds in the arms of his wife, Penelope, and in his family and his palace — in what Aristotle calls his "natural place" in the cosmic order, i.e., the special place in the universe which belongs to him.[49] This idea that each of us once possessed a "natural place" in the cosmos which we have subsequently lost, and the rediscovery of which constitutes the meaning of life, is an idea of profound importance that will come to occupy the center stage of Greek philosophy, particularly in Stoicism.

Thus, the story of Odysseus can be read as the story of someone who is searching for the meaning of life for wisdom, in the sense of *philosophia*. On this account, Odysseus himself is a kind of philosopher, who is engaged in the search for wisdom. In

[49] Hayen André, "La théorie du lieu naturel d'après Aristote: Contribution à l'étude de l'hylémorphisme," *Revue néo-scolastique de philosophie*, 40, no. 53 (1937), 5-43.

his case, wisdom resides in the shift from the chaos of Troy to the harmony of Ithaca and to reconciliation with his kith and kin — as well as to reconciliation with the cosmic order of the world. And this story, as Homer tells it, lasts some 20 years! The grand narrative of his epic has a preliminary to which Homer alludes (cf. *Iliad*, book 24, ll. 25-30) but which he does not develop: a preliminary that explains the origin of Odysseus's philosophical will to pass from chaos to harmony, or from war to peace. This preliminary is the story with which the Trojan War itself begins, i.e., the famous story of the "apple of discord" or the Judgement of Paris, as narrated in the *Cypria*, a lost work of the ancient Greek Epic Cycle which recounted the entire history of the Trojan War in 11 books of dactylic hexameters. Despite the loss of this work, however, the pattern of Homeric (and, in this sense, of all Greek) thought is clear: Wisdom is related to the idea of harmony, expressed in the move away from chaos and discord toward cosmic order and peace.

In his essay *History of the Restoration of the Platonic Theology* (1792),[50] his annotations on his translation (1823) of Porphyry's *On the Homeric Cave of the Nymphs*, [51] and his account in allegorical terms of "The Wanderings of Ulysses" (1823),[52] the English Neoplatonist and translator Thomas Taylor (1758-1835) sought to revive the reading of Homer as allegory proposed by Porphyry in his short treatise *On the Homeric Cave of the Nymphs*. In this short but extremely significant work, Porphyry offered a master class in the allegorical interpretation of the opening lines of Book 13 of the *Odyssey*:

---

[50] Thomas Taylor, "The History of the Restoration of the Platonic Theology by the Later Platonists," in *Oracles and Mysteries* [TTS, vol. 7] (Frome: Prometheus Trust, 2001), pp. 129-244.

[51] "End Notes" to *On the Homeric Cave of the Nymphs*, in Porphyry, *Select Works*, ed. and trans. Thomas Taylor [TTS, vol. 2] (Westbury: Prometheus Trust, 1999), pp. 162-167.

[52] "The Wanderings of Ulysses," in Porphyry, *Select Works*, ed. and trans. Taylor [TTS, vol. 2], pp. 201-224.

High at the head a branching olive grows
And crowns the pointed cliffs with shady boughs.
A cavern pleasant, though involved in night,
Beneath it lies, the Naiades' delight:
Where bowls and urns of workmanship divine
And massy beams in native marble shine;
On which the Nymphs amazing webs display,
Of purple hue and exquisite array,
The busy bees within the urns secure
Honey delicious, and like nectar pure.
Perpetual waters through the grotto glide,
A lofty gate unfolds on either side;
That to the north is pervious to mankind:
The sacred south t'immortals is consign'd.[53]

This text, together with remarks by Plotinus scattered throughout his *Enneads* and material from Iamblichus's treatise *On the Mysteries of the Egyptians, Chaldeans, and Assyrians*, provides the basis for a Neoplatonist reading of Homer.

First, Taylor described Odysseus as a certain kind of hero, not ranking "among the first heroic characters," i.e., those who "descend into the regions of mortality at certain periods [...] for the purpose of benefiting others, and leading them back to their pristine state of perfection" — like such "exalted" heroes as Hercules or Pythagoras or Socrates or Plato.[54] Instead, Odysseus "only benefited himself," an observation confirmed by the fact that all his companions perished before he arrived back at Ithaca.

[53] Porphyry, *Select Works* [TTS, vol. 2], p. 145. For further discussion, see William Franke, "On the Poetic Truth that Is Higher than History: Porphyry and the Philosophical Criticism of Literature," *International Philosophical Quarterly*, vol. 50, no. 44 (December 2010), 415-430.
[54] Taylor, "The Wanderings of Ulysses," in Porphyry, *Select Works* [TTS, vol. 2], p. 201.

Furthermore, Taylor ranked Odysseus "among the middle class of characters that transcend the majority of [hu]mankind," building on Olympiodorus the Younger (c. 495-570) who, in his commentary on Plato's *Gorgias* (47.5), had distinguished between three different types of fate (termed "allotment" or "allocation"), and described as belonging to Zeus/Jupiter, Poseidon/Neptune, and Pluto: "The things within the universe are threefold: the heavens, the earthly realm and the intermediate realm, i.e., things of fire, air and water. The heavens belong to Zeus, the earthly realm to Pluto, and the intermediate realm to Poseidon. Further, through these [divine figures] Powers established over these realms are signified. [...] Hence too they say that some are sons of Zeus, some of Poseidon and some of Pluto, in accordance with the allocation of each of the three," so that "someone with a divine and heavenly character we call a son of Zeus, someone with an earthly character we call a son of Pluto and someone with an intermediate character we call a son of Poseidon."[55] Olympiodorus had placed Odysseus in this third category, arguing: "This is also why they say Odysseus wandered over the sea at the wish of Poseidon," for "thus they signify Odyssean life that is not terrestrial, yet still not heavenly, but intermediate" and "so since Poseidon is lord of the intermediate realm, that is why they say Odysseus wandered by the wish of Poseidon — he belonged to the allotted realm of Poseidon."[56]

Second, Taylor followed Proclus who, in his sixth essay in his commentary on Plato's *Republic* (6.2.4), had argued that "Homer [...] is said to have been deprived of his eyes, because he

[55] Olympiodorus, *Commentary on Plato's "Gorgias": Translated with Full Notes*, trans. Robert Jackson, Kimon Lycos, and Harold Tarrant (Leiden: Brill, 1998), pp. 200-301; cf. Porphyry, *Select Works* [TTS, vol. 2], pp. 201-202; and "Notes to the *Gorgias*," in Plato, *Works*, vol. 4, trans. Thomas Taylor and Floyer Sydenham [TTS, vol. 12] (Westbury: Prometheus Trust, 1996), p. 426.
[56] Olympiodorus, *Commentary on Plato's "Gorgias,"* pp. 300-301; cf. Porphyry, *Select Works* [TTS, vol. 2], pp. 201-202; and "Notes to the *Gorgias*," in Plato, *Works*, vol. 4, p. 426.

has transcended all beauty of the senses and, after investigating the war of souls here, he led himself up to the intellective contemplation of beauty." Citing Socrates's remark in the *Phaedrus* that "vision comes as the sharpest of senses through the body, but it cannot see intelligence [*phronêsis*]" (250d), Proclus associates himself with the more melodramatic view that "the one who has transcended the visible beauty, and turned his own activity to intelligence [*phronêsis*] and the intellective life, has lost his eyes."[57] Furthermore, that intellectual beauty is identified by Proclus with Helen, through whom the myths want to indicate "the whole of that beauty which has to do with the sphere in which things come to be and pass away and which stems from creation," a beauty over which "eternal war rages among souls, until the more intellective are victorious over the less rational forms of life and are brought back to the place from which they came in the first place."[58]

And in his Scholia on the *Phaedrus*, Hermias interpreted the Trojan War as a whole in the following terms: Ilium represents "the generated and enmattered region, having got the name 'Ilium' from 'mud' [*ilus*] and 'matter' [*hulê*], in which there is also war and faction"; the War itself pits the Trojans (as "the enmattered forms and all the life-styles associated with bodies") against the Greeks (as "the rational souls travelling from Greece, that is to say, from the intelligible [realm] into matter"); and Helen, over an apparition (*eidôlon*) of whom battle breaks out between the Trojans and the Greeks (cf. *Iliad*, Book 5, ll. 451-451, which actually refers to the image that Apollo made of Aeneas to save him from Diomedes),

[57] Proclus, *Commentary on Plato's "Republic,"* vol. 1, *Essays 1-6*, ed. and trans. Dirk Baltzly, John F. Finamore, and Graeme Miles (Cambridge and New York: Cambridge University Press, 2018), p. 287; cf. *Proclus the Successor on Poetics and the Homeric Poems: Essays 5 and 6 of His "Commentary on the Republic of Plato,"* ed. and trans. Robert Lamberton (Atlanta, GA: Society of Biblical Literature, 2012), p. 253.

[58] *Proclus the Successor on Poetics and the Homeric Poems*, ed. and trans. Lamberton, p. 253; cf. Proclus, *Commentary on Plato's "Republic,"* ed. and trans. Baltzly, Finamore, and Miles, p. 287.

signifies "intelligible beauty, which is a kind of 'attractor of intellect' [*helenoê*] that draws the intellect to it."[59] Thus, under the allegorical form of a military adventure, the Trojan War relates what is essentially a *spiritual* struggle:

> An emanation of this intelligible beauty then has been granted to matter through the agency of Aphrodite, over which emanation of beauty the Greeks fight as though over a human being. And some, prevailing over matter and successfully rising free [*katexanistasthai*] of it, depart to the intelligible [realm], their true homeland, while others are held fast in it, which is the life of the many.[60]

Within this overall allegorical framework, individual episodes acquire a precise meaning. Odysseus's first adventure with the Lotus eaters in Book 9, for example, can be read as signifying the attraction of those "false and boasting speeches and opinions" which, in the absence of "fair studies and practices and true speeches," are said by Socrates in the *Republic* to run up and occupy "the acropolis of the young man's soul" (560b-c). Then again, the Cyclops whom Odysseus tricks and blinds can, on Taylor's reading of Porphyry, be read as representing Odysseus's own "natal daimon": because he has "many laborious wanderings to accomplish, and many difficulties and dangers of no common magnitude to sustain," Odysseus is "departing from a sensible to an intellectual life, though circuitously and slowly," and hence, he is represented in so doing as "blinding and irritating his natal daimon" (as opposed, that is, to his "essential" daimon) — "for he who blinds the eye of sense, and extinguishes its light, after his will

[59] Hermias, *On Plato: Phaedrus 227A-245E*, trans. Dirk Baltzly and Michael Share (London: Bloomsbury, 2019), pp. 77-78.
[60] Hermias, *On Plato: Phaedrus 227A-245E*, trans. Baltzly and Share, p. 78.

has profoundly assented to its use, must expect punishment for the deed," just as Porphyry's words Odysseus deprives the Cyclops of his sight in order that "he might by this means while sailing over the stormy ocean be reminded of his sins, till he was safely landed in his native country."[61]

The episode where Aeolus tries to ensure a safe return home by giving Odysseus a leather bag with all the winds except the west wind, only for the sailors (thinking it contains gold) to open it while Odysseus is asleep just at the very moment when Ithaca comes into sight, can be read as signifying "that providence of divinity which is of an elevating and guardian nature, the influence of which, when properly received by the subjects of it, enables them to pass with security over the stormy sea of life to their native land; but when this influence is neglected through the sleep of reason, the negligence is followed by a temporary destruction of hope" (205). Then, the episode of the Laestrygonians, the man-eating giants who eat many of Odysseus's men and destroy 11 of his 12 ships by throwing rocks at them from high cliffs, represents Odysseus "flying from veracity, and fierce and savage manners," a flight that is necessary as "preparatory to his attainment of the higher virtues" (206).

In the case of Circe, whom Odysseus visits on her island of Aeaea only for her to change most of his crew into swine (in an episode that is said to contain "some deep arcana of philosophy"), Taylor says that we should understand her as representing "the goddess of sense" (206). In a passage found in Stobaeus, vol. 1, 445.14-448.3, which is attributed to Porphyry (but is now thought to be by Plutarch),[62] and offers an allegorical interpretation of

[61] Taylor, "The Wanderings of Ulysses," in Porphyry, *Select Works* [TTS, vol. 2], pp. 204-205; citing Porphyry, *On the Homeric Cave of the Nymphs*, p. 161.

[62] Christoph Helmig, "Plutarch of Chaeronea and Porphyry on Transmigration: Who Is the Author of Stobaeus I 445.14-448.3 (W.-H.)?", *The Classical Quarterly* [NS], vol. 58, no. 1 (May, 2008), 250-255.

Odyssey, Book 10, ll. 239-240, Circe is associated with the doctrine of the transmigration of souls (206). In his Scholia on the *Cratylus*, Proclus identifies Circe with a demiurgic deity who is responsible for distinguishing life in its four orders descending from the intelligible via the intelligible-intellectual and then the intellectual, into the realm of soul (cf. *Theology of Plato*, Book 4, §2, 15-20). For Circe "weaves all of life in the four classes and at the same time makes the region under the moon harmonious with songs"; indeed, "golden" Circe, as she is called — assigned to the weaving deities by those theologians who "thereby indicate her intellectual and immaculate essence" — has the function of "discriminat[ing] the things that are at rest from those that are in motion, and to separate them according to divine differences."[63]

In Book 11, Odysseus undertakes a descent to the underworld, or katabasis (κατάβασις), in order to consult Tiresias, the blind prophet. Of the many souls whom Odysseus sees (including Achilles), Olympiodorus comments in particular on the significance of the fates facing Tityos (whose punishment for his attempted rape of Leto was to be stretched out in Tartarus and to be tortured by two vultures that devoured his liver signifies that he "had lived by the appetitive part of the soul" while "the earth signifies his earthly designs"), Sisyphus (whose perpetual rolling of the stone reflects "the harsh and stubborn nature of his life"), and Tantalus (whose punishment for having offended Zeus by stealing nectar and ambrosia from the table of the gods on Olympus was to be forced to stand in a pool of water with a fruit tree whose branches always eluded him; here the water he could never drink

[63] Proclus, *On Plato Cratylus*, ed. and trans. Brian Duvick and Harold Tarrant (London and New York: Bloomsbury, 2007), pp. 30 (and 127, n. 125); cf. Taylor, "The Wanderings of Ulysses," in Porphyry, *Select Works* [TTS, vol. 2], p. 206; and "Extracts from the MS. Scholia of Proclus on the *Cratylus*," in Plato, *Works*, vol. 5, trans. Thomas Taylor and Floyer Sydenham [TTS, vol. 13] (Westbury: Prometheus Trust, 1996), pp. 542-614 (p. 553).

signifies "a life of imaginings" while the fruit denotes "something slippery and insubstantial and soon to come to an end") (50.1).[64]

Further adventures show how, in Taylor's words, Odysseus passes "from sense to imagination" (207). These include his encounter with the Sirens, those half-birdlike, half-female creatures whom Proclus, in his commentary on the *Cratylus*, describes as being categorized into three kinds: the celestial (under Zeus/Jupiter), the generative (under Poseidon/Neptune), and the purificatory or cathartic (under Hades/Pluto). While the soul in heaven is united by their song with the ways of life there, and the soul in Hades is attached to this god through their intellectual thoughts, souls living "in generation" should (in the words of the *Phaedrus*) "sail past them" (259a), lest they be "lured astray by generation," of which the sea is an image.[65] In Taylor's words, as Odysseus now proceeds "to a life which is under the dominion of imagination, but which is superior to a life consisting wholly in sensitive energies," so he "abandons those alluring and fraudulent pleasures of sense, which charm the soul with flattering and mellifluous incantations" (208). Odysseus's ruse of getting his sailors to plug their ears with beeswax and to tie him to the mast so that he may hear the Sirens' song is described by Taylor in terms of "restrain[ing] the corporeal assaults by the bands of morality," "employ[ing] the senses without yielding to their impetuous invasions," and "experienc[ing] delight without resigning the empire of reason to its fascinating control" (208): a very different kind of reading of this episode from the one presented by Theodor W. Adorno and Max Horkheimer in their *Dialectic of Enlightenment*!

Next, Odysseus must pass between the rocks of Scylla and Charybdis, legendary monsters that signify, in Taylor's words, "the passions of anger and desire, and their concomitants, that compress

[64] Olympiodorus, *Commentary on Plato's "Gorgias,"* pp. 316-317; cf. Plato, *Works*, vol. 4 [TTS, vol. 12], p. 431; and Porphyry, *Select Works* [TTS, vol. 2], p. 207.
[65] Proclus, *On Plato Cratylis*, ed. and trans. Duvick and Tarrant, pp. 88-89.

human life on both sides" and are experienced by everyone who, like Odysseus, proceeds "in a regular manner to an intellectual state of existence" (208). On the island of Thrinacia, the crew ignores the warnings of Tiresias and Circe, and hunt the sacred cattle of Helios: a sacrilegious act for which the sun god insists that Zeus punish them. This episode is said to show how "punishment attends the sacril[e]gious and the perjured," teaching us how we should "perpetually reverence divinity, with the greatest sanctity of mind, and be cautious how we commit anything in divine concerns contrary to piety of manners and purity of thought" (209-210).

Driven back toward Scylla and Charybdis, clinging to his raft which is all he can rescue from his boat in a terrible storm, Odysseus survives when his raft is swallowed up by Charybdis by clinging to a wild fig tree on the summit of her rock. Uncovering the "secret meaning" of this allegorical episode, Taylor interprets the fig tree as a symbol of the will, which, "like the wild fig-tree, affords the best refuge to the soul struggling with the billows of base perturbations" (210). Having followed Odysseus thus far in his voyage "over the turbulent and dangerous ocean of sense," in which we see him "struggling against the storms of temptation, and in danger of perishing through the tempestuous billows of vice" (211), we now find him in "the region of imagination," symbolized by the enchanted island of Calypso, a nymph who lives on the island of Ogygia, where she detains Odysseus for seven years. The allegorical symbolism of this episode turns out to be particularly rich.

Calypso, whose name is derived from *kalyptō* (καλύπτω), i.e., to cover with a veil (and, according to the *Etymologicum Magnum*, means *kalýptousa to dianooúmenon* (καλύπτουσα το διανοούμενον), i.e., "concealing the knowledge"), lives on Ogygia (i.e., *Ōgygíā* = Ὠγυγία), which derives from *Ogygios* (Ὠγύγιος), i.e., "ancient" or "archaic," a remote island in the middle of the mighty ocean; she dwells in a cave illuminated by a great fire, surrounded by a thick wood, and sustained by water from four fountains. The ocean by which this island is surrounded signifies "a corporeal nature for ever flowing, without admitting any periods of repose"; the fire represents the luminous power of the phantasy or the "imaginative spirit"; the wood corresponds to the material body, in which phantasy takes form; and the four fountains signify the four "gnostic powers of the soul," i.e., sense, opinion, the discursive energy of reason, and intellect (211). Indeed, the fact that Zeus sends Hermes/Mercury to tell Calypso to set Odysseus free symbolizes the intervention of reason and the abandonment of "the delusive and detaining charms of imagination" (212), while the passage in which Odysseus departs from Calypso and sets sail by night, contemplating "the order and the light of the stars" (Book 5, ll. 269-277), is read as compatible with Plato's "signature allegory" — that is, the allegory of the cave in Book 7 of the *Republic*.

In that allegory, the individual is led up from the cave into the light of day, i.e., "from a sensible to an intellectual life," described by Socrates as a turn to "beholding the things in heaven and heaven itself, more easily at night — looking at the light of the stars and the moon — than by day — looking at the sun and sunlight" (516b; trans. Bloom, p. 195), a turn which Taylor follows Proclus (in his commentary on the *Republic*) in interpreting as signifying "the contemplation of intelligibles, of which the stars and their light are the imitations" (213). On this reading, Odysseus is "hastening to an intellectual life" and so "contemplates these lucid objects with vigilant eyes, rejoicing in the illuminations and assistance they afford him while sailing over the dark ocean of a sensible life" (213).

On learning that Odysseus has escaped from Calypso's island, however, Poseidon/Neptune is angered and wrecks his raft. Thanks to the assistance of the sea nymph Ino, who appears as an aspect of the ancient sea goddess Leucothea, Odysseus eventually lands on Phaeacia, the island of the Phaeacians. Just as Odysseus leaves "the delusions of imagination" and turns to "the more intellectual light of the rational energy of the soul," the island of Phaeacia represents the capacity for *dianoia*, or "the power of reasoning scientifically, deriving the principles of its discursive energy from intellect" (213). Phaeacia is one of the Blissful (i.e., Blessed or Fortunate) Islands, interpreted by Olympiodorus in his commentary on the *Gorgias* as signifying "that polity [or condition of being] which transcends the present [or corporeal] life."[66] Homer's description of the palace of Alcinous (i.e., *Alkínoös* = Ἀλκίνοος, or "mighty mind"), the happy ruler of the Phaeacians, indicates the splendid light of reason (Book 7, ll. 84-94 and 100-103), thereby indicating its agreement with Mercury, the deity of rational energy whom Proclus describes as "unfold[ing] into light intellectual gifts, fill[ing] all things with divine *reasons*, elevat[ing] souls to intellect, [...] and bring[ing] them to a blessed life."[67] And Homer's account of the excellence of the ships made by the Phaeacians (Book 8, ll. 57-62) is said to confirm this reading of the island of Phaeacia as the "dominion of reason" (215). The earlier praise of the Phaeacians' ships, placed in the mouth of Pallas Athene (Book 7, ll. 34-36), even includes the phrase "as swift as any wing or thought."[68] In the palace of Alcinous, Odysseus behaves as befits someone "passing in a regular manner from the delusions of sense, to the realities of intellectual enjoyment" (216); hence, when Demodocus sings at a feast about the disagreement between Odysseus and Achilles at Troy, Odysseus is right to burst into tears, for "to the man who is making a proficiency in virtue, the recollection of his former

[66] Plato, *Works*, vol. 4 [TTS, vol. 12], p. 426; cf. Porphyry, *Select Works* [TTS, vol. 2], p. 214.

[67] Proclus's commentary on the first book of Euclid's *Elements* (book 1, chapter 15), cited in Porphyry, *Select Works* [TTS, vol. 2], p. 215; cf. Proclus, *Commentary on the First Book of Euclid's "Elements,"* trans. Thomas Taylor [TTS, vol. 19] (Sturminster Newton: Prometheus Trust, 2006, p. 132).

[68] Homer, *Odyssey*, ed. and trans. Albert Cook, 2nd edn (New York and London: Norton, 1993), p. 71.

conduct is both pleasing and painful; pleasing, so far as in some instances it was attended with rectitude, but painful so far as in others it was erroneous" (217). Indeed, Odysseus's decision to relate his past wanderings to the king — a decision to which the *Odyssey* as a work owes much of its narrative structure — confirms the hero's ascendency to "the intellectual light of the reasoning power," as he undertakes to "review his past conduct, faithfully enumerate the errors of his life, and anxiously solicit a return to true manners and perfect rectitude of mind" (217). Tellingly, then, when Odysseus finally leaves the Phaeacians and sets sail again for Ithaca, and catches his first glimpse of the island, Homer describes it as appearing to the returning seafarer as does the morning star when it emerges from the darkness of night (Book 13, ll. 93-95; 217).

On Ithaca, Odysseus is advised by Athena or Minerva, the goddess of wisdom, how he might "banish the various perturbations and inordinate desires, which yet lurk in the penetralia of his soul," hence his relinquishing of all external possessions and his embrace of poverty (217; cf. Book 13, ll. 372-381 and ll. 397-403). His son, Telemachus, is said to represent "a true scientific conception of things"; the suitors, "those baneful passions which are secretly attempting to subvert the empire of his mind"; and Penelope, the image of philosophy (219). When Penelope does not recognize Odysseus, even after he has dispatched the suitors (Book 23, ll. 88-95), Homer is said to illustrate how "Philosophy, through her long absence from the soul [...], is a stranger to it" (220). But when, thanks to Athena or Minerva, Odysseus reacquires his former dignity (Book 23, ll. 130-134), that is, he "renders all pure and harmonious within the recesses of his soul," he is now described as stepping from the bathtub "*in form like the immortal gods*" (ll. 160-161). Having "completely destroyed the domination of his passions," having "purified himself, through the cathartic virtues, from their defiling nature," and having been "assimilated to divinity," only now is Odysseus in a fit state to "become entirely known to Philosophy, that chaste Penelope of the soul" (220). And so he makes himself known to her by relating "the secrets of their mystic union," that is, by recognizing "the bower of intellectual love," which leads to "perfect recollection" — to "transports of assurance," as well as to "tears of rapturous delight" (220).

In his "various wanderings and woes," that is, through the *cathartic* virtues, Odysseus succeeds in "recover[ing] the ruined empire of his soul" (220). Yet there is a further step: Now he must "possess and energize according to the theoretic or contemplative virtues," a process which will lead to "a union with deity" — insofar as this is possible in this present life. This union is signified by Odysseus first seeing his father, Laertes, then embracing him with ecstatic delight (Book 14), a union whose enactment in solitude is emphasized by the reference to Odysseus, acting *alone*, going to his father, who is *alone*. This emphasis on being *alone* in order to accomplish "a union with [...] the true father of the soul," with "the ineffable *one* of the Demiurgus," echoes the famous phrase found in Plotinus about the union of the soul and the deity as "a flight of the alone to the Alone,"[69] and the commentary by Proclus on a line from Plato's *Timaeus*, "The maker and father of this universe it is a hard task to find, and having found him it would be impossible to declare him to all [hu]mankind" (28c),[70] as follows: "But it is also necessary for the soul, after becoming an intellective cosmos and assimilating itself to the extent possible to the entirety of the intelligible cosmos, to make its approach to the Maker of the universe, and from this approach to become familiar with him somehow through its continual concentration [...] and through this

[69] Plotinus, "The Good or the One," in *Enneads*, VI.9 [9], §11; in *The Essential Plotinus: Representative Treatises from the Enneads*, ed. and trans. Elmer O'Brien, SJ (Indianapolis, IN: Hackett, 1964), p. 88.

[70] Francis MacDonald Cornford, *Plato's Cosmology: The "Timaeus" of Plato* (Indianapolis, IN: Hackett, 1997), p. 22.

familiarity to stand at the gate of the Father and be unified with him."[71] Indeed, Proclus's commentary on this line from the *Timaeus* could stand *pars pro toto* for the overall Neoplatonic meaning discerned in the *Odyssey*:

> For it is only when the soul has passed beyond the distraction of birth and the [process of] purification and beyond the illumination of scientific knowledge that its intellective activity and the intellect in us lights up, anchoring the soul in the Father and establishing it immaculately in the demiurgic thoughts. [...] This is the Paternal harbour, the discovery of the Father, the immaculate unification [*henôsis*] with him.[72]

The humble attire of Laertes, solitarily engaged with his agricultural work (Book 24, ll. 225-231), is said to recall what Proclus says in his commentary on Plato's *Parmenides* about how divine beings "have their foundation in the simplicity of the One, who fervently rejoice in 'unadorned beauty' (as one of the experts in divine matters says) and extend it to those capable of looking at the divine,"[73] and to exemplify how "ancient mythologers" intimated "the transcendency of divine natures" by "things preternatural," suggested "a power more divine than all reason" by "things irrational," and by "apparent deformity" evoked "a beauty which surpasses every thing corporeal" (223).

Odysseus's intimation of his mortality in conversation with Penelope (Book 23, ll. 281-284), echoing the prophetic words of

[71] Proclus, *Commentary on Plato's "Timaeus,"* vol 2, *Book 2: Proclus on the Causes of the Cosmos and its Creation*, trans. David T. Runia and Michael Share (New York: Cambridge University Press, 2008), p. 156.

[72] Proclus, *Commentary on Plato's "Timaeus,"* vol. 2, p. 157.

[73] Proclus, *Commentary on Plato's "Parmenides,"* trans. Glenn R. Morrow and John M. Dillon, ed. John M. Dillon (Princeton, NJ: Princeton University Press, 1987), p. 38 (book 1, 645).

Tiresias (Book 11, ll. 122-137) with its reference to the twin gesture of carrying a winnowing shovel on one's shoulder and sticking the shaft of an oar into the ground,[74] recalls for Taylor the remark by Porphyry in his treatise on the cave of the nymphs that, even if someone should "recover the ruined empire of his soul," no one is "freed from molestation, till he has entirely passed over the raging sea, and taken a long farewell of its storms,"[75] that is, has become "impassive to the excitations of the irrational life" — an impassivity or perfect subjugation of the passions to reason that constitutes the *apatheia* (i.e., ἀπάθεια) of Stoicism and Platonism, symbolized by Tiresias's words about "men who do not know / The sea and eat a food that has not been mixed with salt" (Book 11, ll. 122-123) — "and is entirely abstracted from external concerns" (223). To underscore both the core message and the methodological possibility of this kind of allegorical reading of Homer's epic, Taylor reminds us of the passage in Plotinus's *Ennead* on beauty, which quotes from the *Iliad*, "Let us fly then to the beloved Fatherland,"[76] and interprets it as a call for us to "close our eyes and invoke a new manner of seeing, a wakefulness that is the birthright of us all, though few put it to use."[77]

The Neoplatonists' reading of Homer as synthesized by Taylor in 1823 was revived by the Canadian esotericist Manly P. Hall (1901-1990) in a series of five lectures presented to the

---

[74] For discussion of the gesture of carrying a winnowing shovel and sticking the shaft of an oar into the ground, see David A. Beardsley, *The Journey Back To Where You Are: Homer's "Odyssey" as Spiritual Quest* (Highland Park, NJ: Ideograph Media, 2014), pp. 302-304; and Gregory Nagy, *The Ancient Greek Hero in 24 Hours* (Cambridge, MA, and London: Belknap Press of Harvard University Press, 2013), pp. 336-337 and 340-344.

[75] Porphyry, "On the Homeric Cave of the Nymphs," in *Select Works* [TTS, vol. 2], p. 161.

[76] *Iliad*, Book 2, l. 140. This quotation comes from a quite irrelevant context, although there are reminiscences of *Odyssey*, Book 9, ll. 27-29 and Book 10, ll. 483-484; see Plotinus, *Porphyry on Plotinus; Ennead I*, trans. A.H. Armstrong (Cambridge, MA, and London: Harvard University Press, 1995), p. 257.

[77] *Enneads* I.6 [1], §8; in *The Essential Plotinus*, p. 42.

Philosophical Research Society in Los Angeles in 1983.[78] When, in his fourth lecture on Porphyry on the wanderings of Odysseus (or, as he calls, him, Ulysses), Hall attributes to Olympiodorus the view that Homer's "fable" should be considered as having "a secret and mystical meaning" (113), he might be thinking of the passage in the commentary on the *Gorgias* (46.4) where Olympiodorus introduces the distinction between philosophical and poetic myths.[79] Poetic myths have the advantage, Olympiodorus argues, that "its content is such that even one who happens not to believe it nevertheless proceeds to a concealed truth," that is, it has the advantage of "saying the sort of things that does not allow us to stay with the surface meaning but makes us seek a concealed truth" (291). The *disadvantage* of poetic myth, however, is that it can be deceptive, and this is why, in the *Republic*, Plato expels Homer from the *polis* (*Republic*, Books 2-3 and Book 11), referring to the existence of an ancient quarrel between philosophy and poetry. On Olympiodorus's account (46.5), the young in particular should not listen to these myths, as they are incapable of allegorical interpretation and hence cannot judge their "hidden sense," with the result that their misunderstandings become "hard to eradicate" (*Republic*, 378d-e). Then again, philosophical myths share with the poetic kind the characteristic of being constructed "so as not to transmit doctrines indiscriminately," acting as "screens for doctrines" so that they are "not uncovered and accessible to anyone who wants," just as "in temples the sacred objects and mysteries are behind screens, so that the unworthy do not see them indiscriminately" (292). Unlike poetic myths, however, philosophical ones have the feature that, "even if one stays with the surface meaning, one is not harmed," although they have the *disadvantage* that, "since their surface meaning is not harmful, we often stay right there and do not seek the truth"

[78] Manly Palmer Hall. *Neoplatonism: Theology for Wanderers in the New Millennium* (Los Angeles, CA: Philosophical Research Society, 2010).
[79] Olympiodorus, *Commentary on Plato's "Gorgias,"* pp. 292-293.

(292). Moreover, philosophical myths address themselves to "the three [cognitive] activities of the soul," rather than the "imaginative faculty," raising the question: Why do we need myths at all? Why not always "deal with intelligibles"? The answer is that, if our entire selves were mind alone, we would not need myths, just as, if we were without reason and lived in accordance with imagination, we would "live all our life as if in a myth." Because, however, we have intellect and opinion and imagination, we require demonstrations for intellect, the evidence of sound persons for opinion, and myths that stimulate the imagination (293).

Hence it is open to us, Hall argues, to read Homeric epic as "a highly allegorical and symbolical poem," and as possibly even revealing Orphic (or some other) mysteries (113). How did Homer's works acquire this meaning? On the one hand, does it mean that Homer himself had been in possession of "a knowledge not generally accessible to the Greeks of his time"? Or that the later Greeks interpreted this meaning "*into* the writings of Homer by a fortuitous method of reasoning and interpretation" (114; my emphasis)? Or, on the other hand, do these works rather draw "*out of* their interpreters certain secret knowledge locked within the mind and hearts of the interpreters," so that poems which were not "*consciously* intended to have a message" nevertheless may "*release* a message from the psychic life of the reader of the poem" (114; my emphasis)? (This power of *releasing* a message in their readers is surely one that also characterizes the four works by Wolfram, Goethe, Nietzsche, and Jung.)

On Hall's synthesizing account, Odysseus represents the heroic aspect of the human soul, inasmuch as the hero belonged to a separate order between the human and the divine — semidivine or superhuman, one might say. In accordance with this view, the hero may be defined as "a human being who has at some time or another, either in the present life or a preceding life, made the final commitment of his consciousness to the process of growth";

someone who "is no longer merely living for the gratification of the whims and passing fancies of external life"; someone who "has a motion, a pressure, a dynamic within himself by which he is being moved throughout all the ensuing cycles of his existence in a direct and positive motion toward the fulfillment of his essential destiny" (117-118). Thus, the entire story of Odysseus's journey involves "the problem of sensation and [...] the development of the sensory perceptions and internal psychic instincts" (120), and the *Odyssey* thereby acquires a profound and universal meaning:

> The sensory world, as it was understood by the Greek philosophers, was a world which resulted in the polarization of the psychic nature in a middle distance between a spiritual and a material state. In other words, in the strangely symbolical meaning, the Greeks [...] recognized that the hero was almost the true human being but that man as he knows himself now cannot be truly human until he is born again through the mystery of heroic attainment. (123)

On this reading, the Homeric hero represents "the integrated human person in whom the psychic nature is in equilibrium," an equilibrium which can only be achieved if the psychic nature "resolve[s] its conflicts and achieve[s] a moderation within itself," a moderation which in turn is achieved through two kinds of discipline — cathartic disciplines or disciplines for "complete and positive possession of the internal nature itself" (123-124).

In this respect, there are important links to texts under study in this series: to Faust, who tells Wagner that there are "spirits in the air, / Who float 'twixt heaven and earth dominion wielding" (*Geister in der Luft, / Die zwischen Erd und Himmel herrschend weben*) (ll. 118-119), that is, we can be drawn by sense "downward into an objectivity" or become "bound by matter," but the soul also possesses a theurgic power, by means of which it can "verge away from matter and toward divine things," causing it to "ascend or rise toward the gods" (124). And there is a link to the legend of Parzival in its operatic treatment by Wagner. In Homer, the episode with Circe can be read in terms of being captured in the snares of the imagination, a predicament that Hall relates to Eliphas Lévi's notion of "astral light" as a beautiful garden in which, around the stem of each flower, a deadly serpent is entwined, and to Klingsor's magic garden in Wagner's *Parsifal* (133).

Finally, in connection with the episode of the Sirens and Odysseus's cunning stratagem of being tied to the mast of his ship, Hall comments on the symbol of the ship and its various interesting meanings. In Buddhism, he notes, there is the notion of the "ship of the doctrine," reflected in the Buddha's resolve to "acquire the supreme wisdom, [...] to cause multitudes to go on board the ship of Doctrine and cross the ocean of the round of rebirth, and [...] afterwards to pass into Nirvana";[80] in Christianity, there is the notion of the "ship of Christianity," reflected in the motif of St. Peter's boat on the papal ring (and used by Nietzsche in *Dawn*, §68); all in all, it is said to be a symbol of "the mysteries, the institution, the sacred doctrine itself by which all souls are carried home [...] the purity of the revealed rite, the ancient institutions by means of which the preservation and security of [humankind] is guaranteed" (131).

For his part, Jung similarly reminded his audience during one of his lectures on Nietzsche's *Zarathustra* of how the ship functions "as a symbol," especially in religions (SNZ, vol. 2, 970); and one might add that, in Book 7 of Plato's *Laws*, the Athenian Stranger intriguingly uses precisely this image of shipbuilding in respect of designing education, saying that what he is doing is "much the

[80] Henry Clarke Warren (ed. and trans.), *A Buddhist Reader: Selections from the Sacred Books* [1896; [4]1906] (Mineola, NY: Dover, 2004), p. 14; see Edward J. Thomas, *The History of Buddhist Thought* (London: Routledge & Kegan Paul, 1833), p. 134.

same as what a shipwright does in the beginning of building ships, when he sketches the shape of ships in outline by laying down the keels" (803a).[81] In terms of Christian allegory, Jung remarks, Christ is "at the tiller of the Church" (and, in German, the word *Schiff* means the nave of a church, so that in architectural terms the Church is a ship). Then again, within Buddhism, there are the two schools of the Hīnayāna and the Mahāyāna,[82] or "the little and the great vessel" (970). Indeed, a religious system itself is described by Jung as being "like a safe form, a body of teaching, of principles, of advice and so on, which is destined to help [humankind] to navigate over the troubled waters of the unconscious"; it is "a human contrivance to protect one against the dangers of real life," for "there is no real life without archetypal experiences" (970). We are, he argued, "always exposed to the operations of nature" and therefore we need "a system of thought, or laws, or prescriptions" to act as "a sort of wisdom that would help us to navigate on the sea of the unconscious" (970).

(Where do these teachings come from? According to Jung, all these methods of, so to speak, religious shipbuilding are "not inventions, but […] revelations," expressing "a revealed truth or a perceived truth which has been thought before [the human being] has thought" (SNZ, vol. 2, pp. 970-971). And here we find a deeply Platonic resonance within Jung's thinking: "Before I had that thought it had already been thought, and I merely happened to perceive it once in time; it has been there since eternity, is always there, has always lived, and I just happened in a certain moment to perceive it. […] The helpful thought [is] personified in many forms in many times […]" [971].)

[81] Plato, *The Laws*, ed. and trans. Thomas L. Pangle (Chicago and London: University of Chicago Press, 1988), p. 192.
[82] Nowadays the term Hīnayāna is considered pejorative, and instead the term Nikaya Buddhism is used to refer to early Buddhist schools.

In much the same way, Manly P. Hall (following Olympiodorus's categories) describes Odysseus as a hero of the Neptunian allotment, for "his great adventure, struggle, everything practically concerned with him has to do with the sea": He is making "a long water journey and when it seems that he is almost going to be victorious, then Neptune, the god of the sea, turns upon him and attempts to destroy him" (118). Odysseus himself can, then, be said to represent "the soul that has already been dedicated to the path of progress," and in this sense he belongs "on the level of the dark Neptune"; a Neptune, that is, who is the principle of water or the principle of generation. If, in Heraclitus's words, "the dry soul is the wisest and best" (DK 22 B 118), this is because a soul that becomes involved in generation becomes involved in humidity, drinks of the waters of Lethe, and falls into illusion; water, because of its inconstancy, eternal motion, and mysterious depths, serving the Greeks as a symbol of sensation and the emotional sphere of the human being (120).

As the guardian of the sea, under whose aquatic allotment Odysseus belongs, Neptune himself is described as "a strange and mysterious power governing the middle diffusion of the objective universe," and — in accordance with the categorization of Olympiodorus — the patron over the psychic life of the human being, so that if the spirit belongs to Jupiter/Zeus and the body to Pluto/Hades, the soul belongs to Neptune/Poseidon. Representing the psychic sphere, Neptune does not wish Odysseus to escape, and so "in the long journey through this fluidic element, the psychic life, […] Neptune brings the great tempest to bear upon him," and there is a universal message here:

> Thus, along the great journey of life, the individual is beset with hardships, the storm of life threatens to close over him and the psychic stress threatens to engulf him. In this emergency that he must fare, Minerva [or Pallas Athene] appears giving him the internal experience of

> security. She bestows upon him the vision or the internal participation in Reality. Minerva therefore brings with her, so to say, the mystical experience, the sign, the proof, the evidence that the powers of darkness shall not prevail. Thus strengthened, [Odysseus] is able to escape the wrath of Neptune and to continue on his journey home. (135-136)

In this respect, Minerva, or Pallas Athene, represents an intervention from the outside, whether in the form of an intervening deity or access to a realm or a repository that lies outside or beyond the individual. It finds a corresponding motif in the will of the heroic individual, represented (as Thomas Taylor noted) in the form of the wild fig tree that grows on the summit of the rock over her lair — a symbol of "the human will which was called upon in emergency and gave the individual strength to survive the damages and dangers of this hazardous journey he must take" (138).

Originally formulated by (among others) Porphyry in his treatise *On the Homeric Cave of the Nymphs*, by Plotinus in various allusions, and by Proclus in his sixth essay in his commentary on Plato's *Republic*, and repackaged in the late 18th and early 19th centuries by Thomas Taylor and in the 20th century by Manly P. Hall, this Neoplatonic reading of Homer has its representative in our own century in David A. Beardsley's *The Journey Back To Where You Are: Homer's Odyssey as Spiritual Quest* (2014). As Beardsley has suggested, if all Western philosophy is, as Alfred North Whitehead says it is, a series of footnotes to Plato,[83] one could equally say that all Western literature is a series of spinoffs from Homer.[84] For as

[83] A.N. Whitehead, *Process and Reality: An Essay in Cosmology*, ed. David Ray Griffin and Donald W. Sherburne (New York: The Free Press, 1979), p. 39.
[84] Beardsley, *The Journey Back to Where You Are*, p. 240; cf. Robert Lamberton, *Homer the Theologian: Neoplatonist Allegorical Reading and the Growth of the Epic Tradition* (Berkeley, Los Angeles, and London: University of California Press, 1986).

Werner Jaeger (1888-1961) argued in his influential three-volume study, *Paideia: The Ideals of Greek Culture* (1933-1947), art has "a limitless power of converting the human soul — a power which the Greeks called *psychagogia*," for "art alone possesses the two essentials of educational influence — universal significance and immediate appeal."[85] Now the immediate appeal of epic drew in no small measure from hearing it as it was performed by professional rhapsodes; in Greek, the word *kleos*., i.e., the glory associated with the hero, derived from *kluein*, i.e., "to hear" (241). Thus, the hearer of epics was imagined as being enabled to participate in the glory of the hero, an idea to which Plato alludes in the *Ion*:

> **Socrates:** Stop now and tell me, Ion, without reserve what I may choose to ask you: when you give a good recitation and specially thrill your audience, either with the lay of Odysseus leaping forth on to the threshold, revealing himself to the suitors and pouring out the arrows before his feet, or of Achilles dashing at Hector, or some part of the sad story of Andromache or of Hecuba, or of Priam, are you then in your senses, or are you carried out of yourself, and does your soul in an ecstasy suppose herself to be among the scenes you are describing, whether they be in Ithaca, or in Troy, or as the poems may chance to place them?
>
> **Ion:** How vivid to me, Socrates, is this part of your proof! For I will tell you without reserve: when I relate a tale of woe, my eyes are filled with tears; and when it is of fear or awe, my hair stands on end with terror, and my heart leaps. (535b-c; trans. W.R.M. Lamb)

[85] Werner Jaeger, *Paideia: The Ideals of Greek Culture*, vol. 1, *Archaic Greece: The Mind of Athens*, trans. Gilbert Highet, 2nd edn (New York and Oxford: Oxford University Press, 1965), p. 36.

As Plato makes clear, however, the rhapsode must be aware of affect of recitation on his audience (even if, in so doing, his motives are not purely artistic) (241):

> **Socrates:** And are you aware that you rhapsodes produce these same effects on most of the spectators also?
>
> **Ion:** Yes, very fully aware: for I look down upon them from the platform and see them at such moments crying and turning awestruck eyes upon me and yielding to the amazement of my tale. For I have to pay the closest attention to them; since, if I set them crying, I shall laugh myself because of the money I take, but if they laugh, I myself shall cry because of the money I lose. (535d-e; trans. Lamb)

Nowadays, as Beardsley recognizes, we know the *Odyssey* mainly from reading it, not hearing it (241), and even if Wolfram's *Parzival* still retains something of the performativity of ancient epic, our approach to it and the three other works discussed here is largely, if not entirely, textual. Be that as it may, we can nevertheless understand both the *Odyssey* and *Parzival*, *Faust*, *Zarathustra*, and *The Red Book* in an inductive way as a guiding myth, showing us the steps involved in the spiritual journey; if, as Beardsley suggests, we can set aside the discursive tools of the discursive mind (whose use began with Aristotle) and enter into their imaginary worlds.

Why these four works?

Although the significance of at least three of these four works could be said to be "canonical," in recent years the very notion of the canon itself has become increasingly controversial, leading the American critic Harold Bloom (1930-2019) to publish in 1994 his book titled *The Western Canon: The Books and School of the Ages*. (One might note that of the works discussed here, oddly only one — Goethe's *Faust* — is included in Bloom's study.)

Although the notion of a work being considered a "classic" goes as far back as Aulus Gellius who, in the second century in his *Noctes Atticae* (19, 8, 15), refers to a writer as a *classicus scriptor, non proletarius* ("a distinguished, not a commonplace writer"), the idea of the canon has become so problematic within the academy that not only has the notion itself fallen into disuse, but many of the works usually recognized as canonical have been removed from the syllabus and are no longer taught or read. Nowhere is this more the case than in German studies in the U.K., where Goethe's *Faust*, once a core part of an undergraduate curriculum, is rarely studied (and, if so, in the form of the *Urfaust*, with little or no opportunity to look at the second part). Even in Germany, *Faust* is increasingly rarely read; one cannot take for granted, if making an allusion to this work, that everyone will recognize it or appreciate its significance.

Yet these works —*Parzival*, *Faust*, *Zarathustra* — simply will not go away; and no figure is better placed to allow us to approach them in the 21st century than Jung, whose *Collected Works* constitute a veritable education in their own right,[86] and whose *Red Book* represents (so I shall argue) a continuation of a tradition exemplified by those earlier works. Of course, Jung himself remains a marginal figure in the arts and humanities, at least within academic circles. Could this be, in part, precisely because of his deep-rootedness in the texts and cultures of the past? One has only to think of the amazing erudition displayed across his works: from *Symbols and Transformations of the Libido* (1911-1912) with its mythological references and allusions to Longfellow's

[86] For further discussion, see the essays collected in *How and Why We Still Read Jung: Personal and Professional Reflections*, ed. Jean Kirsch and Murray Stein (London and New York: Routledge, 2013), including Paul Bishop, "On Reading Jung in German: Jung's Significance for *Germanistik*" (pp. 66-85).

Hiawatha, Goethe, Hölderlin, and Nietzsche, via *Psychological Types* with its discussions of the problem of types in the history of classical and medieval thought (the Gnostics, Tertullian, and Origen; the theological disputes in the ancient Church; the problem of transubstantiation; nominalism and realism; and the controversy about Holy Communion between Luther and Zwingli), in Schiller's *Letters on the Aesthetic Education of Humankind* and *On Naïve and Sentimental Poetry*, and in Nietzsche's *The Birth of Tragedy* and its concepts of the Apollonian and the Dionysian, not to mention his discussions of John Furneaux Jordan (1830-1911), Carl Spitteler (1845-1924), and William James (1842-1910), to *Answer to Job* (1952) with its close reading of a biblical text and *Mysterium coniunctionis* (1955-1956) with its astonishing range of references (thanks, in part, to his collaboration with Marie-Louise von Franz) to a vast body of alchemical texts.[87]

Jung's writings represent a concerted effort to recover and to make sense of the past, as Peter Kingsley has shown.[88] Small wonder, then, that Jung is regarded with suspicion, even loathing, by those wishing to smash patriarchy, erase hierarchy, and in various other ways "deconstruct" texts for political causes with which one might, in fact, not necessarily disagree, other than that these great texts should not be instrumentalized for the purposes of individual (or even collective) *parti pris*. If the notion of the archetype means

[87] As Philip Rieff insightfully observed, Jung is "the latest in a line of great erudites," and may even be "the last as well as the latest of all the erudites," inasmuch as "in him Protestant erudition has completed a full circle, to attack rationalism itself" (Philip Rieff, *The Triumph of the Therapeutic: Uses of Faith After Freud* (Harmondsworth: Penguin, 1973), pp. 108-109). For the third volume of *Mysterium coniunctionis* (not included in the English *Collected Works*) see Marie-Louise von Franz (ed.), *"Aurora consurgens": Ein dem Thomas von Aquin zugeschriebenes Dokument der alchemistischen Gegensatzproblematik* [*Gesammelte Werke*, vol. 14/3] (Olten und Freiburg im Breisgau: Walter-Verlag, 1971).

[88] Peter Kingsley, *Catafalque: Carl Jung and the End of Humanity*, 2 vols (London: Catafalque Press, 2018).

anything, it is that Jung speaks to us of our present concerns by way of a detour through the — sometimes, very ancient — past.

So, this study in four volumes does not so much propose a "Jungian" reading of Wolfram von Eschenbach, Goethe, and Nietzsche, as offer a way into discovering (or rediscovering) these works and establishing the position of Jung's *Red Book* as belonging to this quasi-canonical epic tradition in German. While the case for understanding the significance of Jung's reception of Nietzsche and of Goethe has been made elsewhere,[89] the idea of including *Parzival* was prompted (at least, in part) by Jung's suggestion in *The Red Book*: "I must catch up with a piece of the Middle Ages — within myself. We have only finished the Middle Ages of — others" (RB, 330). The occasion for beginning work on this series of four books was the first lockdown due to the coronavirus crisis in April 2020, when focusing on the essential things, on what really matters, seemed the order of the day. The five weeks of lockdown were an opportunity to read systematically through Jung's seminar on Nietzsche's *Zarathustra* and *The Red Book*; I had refreshed my memory of *Parzival* by reading it through in the preceding summer while a visiting lecturer in the Traumkolleg at the University of Saarbrücken; and for the discussions of *Faust* and *Zarathustra,* I have drawn on notes for when I used to teach these texts at the University of Glasgow. The invitation to contribute to a volume on narratives of individuation edited by Raya Jones and Leslie Gardner offered a chance to undertake an initial exploration of some of the structural parallels across three of these texts.[90]

---

[89] See Paul Bishop, *The Dionysian Self: C.G. Jung's Reception of Friedrich Nietzsche* (Berlin and New York: de Gruyter, 1995); and *Analytical Psychology and German Classical Aesthetics*, 2 vols (London and New York: Routledge, 2008-2009).

[90] Paul Bishop, "Telling Stories: Jung's *Red Book* as an Exercise in Narrative," in Raya A. Jones and Leslie Gardner (eds), *Narratives of Individuation* (New York and London: Routledge, 2019), pp. 111-131.

As far as recommended editions are concerned, this is not always easy. *Parzival* is available in a superb two-volume edition (translated into modern German by Dieter Kühn with extensive commentary by Eberhard Nellmann) in the Deutscher Klassiker Verlag series; and a parallel MHG-modern German edition in two volumes was published by Wolfgang Spiework using the text established by Karl Lachmann in two Reclam volumes in 1981, drawing on a translation previously published in the GDR in 1977. The work has been translated in 1980 in a sparsely commented edition by A.T. Hatto (1910-2010), professor of German at the University of London; and (together with *Titurel*) in 2004 as volume 56 of the *Arthurian Studies* series (and subsequently as an Oxford World's Classics paperback in 2006) by Cyril Edwards, a lecturer in German at St Peter's College, Oxford; to capture something of the "epic" flavor, however, I have decided to cite from Jessie L. Weston's translation of 1894. A number of useful (if, these days, rather out-of-date) essays on *Parzival* are collected in the volume of *Wege der Forschung* dedicated to Wolfram von Eschenbach published in 1966; while a Camden House *Companion* volume to *Parzival*, edited by Will Hasty and published in 1999, and a two-volume *Handbuch* to Wolfram, edited by Joachmin Heinzle and published in 2011, offer a range of more recent critical perspectives.[91]

For Goethe's *Faust*, I would recommend the one-volume edition edited by Erich Trunz as part of the 14-volume *Hamburger Ausgabe* of Goethe's works, the two-volume edition edited by Albrecht Schöne in the Deutscher Klassiker Verlag (2005), or the three-volume edition edited by Ulrich Gaier for Reclam (1999);

---

[91] Will Hasty (ed.), *A Companion to Wolfram's "Parzival"* (Rochester, NY, and Suffolk: Camden House, 1999); and Joachim Heinzle (ed.), *Wolfram von Eschenbach: Ein Handbuch*, 2 vols in 1 [vol. 1, *Autor Werk, Wirkung*; vol. 2, *Figuren-Lexikon, Beschreibendes Verzeichnis der Handschriften, Bibliographien, Register, Abbildungen*] (Berlin and Boston: de Gruyter, 2011).

while I prefer the translation made in two volumes by David Luke (1921-2005) of Christ Church, Oxford, for Oxford University Press, a more useful commentary and interpretative apparatus is available in the translation made by Walter W. Arndt (1916-2011) and edited by Cyrus Hamlin (1936-2011) in a Norton Critical Edition: the best single-volume, "one-stop-shop" edition available (the first edition in 1976 was revised for a second edition in 2001).

Although numerous (and mostly very good, even excellent) translations of Nietzsche's *Thus Spoke Zarathustra* exist (from those of R.J. Hollingdale or Walter Kaufmann to the more recent ones by Graham Parkes, Adrian Del Caro, etc.), the best commentary has yet to appear — the one in the series titled *Historischer and kritischer Kommentar zu Friedrich Nietzsches Werken*, edited by the Heidelberger Akademie der Wissenschaften. (Across the two collections of Nietzsche's works as translated by Walter Kaufmann, the Viking Penguin *Nietzsche Reader* and the *Basic Writings* published in the Modern Library series, the reader has access to almost the entirety of Nietzsche's works, while the critical edition of Giorgio Colli (1917-1979) and Mazzino Montinari (1928-1986), including the whole of the *Nachlass*, is currently being translated for Stanford University Press edition of the complete works.)[92]

Finally, thanks to the editorial efforts of Sonu Shamdasani and his two fellow translators, Jung's *Red Book* was published with an extensive commentary in a facsimile edition in separate German and English editions in 2009, with a shorter (because unillustrated) Reader's Edition in 2012. For convenience's sake, this is the edition referred to here, while for copyright reasons (and also out of a

[92] For a useful discussion of the challenges posed by translating *Zarathustra*, see Paul S. Loeb and David F. Tinsley, "Translators' Afterword," in *Unpublished Fragments from the Period of "Thus Spoke Zarathustra" (Summer 1882 – Winter 1883/84)*, trans. Paul S. Loeb and David F. Tinsley [*Complete Works of Friedrich Nietzsche*, vol. 14] (Stanford, CA: Stanford University Press, 2019), pp. 717-797.

certain affection for them) *Parzival* is quoted from the translation by Jessie L. Weston (1850-1928); *Faust* is quoted in English from the edition by Albert G. Latham (1864-1940), the first Professor of Modern Languages at Newcastle University, published in the Everyman series in 1908; and *Thus Spoke Zarathustra* from the translation by Thomas Common (1850-1919), published in 1909 as part of the project (initiated by Alexander Tille (1866-1912) with his own translation of *Zarathustra* in 1896) overseen by Oscar Levy (1867-1946) to produce a complete English edition of Nietzsche's works. (This was also the translation used by Jung in his seminar on *Zarathustra*, held in Zurich between 1934 and 1939). Where necessary or appropriate I have corrected or adapted these translations, especially in respect of gender inclusivity.

Conclusion

According to Jung, self-knowledge, or *Selbsterkenntnis,* lies in extending the range of human consciousness, while simultaneously acknowledging the power of the unconscious — the way that "the life, that has been repressed, forces its way into the open through all the cracks" (CW 14 §742). And this kind of self-knowledge is what Jung understood by culture, a position summed up in *Memories, Dreams, Reflections* as "attainment of consciousness is culture in the broadest sense, and self-knowledge is therefore the heart and essence of this process" (*Bewußtwerdung ist Kultur im weitesten Sinne und Selbsterkenntnis daher Essenz und Herz dieses Vorgangs*) (MDR, 356). This emphasis on the link between understanding and culture is comparable with the remark made by another inheritor of the German literary tradition, Thomas Mann (1875-1955) — whose novels reflect a profound engagement with medieval literature (*Gregorius*), as well as with Goethe's *Faust* and with Nietzsche (*Doktor Faustus*) — in a letter to Klaus Mann of 22 July 1939: "To inherit is an art in itself; for inheriting, in the final analysis, is culture" (*Aber schließlich, zu erben muß man auch verstehen, erben, das ist am Ende Kultur*).[93]

According to Jung, this self-knowledge involves insight into the dynamic of *transformation*; after all, the work with which Jung broke with Freud was titled *Transformations and Symbols of the Libido* (1911-1912), and he regarded the work as so important that, after reissuing it essentially unchanged in its second and third (German) editions in 1925 and 1938, he entirely reworked it for its fourth (Swiss) edition in 1952, retitling it *Symbols of Transformation* (CW 5). So a work about transformation — originally a product of Jung's 36th year, which "marks the beginning of the second half of life, when a metanoia, a mental transformation, not infrequently occurs" (CW 5 p. xxvi) — itself underwent transformation: "Much pruning had to be done, many gaps filled [...] I had to incorporate many things that I found out only many years later," as Jung put it in his foreword (xxv). In this respect, *Symbols of Transformation* is a self-performative work: It examines the symptoms of the case of Miss Frank Miller, which "form the Ariadne thread to guide us through the labyrinth of symbolistic parallels" — that is to say, through the "amplifications" which are "absolutely essential" if one wishes to establish "the meaning of the archetypal context" (xxv); it emerges from the metanoia of Jung's own "midlife crisis" (about which, thanks to *The Black Books* and *The Red Book*, we now know a lot more); and it undergoes major editorial transformation when the original text of *Symbole und Wandlungen der Libido* is revised as *Symbole der Wandlung* (or when, so to speak, Supplementary Volume B becomes CW 5).

[93] Thomas Mann, *Briefe, 1889-1955*, ed. Erika Mann, 3 vols (Frankfurt am Main: Fischer, 1961-1965), vol. 2 (1963), p. 107. Here I am quoting the "official English translation" as apparently confirmed by email by the Buddenbrookhaus on 6 March 2006 and subsequently quoted as an epigram to Regine Andersen, *Governing Agrobiodiversity: Plant Genetics and Developing Countries* (London and New York: Routledge, 2016)!

And the theme of transformation runs through the works proposed in this and the following three volumes like the letters of a name of a seaside resort through a stick of rock. In Wolfram's *Parzival*, the Grail serves as a symbol of the transformative power of God's grace, healing Anfortas and leading to Parzival's discovery of his true identity as the Grail King; in Goethe's *Faust*, we find a work that is replete with all kinds of transformation, from the transformation of Faust from elderly scholar into a much younger (and, in Gretchen's eyes, attractive) man, the transformation of Mephistopheles into the hideous Phorkyas and back again, and the disastrous (from the point of view of Philemon and Baucis) transformation of the geological landscape in Faust's land reclamation project in the final Act of Part Two; in Zarathustra's impassioned call for human beings to transform themselves into *Übermenschen* in Nietzsche's *Thus Spoke Zarathustra*; and in *The Red Book*, we follow Jung as he undergoes a series of transformations: notably (or notoriously) in *Liber Primus* into the Deus Leontocephalus of the Mithraic mysteries: "At the foot of the cross the black serpent coils itself [...] I am held fast and I spread my arms wide [...] The serpent has wound itself around my whole body, and my countenance is that of a lion" (RB, 197), and in *Liber Secundus* into a Green Man, "a laughing being of the forest, a leaf green daimon, a forest goblin and prankster [...] a greening tree being, who loved nothing but greening and growing [...], utterly inconstant and superficial, and yet reaching deep down, down to the kernel of the world" (RB, 272-273) and into Odin, "hang[ing] high above the ground on the swaying branch of the divine tree, for whose sake the original ancestors could not avoid sin," "hands [...] bound and [...] completely helpless" (RB, 443; cf. 449).

(This is to say nothing of the transformations that God undergoes in these works: in *Parzival*, God's grace takes the form of the white dove that descends on Good Friday with the white host in its beak; in *Faust*, God is shown as being on disturbingly good terms with the Devil and, at the end of the work, is displaced by the Magna Mater; in *Zarathustra*, where he is announced as being dead, killed by a humankind that does not yet realize what it has done and has barely begun to realize that the *Übermensch* must take the place of God; and in *The Red Book*, where Izdubar is squeezed into the size of an egg and placed in Jung's pocket in order that he should find healing — "Thus my God found salvation" [RB, 295].)

Of all these works, Jung's alone recognizes itself as being the book of its author's "most difficult experiments" (BB2, 171), yet this term could equally well be applied to all of them. By reading them in a sequence, the connections and interrelations between them should, it is hoped, become clear, along with their forceful call — albeit expressed in different ways — that we should, as their readers, transform ourselves as well. Having read and studied these books over several decades, I am convinced that this call still resounds from them as strongly as — and more urgently than — ever before.

Chapter 2

Wolfram's *Parzival*

Up until 1877, the composer Richard Wagner had followed the medieval spelling of the German version of the French name *Perceval*, but he changed its spelling from *Parzival* to *Parsifal* on discovering that the name allegedly derived from "foolish Parsee" or "pure fool," i.e., *Parsi* (or *Parseh*) *Fal*.[1] On another account, however, *Parzival* derives from *Parsi-wal*, meaning "Persian flower,"[2] while in the work itself, *Parzival* is said to mean "to-pierce-through" (§140, l. 16), as its French origin — *Perceval*, or "pierce-through-the-valley" — would suggest. Which of these etymological derivations is true? Ultimately, it seems, the origin of the name is uncertain, and uncertainty — or, in Middle High German, *zwîvel* = "doubt," "undecidedness," "vacillation" — occurs in the first line of Wolfram von Eschenbach's *Parzival*, announcing its importance as a key theme in this work.

As an epic work, *Parzival* revolves around two questions, one asked and one unasked: What is God? and why is Anfortas suffering? By the end of the work, we have learned the answer to the second question, but it is by no means quite so clear that we ever really learn the answer to the first, posed twice by Parzival. Nor is Parzival

---

[1] Richard Wagner, *Das braune Buch: Tagebuchaufzeichnungen 1865 bis 1882*, ed. Joachim Bergfeld (Zurich and Freiburg im Breisgau: Atlantis, 1975), p. 22; cf. Johann Joseph von Görres (ed.), *Lohengrin, ein altdeutsches Gedicht* (Heidelberg: Mohr & Zimmer, 1813), p. vi. See *Parsifal*, Act 2, Scene 2: "You I named, you foolish pure one, / 'Fal parsi' — / You, the pure fool, 'Parsifal'" (*Dich nannt' ich, tör'ger Reiner, / "Fal parsi" / — Dich, reinen Toren "Parsifal"*) (Richard Wagner, *Sämtliche Schriften und Dichtungen: Volks-Ausgabe*, 16 in 8 vols (Leipzig: Breitkopf & Härtel/Siegel, 1911), vol. 10, p. 355).

[2] Max Unger, "The Persian Origins of 'Parsifal' and 'Tristan,'" *The Musical Times*, 73, no. 1074, (1 August 1932), 703-770.

alone in asking this question: for, according to one of his earliest biographers, Petrus Calò (d. 1348), when St. Thomas Aquinas was a boy of 5 or so, he would pester his tutor with the question, *quid est Deus* — what is God?[3] As a theologian, Aquinas would devote thousands of pages in his *Summa theologica* — a work in three parts of some 512 questions, 2,669 articles, and around 10,000 objections and replies — to answering the question, and whether he did so successfully is a matter still open for debate. For our own purposes, let us note that the question "what is God?" is taken up again in Goethe's *Faust*, where the work's theological framework leads to the replacement of the Judeo-Christian God by the goddess-like figure of the *Mater gloriosa*; in Nietzsche's *Zarathustra*, where we are reminded of the pronouncement in *The Gay Science* (§125) that "God is dead"; and in Jung's *Red Book*, where Philemon proclaims, "God is not dead. He is as alive as ever" (RB, 516).

A note on translation

Modern German editions of *Parzival*, such as those published by Reclam and by the Deutscher Klassiker Verlag, offer parallel versions, printing the Middle High German text on one page (as edited in the 19th century by Karl Lachmann (1793-1851) and a modern German translation (by Wolfgang Spiework in the case of Reclam, and by Dieter Kühn in the case of the DKV) on the opposite page. Although most commentators outside the field of *Germanistik* refer to the English translation by the scholar of German studies A.T. Hatto (1910-2020) (published by Penguin in 1980), I have chosen a version usually eschewed by *Germanisten* and I shall use the translation published in 1894 by Jessie L. Weston (1850-1928), an independent English scholar and medievalist who

[3] Petrus Calò, *Vita S. Thomae Aquinatis*, §3, 191 cited in Stephen L. Brock, *The Philosophy of Saint Thomas Aquinas: A Sketch* (Eugene, OR: Cascade, 2015), p. xv.

is otherwise perhaps known for her work on the Arthurian tradition *From Ritual to Romance* (1920). I have done so for three reasons.

First, because Weston dedicated her translation "to the memory of Richard Wagner, whose genius has given fresh life to the creations of mediæval romance."[4] In her introduction, Weston expressed the hope that her translation should "encourage others to study that [Middle High German] original for themselves," adding that if they should "learn to know Wolfram von Eschenbach, while at the same time they learn better to understand Richard Wagner," she should feel herself "fully repaid" (vol. 1, p. xiv). Everything about this dedication and about this ambition is characteristically generous; and the wish to return the reader to Wolfram and Wagner alike is very much shared!

Second, because Hatto's version — like the earlier translation by Helen M. Mustard and Charles E. Passage published by Random House in 1961 as *Parzival: A Romance of the Middle Ages* and the later translation by Cyril Edwards published in 2004 by D.S. Brewer as *Parzival: With Titurel and the Love Lyrics* (subsequently republished in shortened form in 2006 as a paperback in the Oxford World's Classic series as *Parzival and Titurel*) — is in prose. By contrast, Weston's version is in verse — albeit in an entirely different meter from the one used by Wolfram. For Weston transformed Wolfram's text of some 25,000 lines, written in an irregular meter and in rhyming couplets, into much longer lines of a regular meter, which enabled her to retain the rhyming couplets. "As a general rule," Weston wrote, "one line of the English version represents two of the German poem," adding that "the difference of language has occasionally demanded expansion in order to do full justice to the poet's meaning" (vol. 1, p. xiv). Nevertheless, Weston goes on to enunciate the following methodological principle: "Throughout,

[4] As well as writing an opera about the Perceval/Parzival story in *Parsifal* (1882), Wagner had given a prominent role to the figure of Wolfram von Eschenbach in his earlier opera *Tannhäuser* (1845).

the translator's aim has been to be as literal as possible, and where the differing conventionalities of the thirteenth and nineteenth centuries have made a change in the form of expression necessary, the *meaning* of the poet has been reproduced, and in no instance has a different *idea* been consciously suggested" (xiv).

Finally, the antiquated diction of Weston's translation reminds us of the distance not just between the late 19th century and our age, but between the 13th century and the 21st, and the stylistic alienation of Weston's version subtly yet strongly reinforces the sheer strangeness of Wolfram's Middle High German original. That stylistic strangeness is, at the same time, not the last of the many links between this work and others in the German tradition such as *Faust* or *Zarathustra* — or, indeed, *The Red Book*.

Although Weston used the version of *Parzival* edited in 1870-1871 by the German medievalist Karl Bartsch (1832-1888), most readers and critics regard as authoritative the critical edition of 1833 by the German philologist Karl Lachmann. On the basis of a medieval manuscript in St. Gallen (known as Codex sangallensis 857, which is a complete collection of 13th-century epics), Lachmann organized the text by dividing it into 16 books, offering a general orientation (Book 3 tells the story of Parzival's youth, Book 5 relates his visit to the Grail Castle, while Book 9 contains the conversation with Trevrizent about religion). The books are then subdivided into groups of 30 lines; consequently, Lachmann's enumeration allows for a universal system of reference, according to which one can identify any given line by its position within a particular section. (So §1, ll. 1-2 means lines 1-2 in section 1; the volume number and page reference refer to the Weston translation.) As a result, any quotation can be located in an edition that uses Lachmann's numbering of the lines.[5]

[5] Jung owned the following editions of Wolfram's *Parzival*: (a) *Parzival*, ed. Wilhelm Hertz and Gustav Rosenhagen (Stuttgart: Cotta, 1911); (b) *Parzival und Titurel*, ed. Karl Bartsch, 2 vols (Leipzig: Brockhaus, 1870-1871); and (c) *Parzival und Titurel*, ed. Ernst Martin (Halle/Saale: Buchhandlung des Waisenhauses, 1920).

Prologue

Book 1 opens with a prologue, one of the conventions of Middle High German and Old French epic literature. Wolfram addresses us by making the following declaration: "If unfaith in the heart find dwelling, then the soul it shall reap but woe" (§1, l. 1-2; vol. 1, p. 3). It would not be wrong to regard this a key statement for the action that follows, but what is the *zwîvel*, that is, "unfaith" (Weston), "vacillation" (Hatto), or "doubt," of which it speaks? Does it mean ethical uncertainty, for example, Parzival's failure to ask the question that would bring redemption? Or "lack of belief," for example, Parzival's rejection of God? Or "despair," in the sense of *desperatio*?[6] Right in the very first rhyming couplet of the work, we are confronted with doubt of a hermeneutic kind — and with existential ambiguity. The prologue continues:

> And shaming alike and honour are his who such doubt shall show,
> For it standeth in evil contrast with a true man's dauntless might,
> As one seeth the magpie's plumage, which at one while is black and white.
> And yet he may win to blessing; since I wot well that in his heart,
> Hell's darkness, and light of Heaven, alike have their lot and part.
> But he who is false and unsteadfast, he is black as the darkest night,
> And the soul that have never wavered stainless *its* hue and white!
>
> (§1, ll. 3-14; vol. 1, p. 3)

[6] DKV, vol. 2, pp. 445-446.

In these lines, Wolfram's narrator continues the thought of the initial opening lines by distinguishing between three kinds of people.[7] First, there are those who are *staete*, that is, "the soul that hath never wavered" (Weston) or "the man of loyal temper" (Hatto), whose color is white. Second, there are those who are *unstaete*, that is, "[whoever] is false and unsteadfast" (Weston) or "infidelity's friend" (Hatto), whose color is the blackness of Hell. And third, there are those who are "motley" (Hatto) or "at one while [...] black and white" (Weston), who are like checkered cloth (cf. *parrieren*) or the magpie (in MHG, *agelstern*), and whose destiny is undecided between Heaven and Hell. But again, questions arise: Does black also correspond to *zwîvel* and white to those who are *unverzaget*, that is, "steadfast" (Hatto) or "dauntless" (Weston), in which case *zwîvel* and being *unstaete* would amount to the same thing? Or does black correspond to despair, to being *verzaget*? Or can the *unverzaget man*, the "steadfast" or "dauntless" individual, be both *staete* and *unstaete*? Here is another question which is, for now, left open.

And what about Parzival himself? Is he, like a magpie, colored black and white? The quality of *unverzaget mannes muot*, that is, "the courage of a steadfast man" (Hatto) or "a true man's dauntless might" (Weston), is repeatedly applied to Parzival; for example, *küenes herzen* [...] / *unt wâriu zuht bî manheit* (§319, ll. 4-5), *belîp des willens unverzagt* (§502, l. 28). More important, the color symbolism of black-and-white forms part of the symbolism of light and dark that echoes the opening of the First Epistle of John (1:5-7 and 2:9-11) (see below). And the confidence expressed by the narrator that whoever maintains an inner steadfastness will cleave to the light color of heaven will later be restated in the prologue to another work, namely, in the "Prologue in Heaven" in *Faust I*, where the Lord declares: *Ein guter Mensch in seinem dunklen Drange / Ist sich des rechten Weges wohl bewußt* ("a good man, by

[7] DKV, vol. 2, pp. 446-447.

his dim impulse driven, / Of the right way hath ever consciousness") (ll. 328-329).[8]

At this point, Wolfram's narrator makes a self-reflexive move: "This my parable so fleeting too swift for the dull shall be" (§1, ll. 15-16), thus thematizing the *tumben*, that is, those who are "dull" (Weston) or of "unripe wits" (Hatto), and the quality of *tumb*-ness is later applied to Parzival himself. Even though he laments how his "parable so fleeting too swift for the dull shall be," Wolfram's narrator then goes on:

> Ere yet they may seize its meaning from before their face 'twill flee,
> As a hare that a sound hath startled: yea, metal behind the glass,
> And a blind man's dream yield visions that as swift from the eye do pass,
> For naught shall they have that endureth! And at one while 'tis bright and sad,
> And know of a truth that its glory but for short space shall make ye glad.
> And what man shall think to grip me, where no hair for his grasp shall grow,
> In the palm of mine hand? The mystery of a close clasp he sure doth know!
>
> (§1, ll. 20-28; vol. 1, p. 3)

[8] In theological terms, Gottfried Weber (1897-1981) argued that *Parzival* represents a shift from an Augustinian view that the highest ideal (represented by the Grail) can be *passively* gained thanks to the grace of God to the Thomistic view that *active* striving on the part of the individual is required as well as God's grace in order to attain that ideal. Concomitantly, this shift from St. Augustine to St. Thomas Aquinas involves a shift from a feudal concept of God to a new conception of God — as a God of unconditional love. See his *Der Gottesbegriff des Parzival* (Frankfurt am Main: Diesterweg, 1935) and *Parzival, Ringen und Vollendung: Eine dichtungs- und religionsgeschichtliche Untersuchung* (Oberursel: Kompaß-Verlag, 1948).

Here the images of the mirror and of the blind man's dream are used to capture a failure to understand and a lack of insight; this fleeting reflectivity might be contrasted with the moment of visionary insight experienced by the German philosopher and mystic Jakob Böhme (1575-1624) when one day in 1600 he observed a beam of sunlight reflecting on a metal dish: "Sitting one day in his room, his eye fell upon a burnished pewter dish, which reflected the sunshine with such marvellous splendour that he fell into an inward ecstasy, and it seemed to him as if he could now look into the principles and deepest foundations of things"; believing it to be "only a fancy, and in order to banish it from his mind, he went out upon the green," but "he remarked that he gazed into the very heart of things, the very herbs and grass, and that actual nature harmonized with what he had inwardly seen."[9] Likewise, Wolfram's narrator expresses the wish that his audience learn the deeper meaning of the story he is about to tell:

> If I cry aloud in such peril, it 'seemeth my wisdom well.
> Shall I look for truth where it fleeteth? In the fire that the stream doth quell,
> Or the dew that the sun doth banish? Ne'er knew I a man so wise,
> But that was fain to learn the wisdom my fable doth ill disguise,
> And the teaching that springeth from it [...].
>
> (§1, ll. 27-§2, l. 8; vol. 1, pp. 3-4)

[9] Hans Lassen Martensen, *Jacob Boehme: His Life and Teaching, or Studies in Theosophy*, trans. T. Rhys Evans (London: Hodder and Stoughton, 1885), p. 7. In Böhme's experience Colin Wilson has seen a confirmation of Paracelsus's principle that "we may look into Nature in the same way that the sun shines through a glass" (Colin Wilson, *Religion and the Rebel* [1957] (Bath: Ashgrove Press, 1984), pp. 153-154).

The tale that is about to be narrated is described as an *âventiure*, invoking a central concept of courtly literature since the time of Hartmann von Aue (c.1160-70 to c. 1210-1220) (see below).[10] It is said to be a tale *von liebe und von leide*, it "telleth tidings of love, and anon of woe," and it will bring *vröude und angest*, "joy and sorrow" (§3, l. 30 and §4, l. 1). To tell it will require *wilder vunt*, that is, "unbridled inspiration" (Hatto) or extraordinary poetic imagination, and Wolfram's narrator wishes he were not one just man, but three!

> […] 'Stead of *one* man if *three* ye know,
> And each one of the three hath wisdom and skill that outweigh my skill,
> Yet o'erstrange shall they find the labour, tho' they toil with a right good-will
> To tell ye this tale, which I think me to tell ye myself, alone,
> And worn with their task and weary would they be ere the work was done.
>
> (§4, ll. 2-8; vol. 1, p. 5)

The tale is said to revolve around the concept of *triuwe*, that is, "fidelity" (Hatto), both a legal concept (i.e., the contractual loyalty of the vassal to his lord) and a theological one (i.e., faithfulness to God). This *grôze triuwe* comes close to being a metaphysical concept, glossed by the German medievalist Joachim Bumke (1929-2011) as "the honesty and steadfastness of human bonds as such, and the love for God and God's love for humankind."[11]

---

[10] DKV, vol. 1, p. 451.

[11] Joachim Bumke, *Courtly Culture: Literature and Society in the High Middle Ages* [*Höfische Kultur: Literatur und Gesellschaft im hohen Mittelalter*, 1986], trans. Thomas Dunlap [1991] (Woodstock, New York, London: Overlook Duckworth, 2000), p. 303 (cited in DKV, vol. 2, p. 453). Cf. §462, l. 19: "since God himself is *ein triuwe*" (*sît got selbe ein triuwe ist*).

The story of Parzival begins while he is *noch ungeborn*, that is, "as yet unborn," and the story of his father, Gahmuret, takes up the rest of Book 1 and the whole of Book 2. Blood relations are of immense significance in courtly literature, and *Parzival* is no exception. Gahmuret's lineage can be traced back through Gandin (King of Anjou), Addanz, and Lazaliez to Mazadan, a fairy and an ancestor of the House of Anjou and of Arthur's line, who is seduced by and marries Terdelaschoye, another fairy. (In Book 2, we are reminded that Gahmuret "came of the fairy race / That aye loveth, or sweet love seeketh" [§96, ll. 20-21; vol. 1, p. 54].)[12] Parzival is, then, descended from a fairy, which both illustrates (in the words of Gahmuret) how *diu minne wirt sîn vrouwe*, "Love will be his mistress" (§56, l.2), and points to a parallel between Parzival and Aeneas, the Trojan hero whose divine mother was the goddess Aphrodite (or Venus).[13] Another line descends from Mazadan and Terdelaschoye, descending through Brickus and Utepandragun to King Arthur himself. Parzival is thus related, albeit at a distance, to Arthur, and in fact no fewer than three bloodlines inform the story: the Arthurian, the Angevine (i.e., the House of Anjou), and the Grail Line. Like much courtly literature, *Parzival* insists on the importance of ancestors; in the world of *Parzival*, the past is immensely important for understanding the present.

[12] Fairies, along with elves, gnomes, and masked dwarves, belong to the imaginal world of Goethe's *Faust*, Part Two, where — along with other "elusive, contradictory, shape-shifting" beings — they can be read as "root metaphors for certain central aspects of modern Western culture," which are excluded from it and yet continue to appear in our culture in different forms (Patrick Harpur, *The Philosophers' Secret Fire: A History of the Imagination* (Harmondsworth: Penguin, 2002), p. 7).

[13] See Julius Schwietering, "Einwürkung der Antike auf die Entstehung des frühen deutschen Minnesangs" [1924], in *Philologische Schriften*, ed. Friedrich Ohly and Max Wehrli (Munich: Fink, 1969), pp. 237-253 (p. 245) (cited in DKV, vol. 2, p. 485).

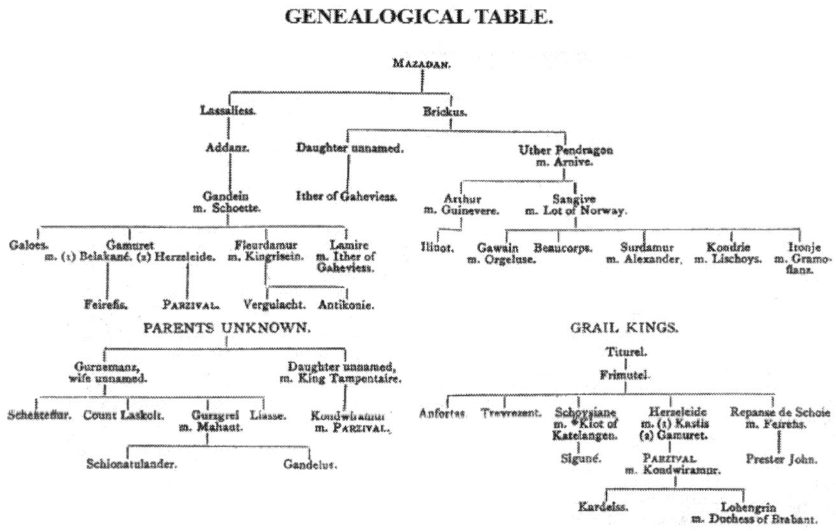

Figure 1: Genealogical Table[14]

Likewise, within the Jungian tradition, the figures of the "ancestors" in general and the Grandfather in particular play an important psychological as well as personal role.[15] In his paper "The Significance of the Father in the Destiny of the Individual" (1909; revised 1927), Jung himself presented an argument about the significance of the archetypal figure of the father that can help illuminate the psychological meaning behind the complex genealogies of *Parzival*:

> The potentialities of the archetype, for good and evil alike, transcend our human capacities many times, and a man can appropriate its power only by identifying with the daimon, by letting himself be possessed by it, thus

[14] This diagram is available online at https://www.gutenberg.org/files/47297/47297-h/47297-h.htm.

[15] For further discussion, see Andreas Jung, "The Grandfather," *Journal of Analytical Psychology*, 56 (2011), 653-673.

> forfeiting his own humanity. The fateful power of the father complex comes from the archetype, and this is the real reason why the *consensus gentium* puts a divine or daimonic figure in place of the father. The personal father inevitably embodies the archetype, which is what endows his figure with its fascinating power. The archetype acts as an amplifier, enhancing beyond measure the effects that proceed from the father, so far as these conform to the inherited pattern. (CW 4 §744)

In the original version of his paper, Jung had summarized his conclusions more modestly as follows, claiming that "in my experience it is usually the father who is the decisive and dangerous object of the child's fantasy, and if ever it happened to be the mother I was able to discover behind her a grandfather to whom she belonged in her heart" (CW 4 §744, footnote).

In his foreword to second edition, Jung noted that he had originally concluded his essay as follows: "It is to be hoped that experience in the years to come will sink deeper shafts into this obscure territory, on which I have been able to shed but a fleeting light, and will discover more about the secret workshop of the daimon who shapes our fate"; and, as well as acknowledging that "experience in later years has indeed altered and deepened many things," he claimed that his work on the mother-complex in *Transformations and Symbols of the Libido* (1911-1912) had in fact revealed to him "what the deeper causes of this complex are" — namely, an archetypal dimension to the incest taboo. In the light of this work, Jung nevertheless stood by the conclusions of his original essay, which he said was not "actually wrong" but "too simple, too naïve," and he endorsed in particular his earlier choice of a quotation from Horace (*Epistles*, §2, ll. 187-189), originally introduced as pertaining to "the secret workshop of the daimon who shapes our fate" and now described as "point[ing] to that deeper, darker background":

Scit Genius, natale comes qui temperat astrum,
Naturae deus humanae, mortalis in unum
Quodque caput, vultu mutabilis, albus et ater.

Why so, the Genius alone knows — that companion
who rules our star of birth,
the god of human nature, though mortal for each
single life,
and changing in countenance, white or black.[16]

In particular, Jung writes that he has gained insight into "how the roots of the psyche and of fate go deeper than the 'family romance,'" to use the expression coined by Freud,[17] and he now understands that "not only the children but the parents, too, are merely branches of one great tree" (CW 4, pp. 301-302 and §744, fn. 26).

Given the complex genealogical relations that inform courtly romance in general and *Parzival* in particular (including the emphasis placed on Gahmuret as the father of Parzival and Feirefiz, the former by Herzeloyde and the latter by Belacane, not to mention the Arthurian line passing from Mazadan and Terdelaschoye to Gawan, the Angevin line passing from Mazadan and Terdelaschoye to Gahmuret, and the Grail line passing from Titurel to Parzival

[16] Horace, *Satires, Epistles, and Ars Poetica*, trans. H. Rushton Fairclough (London; Cambridge, MA: Heinemann; Harvard University Press, 1926), p. 439.

[17] In one of his early papers on psychoanalysis, titled "Family Romances" (*Der Familenroman der Neurotiker*) (1909), Freud had suggested that some neurotics, during their childhood psychological development, entertained the fantasy that their parents were not their biological progenitors, but believed themselves instead to be the offspring of much more (socially) important parents, and this belief centered, in particular, on the figure of the father. Freud's paper was first published in 1909 along with Otto Rank's *The Myth of the Birth of the Hero*; see Freud, *Standard Edition of the Complete Works*, general eds James Strachey and Anna Freud, 24 vols (London: Hogarth Press, 1953-1974), vol. 9, pp. 237-241). In this respect, it is significant that the Fisher King has his "double" or "counterpart," his own father — the Grail King. For further discussion, see Eithne M. O'Sharkey, "The Maimed Kings in the Arthurian Romances," *Etudes Celtiques*, vol. 8, no. 2 (1959), 420-428.

himself and thence to Loherangrin and Kardeiz), Jung's argument about the archetypal aspect of genealogy is an important insight.[18] In sum, "not only the father, but the mother as well, is such an important factor in the child's fate: not because they themselves have this or that human failing or merit, but because they happen to be — by accident, so to speak — the human beings who first impress on the childish mind those mysterious and mighty laws which govern not only families but entire nations, indeed the whole of humanity," which accurately describes the geographical and cultural range of Wolfram's *Parzival*, which is — if not exactly global — nevertheless pan-European, pan-African, and pan-Asian in its scope (not least through Gahmuret's service of the Baruc and the figure of Prester John, the legendary Christian priest-king in India). "Not laws devised by the wit of man, but the laws and forces of nature, amongst which man walks on the edge of a razor" (CW 4 §744, footnote), writes Jung, encapsulating in a single image the existential significance of the story of Wolfram's *Parzival*, symbolized by the quest for the all-powerful, salvific Holy Grail.

The Horatian motif quoted by Jung recurs in *Parzival* in two ways: first, in the opposition in the opening prologue of *lieht* and *swarz*, and the image of "the magpie's plumage, which at one while is black and white" (*swâ sich parrieret* [...] *als agelstern varwe tuot*) (§1, ll. 4 and 6). This contrast does not, however, stand in the way (or might it even be a precondition of?) the individual's salvation, for: "And yet he may win to blessing; since I wot well

[18] Note that, whereas in Chrétien's *Perceval* the (unnamed) king at the Grail procession is the Fisher King's father and the hermit's brother (ll. 6413-6419; cf. *Œuvres complètes*, p. 843, cf. pp. 1372), in Wolfram's *Parzival* he is Anfortas's (and thus Trevrizent's) grandfather (DKV, vol. 2, p. 702). For further discussion, see Clair Hayden Bell, *The Sister's Son in the Medieval German Epic: A Study in the Survival of Matriliny* [*University of California Publications in Modern Philology*, vol. 10, no. 2, pp. 67-182] (Berkeley, CA: University of California Press, 1922); and H.B. Willson, "The Grail King in Wolfram's 'Parzival,'" *The Modern Language Review*, vol. 55, no. 4 (October 1960), 553-563.

that in his heart, / Hell's darkness, and light of Heaven, alike have their lot and part" (*der mad dennoch wesen geil: / wande an im sint beidiu teil, / des himmels und der helle*) (§1, ll. 7-9). And second, it occurs in the figure of Feirefiz, Belacane's son who is both white and black, "as a magpie the hue of his face and hair" (*Als ein agelster war gevar / sîn hâr und ouch sîn vel vil gar*) (§57, ll. 27-28), so much so that when, in Book 16, Loherangrin is taken to his uncle Feirefiz "who was black and white" (*dô der was swarz unde wîz*) (§805, l. 30), he is afraid of him and turns away — much to the amusement of Feirefiz, we are told (who thereby averts an embarrassing social situation. Both the passage from Horace (and its imagery of white and black) and the insight into the symbolic importance of genealogy bring out aspects of the psychological significance of Wolfram's text (and, indeed, the Grail tradition as a whole).

Book 1

In Book 1, Gahmuret finds himself left, as the younger son of Gandin, the king of Anjou, without an inheritance, and he sets out to travel to the East to seek his fortune. He enters the service of the Caliph of Baghdad, known as the Baruc, and then goes to the kingdom of Zazamanc in North Africa. Through knightly contestation against the followers of Isenhart, king of Azagouc, who was a former suitor of Belacane (the black, Moorish queen of Zazamanc), Gahmuret wins the kingship of Zazamanc and he takes Belacane as his bride.

Wolfram's text is insistent on color symbolism: the snow-whiteness of Gahmuret's shield (§18, l. 6), and the black skin of Belacane (§24, ll. 6-11), for instance. And it fits in with the prologue's symbolism of the magpie that Belacane gives birth to Feirefiz, a son who is both white and black:

> Then the queen at the time appointed bare a son, who
> was dark and light,

For in him had God wrought a wonder, at one while
was he black and white.
And a thousand times she kissed him where white as
his sire's his skin.
And she named the babe of her sorrows Feirefis
Angevin.
And he was a woodland-waster, many spears did he
shatter fair,
And shields did he pierce — as a magpie the hue of
his face and hair.

(§57, ll. 15-28; vol. 1, p. 31)

The color symbolism is reflected in Fierefiz's name, which contains the Old French root *vair* or *veir* (i.e., "colorful"), and could be translated as "colorful son," much as Herzeloyde later calls Parzival *bêâ fiz* (i.e., "beautiful son") (§113, l. 4; §140, l. 6).[19]

Although we are told that Gahmuret truly loved Belacane ("Yet his dusky wife was dearer than e'en his own life might be") and are assured of her great qualities ("Ne'er knew he a truer lady whose heart was from falsehood free"), he nevertheless abandons her when she is three months pregnant, largely because of his desire for knightly adventure ("his heart gave him little rest / Since he found there no deeds of knighthood, and gladness forsook his breast"), but ostensibly because she is pagan — as Gahmuret says in the letter he leaves for her, "But this thing I needs must say, / Wert thou, e'en as I, a Christian I ever should weep for thee, / For e'en now I must surely mourn thee") (§54, ll. 21-22, ll. 23-24, ll. 19-20; §56, ll. 24-26). And, stealing away in the dead of night, Gahmuret sets off for Spain and Seville.

[19] Karl Bartsch, "Die Eigennamen in Wolframs *Parzival* und *Titurel*," *Germanistische Studien*, 2 (1875), 114-159 (p. 138) (cited in DKV, vol. 2, p. 487).

On his arrival in Spain, Gahmuret visits his maternal cousin, Kaylet of Hoskurast (king of Spain and of Castile), and eventually arrives at Waleis. Here he participates in a tournament, and as the winner he is entitled to claim the hand of Queen Herzeloyde: "For all do I count my kinsmen, since Adam's flesh we share," she says just before his victory, "Yet Gamuret's hand, I think me, the highest prize hath won" (§82, ll. 1-4; vol. 1, p. 47). This time, Gahmuret has learned his lesson and insists on the freedom to participate in a tournament once a month. When he hears that the Baruc is under siege, Gahmuret returns to the East, and in the service of the Baruc, he is killed near Baghdad by a group of Babylonians, thanks to "heathen guile" (§105, l. 16). But Herzeloyde is 18 weeks pregnant; and, shortly before Gahmuret's death, she has a prophetic dream.

Now in the Middle Ages, dreams were widely regarded as being prophetic, and Herzeloyde's dream combines a number of significant parallels to other recorded dreams: The lightning, thunder, and earthquakes recall the signs of Alexander's birth in the ancient Greek and medieval versions of the Alexander Romance; the prophetic qualities of dreams in Old French epics; the image of the woman and the dragon in the Book of Revelation, Chapter 12; Clytemnestra's dream of a dragon in Aeschylus's *Orestia*; and the dreams involving dragons in the dream (the *Oneirocritica* or *Oneirokritikon*) of Artemidorus.[20]

As A.T. Hatto reminds us, medieval German literature features some notable dreams. In Wernher der Gartenaere's *Meier Helmbrecht*, for instance, the old farmer has four dreams which he interprets as omens of the terrible punishments that will be inflicted on his son if he pursues a life of crime, involving loss of sight, feet, and arms, and finally being hanged: "You were hanging on a tree. Your feet were a fathom from the ground. Above your head on a bough sat a raven, by its side a crow. Your hair was all tangled. On

[20] DKV, vol. 2, p. 509.

the right hand the raven combed your head for you, on the left the crow." In the *Nibelungenlied*, Kriemhild has a dream of a falcon that is killed by two eagles, interpreted by her mother as meaning that Kriemhild's future husband will die a violent death, symbolizing his tragedy and her own. And in Gottfried von Strassburg's *Tristan*, the jealous Marjodoc, Tristan's chief steward, has a dream about a mighty boar that comes out of the forest and into the King's bedchamber where it soils the royal linen with its foam, precisely at the moment when Tristan and Isolde are together.[21]

In *Parzival*, Herzeloyde's dream is even more dramatic:

> So it chanced that the queen one noontide in a restless slumber lay,
> 'Twas as if with a start she wakened and by lightning was borne away,
> And towards the clouds it bare her, and they smote her with mighty force,
> The fiery bolts of Heaven, as they sped on their downward course,
> And sparks sprang from her floating tresses mid the fire of the circling spheres,
> And the thunder crashed loud around her, and the rain-drops were burning tears.
>
> (§103, l. 25-§104, l. 6; vol. 1, p. 58).

[21] A.T. Hatto, "Herzeloyde's Dragon-Dream," *German Life and Letters*, vol. 22, no. 1 (October 1968), 16-31. For further discussion, see Benjamin van Well, "Sprache der Träume – Sprache der Kultur: Ein multiperspektivischer Blick auf den Traum der Herzeloyde in Wolframs von Eschenbach *Parzival*, in *Literaturstraße: Chinesisch-deutsche Zeitschrift für Sprach- und Literaturwissenschaft*, vol. 21, no. 2 (2020), 39-54, as well as Wilhelm Deinert, *Ritter und Kosmos im Parzival: Eine Untersuchung der Sternkunde Wolframs von Eschenbach* (Munich: Beck, 1960); and Steven R. Fischer, *The Dream in the Middle High German Epic: Introduction to the Study of the Dream as a Literary Device to the Younger Contemporaries of Gottfried and Wolfram* (Bern, Frankfurt am Main, Las Vegas: Lang, 1978).

As a dream, this prefigures the death of her husband, yet at the same time it warns of the future loss of her son, symbolized as a dragon, who abandons her, for the most striking aspect of Herzeloyde's dream is the part that comes next:

> For a little space was she conscious, then a grip on her
> right hand fell,
> And lo! it was changed, the vision, and wondrous
> things befell;
> For then did she nurse a dragon, that forth from her
> body sprung,
> And its dragon life to nourish awhile at her breast it
> hung,
> Then it fled from her sight so swiftly she might look
> on it never more:
> And her heart it brake for the anguish, and the terror
> and grief she bore.
>
> (§104, ll. 9-19; vol. 1, p. 58)

According to Artemidorus's *Oneirokritikon*, the loss of one's right hand in a dream means the death of a close relative, while dreams of giving birth to a dragon are by no means unknown in antiquity.[22] Wolfram's narrator describes the beast concerned as *ein trache* and as *ein wurm*. Now a related animal, the black snake, plays a central in the fantasies or visions of *The Red Book*, acting (in Jung's later view) as a "counterpart of the hero" and serving as an indication of a hero-myth (MDR, 206). Moreover, in his seminars on dream

[22] As an archetypal figure, the dragon recalls the great celestial serpent, the *draco caelestis*, of the Babylonians and the Chaldaeans (see Hans Leisegang, "Das Mysterium der Schlange: Ein Beitrag zur Erforschung des griechischen Mysterienkultes und seines Fortlebens in der christlichen Welt (mit 14 Illustrationen)," *Eranos-Jahrbuch*, 9 (1939), 151-250; translated as "The Mystery of the Serpent," in *The Mysteries* [*Papers from the Eranos Yearbooks*, vol. 2], ed. Joseph Campbell (Princeton, NJ: Princeton University Press, 1955), pp. 194-260.

analysis (1928-1930) Jung explains that "these cold-blooded relics [snakes, crocodiles, etc.] are, in a way, uncanny powers, because they symbolize the fundamental factors of our instinctive life, dating from Paleozoic times," and "so whenever life means business, when things are getting serious, you are likely to find a saurian on the way"; when benevolent, this saurian is "a tremendous force of organized instinct and pushes you over an obstacle which you would not believe possible to climb over by willpower or conscious decision," and "there the animal proves to be helpful."[23] In short, the saurian — or the serpent — brings to light the contents of the unconscious in a way that enables us to move forward.[24]

When, in Book 9, Parzival encounters Trevrizent at Fontane la Salvaesche, the hermit interprets the dragon flying away from Herzeloyde as representing Parzival's decision to leave his mother that leads to her death:

> "Ne'er learnt I to deceive,
> Thy mother she died of sorrow in the day thou her side didst leave,
> Such rewarding her love won for her! *Thou* wast the beast that hung
> On her breast, the wingèd dragon that forth from her body sprung,
> That spread its wings and left her: in a dream was it all foretold
> Ere yet the sorrowing mother the babe to her breast did hold!"
>
> (§476, ll. 27-30; vol. 1, p. 274)

[23] C.G. Jung, *Dream Analysis: Notes of the Seminar given in 1928-1930*, ed. William McGuire (London: Routledge & Kegan Paul, 1984), pp. 645-646.

[24] "The contents of all the early manifestations of religion came, not from the mind, but from the sympathetic system. And it is the saurian, the original worm, that brings up the contents of the unconscious" (Jung, *Dream Analysis*, p. 334).

When Parzival is born, he is so strong that Herzeloyde nearly dies when giving birth to him, and she decides to raise him — her *bon fîz, scher fîz, bêâ fîz* — in such a way as to prevent him from learning anything of the world of chivalry. And so she withdraws to a wasteland (*waste*), the forest of Soltane. (This move to the wasteland or the desert is replicated in *Faust* by the scene, "Forest and Cave" (*Wald und Höhle*); in *Zarathustra*, by the prophet's decision to leave his home by the lake and go into the mountains, where he stays for 10 years; and in *The Red Book* by the events of the sixth night in *Liber Primus* when Jung's soul leads him "into the desert," that is: into the desert of his own "self" [RB, 141].)

In *The Truth of the Technological World* (2013), Friedrich Kittler (1943-2011) highlights the distinction made in the Middle Ages between the *clan* — connected by the law of exogamy and linked along the axes of generations and races [*Geschlechter*] — and the *family* (in which norms and imagos are introjected into offspring, subverting binary sexual difference [*Geschlechterdifferenz*]).[25] In the case of Parzival, Wolfram's narrator relates — in a passage which Weston translates euphemistically, "When the queen found sight and hearing she was fain on her child to look, / And her maidens they bare him to her and the babe in her arms she took; / And she saw his limbs soft rounded, and she knew she had born a son, / And her maidens with her were joyful that the earth had a man-child won" (§112, ll. 21-25), but A.T. Hatto does not — how Herzeloyde and her ladies-in-waiting spread the legs of the newly born infant and admire his *visselîn* (his "little piddler," or "willie"), the implications of which are spelled out thus: "As he bare of a man the body, so manly was he of heart, / As a smith did he wield the sword-blade till fire from the helm would start" (§112, ll. 26-30). As Kittler explains: "Coded in terms of sex, the boy receives a

[25] Friedrich A. Kittler, *The Truth of the Technological World: Essays on the Genealogy of Presence* [2013], trans. Erik Butler (Stanford, CA: Stanford University Press, 2014), p. 1.

phallic attribute that symbolically couples desire and power: now he is destined for exogamous alliances and knightly adventures" (1). Noting that "the clan is governed by the metaphor *visselîn* = *swert* ['sword']," Kittler has a swipe at Freud, describing it as "a figure running this way and that — which Freud took up to his own ends and confused with natural fact." Plainly, this is not an accusation that one could level at Jung, who insists on the allegorical or metaphorical dimension of symbols. For Kittler, this phallic symbolic code structures the entirety of the narrative that now enfolds:

> Instead of promoting the play of metaphor, Herzeloyde, out of love and fear, clothes the adventuresome boy in a fool's garb, so that its worldly echoes may bring him back to her. She does so to no avail, however, for an ars amandi and law that are one and the same remove Parzival from the double bond with his mother. Condwiramurs (whose name says what it means — "to conduct love") initiates him into strictly exogamous eroticism — and as *amor de lonh* ("love from afar") at that. Taking the place of Parzival's father, old Gurnemanz prohibits the youth from appealing to childhood and motherly words at all, in order to inscribe him into the axis of succeeding generations. Finally, the boy's uncle on his mother's side — who (as in other cultures) wields greater symbolic power than a biological father precisely because he is not the child's actual sire — articulates, in the capacity of father confessor, debts of blood to relatives [*Verwandtenblutschuld*] and, as a genealogist, the alliances between two clans. Parzival's innocence [*Tumbheit*] ends when the symbolic order, which Herzeloyde has kept silent, is voiced. And because Trevrizent tells Parzival of his expectant mother's dreams,

> which she never revealed to her son, there is no unspoken remainder that might haunt the hero and open the way for psychology or psychoanalysis. The incestuous double bond vanishes without consequence. (1-2)

On Kittler's account, over time these "kinship structures" become detached from "political, juridical, and economic power," so that in modernity "the code governing the conjugal, nuclear family [...] stands opposed to the code of the clan on every point," exemplified in the intellectual bourgeoisie of the 17th century before becoming universal in the 19th (2).

"In terms of discourse analysis," Kitteler goes on to claim, Romantic poetry is "the effect of a semiotechnics that made the conjugal family matrilineal around 1800": this "recoding" (or "coupling" — that is, of "sexuality that derives from cultural coding and of speech that, when it involves self-declaration and self-interpretation, goes by the name of 'poetry'") is said to have been "enacted" by Novalis's novel, *Heinrich von Ofterdingen* (and, in particular, Klingsohr's *Märchen* or "fairy tale" in that work), while "the effects were articulated in the works of Clemens Brentano, Friedrich Schlegel, Ludwig Tieck, Achim von Arnim, and E.T.A. Hoffmann" (2-3). While this may be valid from a psychoanalytic-cum-sociological perspective, this should not lead us to overlook the presence of other universal themes in *Parzival* that persist in our own day — not least the problem of the nature of God.

Waz ist got?

In Book 3, we learn of Parzival's earliest adventures, including his childhood. Stricken with grief at the death of her husband, Gahmuret, and bearing their child, Herzeloyde withdraws to the forest of Soltane and raises Parzival on her own. She is concerned to shield him from as much as possible, especially anything to do with knighthood:

But his mother kept him hidden in the woodland valleys wild,
Nor thought in her love and sorrow how she wronged the kingly child:
Nor knightly weapon she gave him, save such as in childish play
He wrought himself from the bushes that grew on his lonely way,
A bow and arrows he made him, and with these, in thoughtless glee,
He shot at the birds as they carolled o'erhead in the leafy tree.

(§117, l. 30-§118, l.6; vol. 1, p. 67)

(As we shall see in Chapter 3, the image of the bowstring and the arrow serves as a governing metaphor or allegory for the narrative technique of Wolfram's *Parzival*.)

One day, Herzeloyde sees him looking up at the trees and listening to the song of the birds. Suddenly angered, she orders her servants to capture and kill all the birds. Parzival is puzzled and asks her why they are angry with the birds. Herzeloyde regrets her decision, and she explains:

Then the boy spake, "Now sweet my mother, why trouble the birds so sore?
Forsooth they can ne'er have harmed thee, ah, leave them in peace once more!"
And his mother kissed him gently, "Perchance I have wrought a wrong,
Of a truth, the dear God who made them, He gave unto them their song,
And I would not that one of his creatures should sorrow because of me."

But the boy looked up in wonder, "God, Mother? Who
may God be?" [*ôwê muoter, waz ist got?*]
(§119, ll. 1-17; vol. 1, p. 68)

This is, of course, the same question with which, according to one of his earliest biographers, Petrus Calò (d. 1348), St. Thomas Aquinas would, when he was a boy of 5 or so, pester his tutor, namely: *quid est Deus* — what is God? (One might be forgiven for sympathizing with the tutor.) Yet this is precisely Parzival's question, too.

And, in response to his question, Parzival receives from Herzeloyde a basic lesson in theology — and a very basic lesson in a very basic theology at that:

"My son, He is a light beyond all light, brighter than summer's day,
And He bare a Man's Face, that we men might look on His Face always!
Art thou ever in need of succour? Call on Him in thine hour of ill,
And be sure He will fail thee never, but will hear thee, and help thee still.
Yet one there is dwelleth in darkness, and I wot men may fear him well,
For his home is the house of falsehood, and his kingdom the realm of Hell!
Turn thy mind away from him ever, nor waver betwixt the twain,
For he who doubteth, his labour shall ever be wrought in vain."
Thus his mother read him the riddle, the myst'ry of day and night,
The dread and the doom of darkness, and the glory and grace of light!
(§119, ll. 18-§120, l.1; p. 68)

While Herzeloyde's brief catechesis has the function of preparing for Parzival's later comic misunderstandings (§120 and §122), it also recapitulates some key ideas from the opening prologue, notably its opposition of *lieht* and *swarz* and the warning about *zwîvel*:

> If unfaith in the heart find dwelling, then the soul it shall reap but woe;
> And shaming alike and honour are his who such doubt shall show,
> For it standeth in evil contrast with a true man's dauntless might,
> As one seeth the magpie's plumage, which at one while is black and white.
> And yet he may win to blessing; since I wot well that in his heart,
> Hell's darkness, and light of Heaven, alike have their lot and part.
> But he who is false and unsteadfast, he is black as the darkest night,
> And the soul that hath never wavered stainless *its* hue and white!
>
> (§1, ll. 1-14; vol. 1, p. 3)

The insufficiency of this dualistic view of God is borne out by two things that both now and subsequently happen to Parzival. First, there is his confusion when he comes across three knights in the forest and thinks that one of them is God:

> Three knights rode into the clearing, in glittering armour bright;
> From head to foot were they armèd, each one on his gallant steed,

And the lad as he saw their glory thought each one a
god indeed!
[…]
Yet the boy, tho' he spake with a man's tongue, as a
god must account him still;
For he thought how Queen Herzeleide had told him
that God was Light
And dwelleth in Light for ever; and so to his dazzled
sight
This knight, in his shining armour in the glow of the
summer's day,
Was the God of his mother's lesson, and he knelt him
again to pray.

(§120, ll. 24-28 and §121, l. 29-§122, l.1;
vol. 1, pp. 69-70)

The identification of God with light is a key idea in the New Testament, reflected in the First Letter of John, "God is light, and in him there is no darkness" (1 John 1: 5). In Book 9, this idea will be repeated by Trevrizent, when he tells Parzival how Plato and the Cumaean and other Sibyls had foretold the redemption to come and that Parzival must repent of his sins:

Learn faith from the men of old-time, whose rede ever
waxeth new,
For Plato alike and the Sibyls in their day spake words
so true,
And long years ere the time had ripened His coming
they did foretell
Who made for our sin's Atonement, and drew us from
depths of Hell.
[…]

"From the lips of the whole world's Lover came a
message of love and peace,
(For He is a Light all-lightening, and never His faith
doth cease) […]."
(§465, l. 19-28 and §466, ll. 1-4; vol. 1, p. 268)

Second, Herzeloyde's teaching will have to be supplemented by the doctrine supplied by Gurnemanz de Graharz (the grandfather of Schionatulander, the maternal uncle of Condwiramurs, and in effect Parzival's first tutor), when Parzival encounters him in his castle after leaving Arthur's court toward the end of Book 3. Here, Gurnemanz will tell Parzival about the sacraments, teaching him how to make the sign of the Cross and how to attend Mass:

So went our hero witless where to God and the host
they'd sing,
And the prince by the Mass would teach him that
which health to the soul shall bring.
He would rede him well of the Offering — How to
sign himself with the Cross,
And thus work on the Devil vengeance, who seeketh
for aye our loss!
(§169, ll. 15-20; vol. 1, p. 95)

For now, however, Parzival returns home and tells Herzeloyde about his encounter with the knights — and, to her despair, about his decision to become a knight himself and to go in search of King Arthur:

"I met in the woods, sweet mother, four men I deemed
gods indeed,
So light were they all and shining, God Himself ne'er
could brighter be,

And of knighthood they spake and King Arthur, who
might well make a knight of me!"
(§126, ll. 9-14; vol. 1, p. 72)

In this episode, Wolfram evokes the central concept of the story of Parzival's youth, his *tumpheit.*

For Parzival is described as *der knappe tump unde wert*, translated by Weston as "the simple lad and gallant" (p. 72) and by Hatto as "the noble, simple lad" (p. 75). The quality of *tumpheit* is an ambivalent one, combining both *simplicitas* (or "simplicity") as a positive quality and *ignorantia* (or "ignorance") as a consequence of original sin.[26] Hoping to engineer a situation that will persuade Parzival to return, Herzloyde kits out her son to look like a fool:

And she thought her, Queen Herzeleide, "Many folk
thro' the world shall fare
Who love mocking — On his fair body my son shall
a Fool's dress wear,
Then sure when the mockers see him, and to scoff at
his garb are fain,
An he at their hands be smitten, then he cometh to me
again!"
(§126, ll. 24-29; vol. 1, p. 72)

But before he leaves (and before, shortly after his departure, she dies), Herzeloyde gives him some advice about how to deal with women.[27]

That Parzival takes this advice to heart but maybe not for the best is demonstrated later in Book 3 when he comes across

[26] DKV, vol. 2, p. 522.

[27] For a discussion of the complex range of "integral roles" played by women in Wolfram's *Parzival,* see Winder McConnell, "The Denial of the Anima in *Parzival,*" *Quondam et Futurus*, vol. 2, no. 2 (Summer 1992), 28-40.

Jeschute of Karnant, the wife of Duke Orilus, lying asleep in a tent. Remembering his mother's advice about how to "win a lady's ring and greeting," Parzival takes this all too literally, innocently (but nevertheless forcibly) embracing Jeschute and taking her ring. (In the eyes of Jeschute's husband, Orilus, Duke of Lalander, this act disgraces and dishonors her. He decides to punish her by not allowing her new clothes, replacing her horse's bridle with a piece of rope, and smashing her horse's saddle.) They set off on the trail of Parzival, who has traveled on, greeting everyone whom he meets and recalling: "Thus bade me my mother dear" (§138, l. 8; cf. §132, l. 24).

Now Parzival has a second encounter, when he meets his cousin, Sigune, who is grieving over the body of her dead lover, Schionatulander. Before he and Sigune had ever been able to consummate their love, this princely knight-servitor had been slain by Orilus, events recounted in Wolfram's (unfinished) elegiac poem *Titurel* (named after the first king of the Grail in the known line, and Parzival's great-grandfather), which relates the story of the child-love of Sigune and Schionatulander.[28] At first, however, Parzival and Sigune do not recognize each other — and (mis)recognition is a major theme in Wolfram's epic. As D.H. Green has put it, the structure of *Parzival* at large reenacts a task which "confront[s] both the chosen hero and the select listeners, who in their comprehension of the work have to accomplish for themselves what Sigune sees as the obligation

[28] For a translation of the *Titurel* fragments, see Wolfram von Eschenbach, *"Parzival" and "Titurel,"* trans. Cyril Edwards (Oxford and New York: Oxford University Press, 2006), pp. 349-367; and for further discussion, see Margaret F. Richey, "The 'Titurel' of Wolfram von Eschenbach: Structure and Character," *The Modern Language Review*, vol. 56, no. 2 (April 1961), 180-193. Based on Wolfram's fragments, Albrecht von Scharfenberg composed a long poem called *Der jüngere Titurel* (c. 1272); whereas Wolfram uses a special four-line stanza, the so-called "Titurelstrophe," Albrecht uses a more complex, seven-line stanza. *Der jüngere Titurel*, famous for its account of a long inscription of the dog lead (Brackenseil), summarizing chivalric virtues in 54 stanzas (see Tamara Elsner, "Text as thing. The dog lead in Albrecht's 'Jüngerer Titurel,'" in MEMO, 7 (2020) [Textual Thingness / Textuelle Dinghaftigkeit], 81-96.

present in Parzival's name" — namely, "not to remain content with surface impressions, but to think through to the implications behind them," citing in MHG the line found in translation below, *der nam is rehte enmitten durch.*[29] When Sigune asks Parzival what his name is, he replies that his mother called him *bon fils, cher fils, beau fils* (§140, l. 6; cf. §113, l. 4), which fact alone — coupled with his beauty, because "God with skill had wrought him," *er trüege den gotes vlîz* (§140, l. 5) — is enough for Sigune to identify him as Parzival — and to explain the meaning of his name:

"Thou art *Parzival*," she cried,
And thy name it shall mean "*to pierce thro'*," for thy
mother's faithful heart
With furrow of grief was riven when she from her lord
[i.e., Kyot of Katelangen] must part [...]."
(§140, ll. 16-20; vol. 1, p. 79)

Whereas Chrétien's French version of the name, *Perceval,* is explicated in full by Heinrich von dem Türlin in his MHG Arthurian romance, *Diu Crône* (i.e, *The Crown*), as signifying "*parce* means *through*, *val* means *a valley"* (*Krone*, ll. 6390-6391),[30] in Wolfram's epic Sigune only explains the first part of his name, "to-pierce-through," as if to emphasize its directionality — as if describing the trajectory of an arrow shot from a bow, rather than its target?

Parzival promises to seek vengeance against Lähelin (who has stolen part of his kingdom) and Orilus (who has slain Schionatulander and Galoes, Parzival's paternal uncle), but Sigune, fearing for his life, deliberately misdirects him — "but the way

[29] For further discussion of the many encounters in which recognition or non-recognition plays a part, see D.H. Green, *The Art of Recognition in Wolfram's "Parzival"* (Cambridge: Cambridge University Press, 1982), p. 319.
[30] DKV, vol. 2, p. 531.

did she falsely show," *si wîste in unrehte nâch* (§141, l. 30) — and thereby unintentionally assists him in finding the way to King Arthur's court. Parzival rides on, following his mother's advice and greeting everyone he meets (§142, ll. 6-10), until he arrives at the house of a churlish fisherman — a kind of proleptic Anfortas-figure — where he spends the night. The next morning, he is shown the way to Nantes and given directions to Arthur's court — the very same Arthur, of course, that Hartmann von Aue, one of Wolfram's literary rivals, had introduced into German literature in his two Arthurian romances, *Erec* and *Iwein*, and to whom Wolfram in a brief excursus he pays guarded tribute (§143, l. 21-§144, l. 4).

As he rides across a meadow covered with flowers, Parzival meets Ither of Gaheviez, the king of Cucumerlant and a knight of the Round Table who is also (as it turns out) distantly related to Parzival. Because of the color of his red armor — even his horse is dressed in red — Ither is known as the "Red Knight," and he has been described as "the most bafflingly ambiguous of Wolfram's figures."[31] Wolfram's narrator describes this literally colorful figure as follows:

> He was Ither of Gaheviess, "The Red Knight" they called his name.
> All dazzling red was his armour, the eye from its glow gleamed red;
> Red was his horse swift-footed, and the plumes that should deck its head,
> Of samite red its covering; redder than flame his shield;
> Fair-fashioned and red his surcoat; and the spear that his hand would wield
> Was red, yea, the shaft and the iron; and red at the knight's desire

[31] Margaret F. Richey, "Ither von Gaheviez," *The Modern Language Review*, vol. 26, no. 3 (July, 1931), 315-329 (p. 316).

> Was his sword, yet the blade's fair keenness was not
> dimmed by the raging fire.
> And the King of Cumberland, stately, in his mailèd
> hand did hold
> A goblet, with skill engraven, and wrought of the
> good red gold —
> From the Table Round had he reft it — All red was his
> shining hair
> Yet white was his skin, and kindly his speech to the
> lad and fair.
> (§145, l.15-§146, l. 3; vol. 1, p. 82)

Whatever the significance of the color red in the figure of Ither, he has a clear structural function: namely, that of framing Parzival's first meeting with King Arthur himself and with his court.

For Parzival immediately gets caught up in a complicated matter of courtly protocol: When he had ridden to the Round Table to claim his lands, Ither had accidentally spilled a cup of wine into the lap of Lady Ginover, Arthur's wife; and he instructs Parzival to tell the queen that he had not intended to splash her with wine. When he is brought into the presence of King Arthur, Parzival's handsome appearance impresses the court — "And well did they look upon him, for each for himself might see / That never in man or maiden might the fruit of love fairer be. / And in truth it was no ill working that in Parzival God had wrought, / In whom never a sight of terror had awakened of fear a thought" (§148, ll. 22-28; vol. 1, p. 84) — including Queen Ginover. Arthur promises to confer knighthood on Parzival the following day, and Parzival begs to be given Ither's armor; but when Arthur warns Parzival away from the formidable Ither, Keie, who fulfills the role of lord high steward and seneschal at Arthur's court, encourages Arthur to make this gift, hoping to provoke a fight between this young knight-to-be and the Red Knight.

In fact, Keie is a rather troublesome figure, whose scornful and provocative behavior suggests that all is not well at Arthur's court (or, perhaps, simply strikes a realistic note in the depiction of court life). We see this behavior at work in what follows. Now earlier in the episode with Jeschute, Parzival had been told by Orilus, the Duke of Lalander, about his sister, Cunneware, and her curiously prophetic rôle:

> [...] At his court doth she dwell to-day,
> My sister, sweet Kunnewaaré, and grave is her mien alway,
> For her lips may not move to laughter till the day that her eyes shall light
> On him who of all shall be reckoned the fairest and bravest knight.
>
> (§135, ll. 14-18; vol. 1, p. 77)

Now while Orilus — ironically enough — fails to recognize Parzival as this man (cf. §135, l. 19), Cunneware does not make this mistake and, when she sees Parzival riding past, she laughs:

> And the maiden Kunnewaaré she sat there, the fair and proud,
> And never, that man might wot of, had she laughed or low or loud.
> For never she vowed, an she died first, would she laugh ere her eyes might see
> That knight, who of knights the bravest or was, or henceforth should be.
> As the lad rode beneath the window she brake into laughter sweet [...].
>
> (§151, ll. 11-19; vol. 1, p. 85)

Yet her laughter provokes a painful rebuke from Keie, who instantly seizes her hair and roughly pulls her head back, holding her in place to beat her with a stick. When Antanor, a knight who is considered to be dumb, breaks his silence to prophesy that Parzival will one day rob Keie of his joy, he earns himself a beating too, and Parzival, unable because of the crowd to intervene, can only look on while Cunneware and Antanor suffer. He clutches at his javelin, for which he will now find a tragic purpose.

For he now rides out to rejoin Ither on the meadow and demands that he give him his red armor. In his impatience to become a knight, Parzival snatches at Ither's bridle and wonders aloud whether Ither is really Lähelin, the brother of Orilus and Cunneware, about whom his mother had apparently warned him. Ither attacks Parzival, thrusting at him with his lance so that he and his horse fell to the ground. Furious, Parzival — whom the narrator specifically refers to as *der knappe guot*, or "the good lad" (§155, l. 4) — seizes his javelin and throws it so it passes through the gap between Ither's helmet and his visor, and — true to his name? — pierces Ither though his eye and through nape of his neck so that "the knight on the plain lay dead":

> Fierce foe had he been to falsehood; women's sighs,
> true hearts wounded sore,
> Were the fruit of his death, and with tear-drops must
> many an eye run o'er.
> And they whom his love made joyful their gladness
> asunder brake,
> And their joy to the goal of sorrow o'er a rough road
> its way must take.
>
> (§155, ll. 10-18; vol. 1, pp. 87-88)

This fighting prowess — or is it just good luck? — stands in a tension with Parzival's *tumbheit*, as he tries (and fails) to tug off

Ither's armor. In fact, Parzival has to be assisted in his childlike perplexity — *in tumber nôt*, "by his folly was vexed amain" (§156, l. 10) — by Iwanet, a young kinsman of Ginover and a squire, who had befriended him at Arthur's court. Together they succeed in despoiling the dead man of his armor, and Iwanet helps Parzival put on the Red Knight's armor — over the buskins or foolish attire that his mother had dressed him in. This peculiar mixture of clothing — foolish youth beneath, knightly armor on top — symbolizes Parzival's transitory state on his path to becoming a knight — and, more important, to becoming lord of the Grail.[32]

Iwanet refuses, however, to allow Parzival to carry the javelin, claiming that the chivalric code forbids this. Instead, he gives Parzival a sharp sword, teaches him how to draw it, and instructs him never to flee. With a manly vigor that is, we are told, still commended today — "E'en to-day do men speak of his swiftness, and the fame of his might deeds" (§157, ll. 29-30) — Parzival leaps, fully armed, into the saddle. Iwanet instructs him further on the use of the shield, how to hold the lance — *war zuo ist diz vrum?* "What good may that do me?" (§158, l. 7), is Parzival's

[32] From a Steinerian perspective, the Grail path of the Parzival story represents, as Matthew Barton has argued, a "modern initiation in the midst of everyday life" (Rudolf Steiner, *The Mysteries of the Holy Grail: From Arthur and Parzival to Modern Initiation*, ed. and trans. Matthew Barton (Forest Row: Rudolf Steiner Press, 2010), p. 179), and within the tradition of anthroposophical thought the story of Parzival is read as representing different stages of growing up; with, for instance, Parzival's killing of the Red Knight seen as illustrating how "the ninth grader [i.e., the 14- to 15-year-old] may find his impulsiveness overcoming his idealism, while Parzival giving his horse free rein to take it him where it will is "a picture of the adolescent unconsciously allowing his destiny to unfold" (John Wulsin, "Parzival — the journey of adolescence," *Renewal: A Journal for Waldorf Education*, vol. 15, no. 1 (Spring-Summer 2006), 3-5; revised and expanded in *Journal for Waldorf/ Rudolf Steiner Education*, 9 (2007), 9-13). In Steinerian pedagogy, class 11 students (i.e., 16- to 17-year-olds) use Goethe's "The Metamorphosis of Plants" to approach botany, and read Wolfram's *Parzival* as "a tale of profound self-metamorphosis" (Carol Bärtges, "The Journey In, the Journey Out: The Waldorf Elementary and High School Curricula," *Renewal: A Journal for Waldorf Education*, vol. 20, no. 1 (Spring-Summer 2011), 28-32 [p. 30]).

response when he first sees it — and how to thrust the lance through an opponent's shield at a joust. Once his education is complete, Parzival tells Iwanet to return to the court and to pay his respects to King Arthur, to return the golden goblet which held the wine that Ither had spilt over Ginover, and tell him of the deep disgrace that he, Parzival, had suffered when Keie punished Cunneware who had honored him with her laughter. In this way, the two courtly matters that had accompanied Parzival's arrival at Arthur's court are resolved, but the question of how to dispose of Ither's dead body remains.

There are important courtly issues at stake here, too. While alive, Ither had been favored by good fortune, but he had met an undeservedly ignominious end: Rather than from a lance-thrust through his shield in chivalrous combat, he had died from a javelin! Iwanet covers the body with flowers, plants the shaft of the javelin above him, and fashions a cross by placing a stick through the javelin-head. Thus symbolically blessed, Ither's body is then brought to the cart, where his demise is much lamented. Queen Ginover claims to speak for all women when she expresses her grief in these powerful words:

> "Alas! alas! for broken in twain is King Arthur's might,
> For he whom the good Round Table accounted its bravest knight
> Here slain before Nantes he lieth! His heritage did he claim
> Where men gave him death for his guerdon — For naught marred his knightly fame;
> Here long hath he dwelt among us in such wise that never an ear
> The tale of a deed unknightly, or wrong he had done, might hear.

He held him afar from falsehood, to guile was he aye
a foe;
The lock and the seal of knighthood all too soon must
we bury low.
His heart wise in courteous wisdom, and steadfast as
seal and sign,
Taught him ever the fairest counsel that a man's heart
might aye divine,
Whereby with true love and courage a man woman's
love may woo
And show manhood's truth — Fruit-bearing it seedeth
itself anew
The plant of all woman's sorrow! From thy wounds
grief shall ever grow —
So red was thy hair that the blossoms that bloom here
thy corse below
Scarce redder may be with thy life-blood — All
laughter hast thou forbid
To fair women, and joy and gladness by thy death are
for ever hid."

(§160, ll. 3-30; vol. 1, p. 90)

It is one of the peculiarities of Wolfram's epic that Arthur's court is presented as — in the parlance of postmodernism — *always already* deficient in some respect, be it Ither's little wine accident with Ginover, Keie's unprovoked violence toward Cunneware and Antanor, or Parzival's killing of Ither. Structurally, of course, this heightens the contrast between Arthur's court and the world of the Grail; although the Grail, too, will in its turn give rise to questions. The brutal death of Ither at the untutored hands of Parzival raises the question of whether the chivalric ideals to which Parzival aspires are, in fact, already a thing of the past …

While Parzival has fulfilled his wish of acquiring Ither's armor, this has been achieved at great cost: It was the desire of Parzival "in his folly" (*des tumben Parzivâles*) (§161, l. 6), and later in his maturity, Parzival will regret his decision: "Hereafter, when he won wisdom, he scarcely such deed had wrought!" (*sît dô er sich baz versan, / ungerne hete erz dô getân*) (§161, ll. 7-8). In other words, Parzival is still in need of education, and the next step in this educative path is one he will take in the company of Gurnemanz, Prince of Graharz, the pinnacles and tower roofing of whose castle Parzival espies from afar on the evening after he leaves Arthur's court, and whom Parzival meets, sitting alone beneath a spreading lime tree in a green meadow, as he approaches the castle.

In his youthful ignorance or folly (*der tumbe man*), Parzival tells Gurnemanz, "My mother bade me seek counsel [*rât*] from an old man with locks of grey; / For thy rede will I do thee service, for so did my mother speak!" and it turns out that Gurnemanz is more than happy to oblige: "If here thou art come for counsel, and aid at my lips would seek, / Thy favour thou still shalt leave me whatever my counsel be, / If thou will that thy prayer I hearken, and give rede as seem best to me!" (§162, l. 29-§163, ll. 1-2 and §163, ll. 3-6; vol. 1, p. 91).

Just as Herzeloyde's theological teaching requires to be supplemented by Trevrizent (see above), so do her words of practical wisdom. In fact, Gurnemanz explicitly urges Parzival to forget what his mother has taught him —

> "Thou speakest as doth a child,
> Why hold not thy peace of thy mother, and otherwise turn thy speech?
> An thou follow henceforth my counsel far wiser the ways I'll teach!"
>
> (§170, ll. 10-14; vol. 1, p. 95)

— and gives his guest nothing less than a thorough induction or training in how to be a knight. This instruction covers the following topics: modesty; pity for those in need; a prudent approach to property; thoughtfulness in conversation; protection for a defeated opponent; cleanliness after battle; love of women that is without *valschheit* (i.e., with *triuwe*); and a sexual or erotic code.[33] It includes a key concept in courtly ethics, *mâze* — a mixture of *temperentia* (or the Christian concept of moderation) and the *medietas* (or the middle between two extremes).[34] Above all, it includes the fateful words of advice:

> Yield not unto ways discourteous but give to thy hearing heed,
> *Nor be thou so swift to question* — Yet I would not that thou withhold
> An answer good and fitting to the speech one with thee would hold.
>
> (§171, ll. 16-21; vol. 1, p. 96)

This advice given to Parzival by Gurnemanz is put into practice during Parzival's encounter in Book 4 with the beautiful Condwiramurs, whom he frees in his first knightly combat on his arrival in Belrepeire (i.e., the "beautiful place")[35] from the besieging armies of an unwanted suitor, Clamide, King of Iserterre. (Parzival goes on to marry Condwiramurs, who becomes the mother of Loherangrin and Kardeiz. Her name derives from the Old French *conduire amours* or "to guide love," and Parzival's fidelity to her becomes another major theme in the work.) On their first meeting, however, his silence leads to potential confusion:

---

[33] DKV, vol. 2, p. 547.

[34] DKV, vol. 2, p. 547; citing Bumke, *Courtly Culture*: "*mâze* was related to Christian *temperantia* ('moderation') as well as *medietas*, the proper middle between two extremes" (p. 303).

[35] Chrétien calls the city *Biaurepere* (i.e., Beaurepaire) (l. 2408; *Œuvres complètes*, ed. Daniel Poirion et al. (Paris: Gallimard, 1994), p. 745); cf. DKV, vol. 2, p. 551.

And grief to her guest it wrought,
To whose courtesy naught was lacking since
Gurnemanz' side he sought,
And his words had from folly freed him, and had
bidden him questions spare
Save only when they were needful — so he sat by that
lady fair,
And never a word his lips spake, tho' he sat close the
maid beside —
Yet to those who know more of woman such silence
doth oft betide.
Then the queen to herself said softly, "This man
disdaineth me,
He deemeth my fairness faded. [...]"
(§188, ll. 15-27; vol. 1, p. 107).

On the second occasion, however, in the Grail scene in Book 5, the consequences of how Parzival (mis)understands this advice prove to be far more serious.

Around 15 months after winning her hand in marriage and defeating his rival Clamide, King of Iserterre, in battle, Parzival asks leave of Condwiramurs to go and visit his mother — and to seek adventure. One evening at a lake he encounters a fisher, Anfortas, who urges Parzival to find lodging for the night at a nearby castle, Munsaelvaesche (i.e., the savage mountain).[36] As well as promising Parzival a warm welcome, Anfortas specifically warns him, *dâ gênt unkunde wege* ("As thou ridest around the hill / Have a care lest the wood mislead thee"), although Parzival gets safely to the castle ("gaily he took his way, / Nor missed he the path") (§226, ll. 6 and 11-12; vol. 1, p. 130). When Parzival first sees the castle of

[36] On the significance of the name Munsalvaesche (variously interpreted as "wild mountain" or "mountain of salvation"), see DKV, vol. 2, p. 591.

Munsalvaesche, he is impressed by its strength and beauty: "the fortress it lacked not for strength I trow, / As a turner with skill had wrought them stood the turrets in goodly row. / […] And so strong were the towers and the palace that its folk they had held the hall / And mocked at the foe, if all armies thirty years long beset the wall" (§226, ll. 14-19; vol. 1, p. 130). On his arrival at Munsalvaesche, Parzival is greeted by its inhabitants and hosted by Anfortas, who turns out to be its owner (as the Fisher King),[37] and the queen, Repanse de Schoye (again, a name derived from the Old French, Repense de Joie). As well as being the sister of Anfortas, Repanse de Schoye serves as the bearer of the Grail, in a mysterious ceremony that Parzival is allowed to witness.[38]

Lying ill on a bed, Anfortas tells Parzival to come closer; we are not told what Anfortas's illness is, only that *er lebte niht wan töude* ("And his life was but a dying") (§230, l. 20; vol. 1, p. 132). Dining together in a great hall, the knights are all sad and weep at

---

[37] For further discussion of this mysterious figure (and his even more mysterious "double" or "counterpart," i.e., his father), see William A. Nitze, "The Fisher King in the Grail Romances," *Publications of the Modern Language Association of America*, vol. 24, no. 3 (1909), 365-418.

[38] For an extremely helpful tabular overview of the differences between Wolfram's description of the Grail scene and Chrétien's, see DKV, vol. 2, p. 574. The chief differences in the procession of the Grail are:

- Chrétien:
    - white lance which is bleeding
    - golden candelabra
    - golden dish (*graal*)
    - silver carving platter
- Wolfram:
    - lance dripping blood
    - golden candelabra and table pedestals
    - grail is a stone
    - grail placed during the meal on the Fisher King's table

For a more comprehensive comparative analysis, see Karin Elizabeth Nordenhaug, *The symbolism of the Grail: A comparative analysis of the Grail in "Perceval ou Le Conte del Graal" by Chretien de Troyes and "Parzival" by Wolfram von Eschenbach.* BA Thesis, Westhampton College, University of Richmod, 1962. Archived in the UR Scholarship Repository and available HTTP: https://scholarship.richmond.edu/honors-theses/1077.

the sight when a squire comes in, bearing a lance or spear, from the point of which blood issues and runs down the shaft (§231, l. 15-§232, l. 4).[39] Amid much material richness and ceremonial splendor, Repanse de Schoye enters, bearing the wondrous Grail on a green-and-gold cloth:

> And she bare aloft on a cushion of verdant Achmardi
> Root and blossom of Paradise garden, that thing which men call "The Grail,"
> The crown of all earthly wishes, fair fulness that ne'er shall fail!
> Repanse de Schoie did they call her, in whose hands the Grail might lie,
> By the Grail Itself elected was she to this office high.
> And they who would here do service, those maids must be pure of heart,
> And true in life, nor falsehood shall have in their dealings part.
>
> (§235, ll. 20-30; vol. 1, p. 135)

This scene and the action that follows prompt us to ask yet again: What *is* the Grail?[40]

[39] Thus, Wolfram separates two elements, the lance and the Grail, found together in one of Wolfram's sources, Chrétien de Troyes (cf. DKV, vol. 2, pp. 575-576). For Eberhard Nellmann, the motif of the bleeding lance is "one of the greatest mysteries of Gral research"; in some respects, the significance of the lance — understood at the end of the twelfth or the beginning of the thirteenth centuries by the author of a continuation of the Gawain story — lies in its identity with the sacred spear with which the Roman soldier Longinus pierced the side of Christ on the Cross (DKV, vol. 2, pp. 575-576).

[40] For recent scholarship on the Grail that identifies it as the Bamberg Paradise Altar, see G. Ronald Murphy, SJ, *Gemstone of Paradise: The Holy Grail in Wolfram's "Parzival"* (New York: Oxford University Press, 2006); for a summary of the characteristics given by Wolfram to his Grail stone, see pp. 31-36, and see also William C. McDonald, "Wolfram's Grail," *Arthuriana*, vol. 8, no. 1, *The Grail and The Quest* (Spring 1998), 22-34.

daz was ein dinc, daz hiez der Grâl

For a start, it is a thing, *daz was ein dinc, daz hiez der Grâl*, although in Wolfram's poem it is not a dish or a cup or a ciborium, but a stone. Next, it exceeds all earthly wishes, *erden wunsches überwal*. Then, whoever watches over it must preserve purity and renounce falsity, *wol muose ir kiusche sîn bewart, / diu sîn ze rehte solde pflegen: / diu muose valsches sich bewegen*. Finally, it is associated with light, thanks to the six glass vials carried before it: "And lights both rare and costly before the Grail they bore / Six glasses tall, transparent — and wondrous balsam's flame / Burnt within with a strange sweet perfume" (§236, ll. 1-4; vol. 1, p. 135). Now the Grail reveals its remarkable powers, providing endless and delicious food and drink for the assembled company: "As I heard so I tell unto ye, and the truth ye, each one, shall swear, / 'Twas the Grail Itself that fed them, and before the Grail did stand / What of food and drink desiring, each one might stretch forth his hand" (§238, ll. 8-14; vol. 1, p. 136). Consequently, the Grail is described as a source of all earthly delights:

> Such riches ye never on earth shall find,
> So many have said, yet I think me that folly doth rule their mind —
> For the Grail was the crown of blessing, the fulness of earth's delight,
> And Its joys I right well may liken to the glories of Heaven's height!
>
> (§238, ll. 18-24; vol. 1, p. 136)

Not surprisingly, Parzival is amazed at all these wonders, and yet — recalling the advice of Gurnemanz, he does not ask any questions and remains silent:

> And the Grail Itself sustained them, and Parzival wondering saw

The riches and mighty marvels, yet to question his
host forebore.
And he thought, "Gurnemanz he bade me, in truth,
without thought of guile,
To withhold my lips from question — If here I abide
awhile
Methinks it will then befall me as aforetime in Graharz
land,
They will tell me, without my question, how here with
this folk it stands."

(§239, ll. 8-17; vol. 1, p. 130)

Even though Anfortas gives Parzival a valuable sword that he himself used to carry in battle, Parzival *still* does not ask a question. *Ôwê daz er niht vrâgte dô!*, "Ah! woe to the guest that asked not" (§240, l. 3), remarks Wolfram's narrator, hinting at even greater powers of the Grail: "For the host too my heart is heavy, thus tortured by nameless woe, / And a question therefrom had freed him, yet to question his guest was slow" (§240, ll. 7-9; vol. 1, p. 137).[41]

[41] Another — at this point — unresolved puzzle is the identity of the man whom Parzival glimpses in an antechamber to the hall: "And Parzival he gazed after, and lo! thro' the open door / Within an outer chamber, on a folding couch he saw / The fairest of old men ancient whom ever his eyes had seen, / Grey was he as mists of morning […]" (§240, ll. 23-28; vol. 1, p. 137). Later — in conversation with Sigune (§251, ll. 3-6) and with Trevrizent (§474, ll. 10-11, cf. §455, ll. 15-19; and §813, ll. 15-16) — it emerges he is Titurel, the grandfather of Anfortas (and great-grandfather of Parzival) (cf. DKV, vol. 2, pp. 592 and 702). Parzival asks Trevrizent, "Say who shall he be, who lay / Before the Grail? grey was he, yet his face it was as the day!", and Trevrizent explains, "Titurel thou sawest, and he shall grandsire be / To thy mother, first kind and ruler of the Grail and Its knights was he," adding: "But a sickness hath fallen on him, and he lieth, nor findeth cure, / Yet his face on the Grail yet looketh, by Its power shall his life endure!" (§501, ll. 19-30; vol. 1, p. 287). The presence of Titurel is an example of the "double" or "counterpart"; in other versions of the Grail story, this figure appears in triplicate or even quadruple form (see Sharkey, "The Maimed Kings," p. 421)!

Yet this error — this sin, if one will, of omission rather than commission — is made clear to Parzival when he discovers the next morning, after uneasy dreams, that Anfortas and his court have left, and just one squire has remained behind to take him to task (*ir sît ein gans*) for failing to ask his host the all-important question:

> For fain would he ask the meaning, but the squire cried aloud in scorn,
> "Goose that thou art, ride onward, to the sun's hate hast thou been born!
> Thy mouth hadst thou thought to open, of these wonders hadst asked thine host,
> Great fame had been thine — But I tell thee now hast thou this fair chance lost!"
> Then the guest cried aloud for his meaning, but answer he ne'er might win […].
> (§247, l. 25-§248, l. 2; vol. 1, p. 141)

Parzival sets off, following the tracks of those who have departed, until they become fainter and finally disappear. As they do so, he encounters for a second time his cousin Sigune, whom he does not recognize (just as he did not the first time). When he recounts where he has spent the night, Sigune tells him its name, "Monsalväsch I ween its name, / Terre de Salväsch the kingdom where its lord the crown may claim" (§25, ll. 2-4; vol. 1, p. 142), and explains this castle cannot be found intentionally, but can only be discovered by chance (or, in other words, by those considered worthy of the Grail). Explaining further that Munsalvaesche had been bequeathed by Titurel (the first king of the Grail, and the great-grandfather of Parzival) to his son Frimutel, who had four children (Anfortas, Repanse de Schoye, Herzeloyde, and Trevrizent; a fifth child,

Sigune's mother, Schoysiane, is not mentioned, because she died before her father).[42]

And she tells him that, if he had found his way to the castle, he could have redeemed Anfortas from his suffering: "If indeed thou camest to that folk who so sore doth mourn / Then perchance is their kind releasèd from the burden he long hath borne?" (§251, ll. 21-24; vol. 1, p. 143). Parzival's response to this remark is not untruthful, but tactical: "I saw truly great marvels, and many a maid / Of beauty rare" (§251, ll. 26-27), but it is sufficient to bring about a moment of recognition, *bî der stimme erkannte sî den man*, "she knew him by his voice ere the words were said," and she declares: *du bist Parzivâl!* ("Now indeed I know thee, for in sooth art thou Parzival!") (§251, ll. 28-29; vol. 1, p. 143). And she goes on to ask, "Didst thou see the mournful monarch? Didst thou see the wondrous Grail? / Ah! Tell me joyful tidings, may his woe at last be stilled?" (§251, l. 30-§252, l. 2; vol. 1, p. 143). But rather than answer her question, Parzival poses one of his own: "Say, Lady, whence knowest thou me?" (§252, l. 10). When she replies, "I am that maiden who erewhile made her plaint to thee, / I am she who thy name first told thee" (§252, ll. 11-13; p. 143), Sigune refers back to their first encounter in Book 3, where she recognized him and gave an etymology of his name, *deiswâr du heizest Parzivâl. / der name ist »Rehte enmitten durch«*, "Thou art *Parzival* [...] / And thy name it shall mean '*to pierce through*,' for thy mother's faithful heart / With furrow of grief was riven when she from her lord must part" (§140, ll. 16-20; vol. 1, p. 79).[43]

If Parzival did not recognize Sigune the first time because he had never met her before, this time he fails to recognize her because she has cut off her brown locks of hair.[44] He asks, *bistuz Sigûne, diu mir kunt / tet wer ich was, ân allen vâr?*, "Alas! is it thou, Siguné?

[42] DKV, vol. 2, p. 592.
[43] Cf. DKV, vol. 2, p. 531.
[44] DKV, vol. 2, pp. 592-593.

[…] That gave me to wit so truly who I was?" and he laments the loss of her red lips, *ôwê war hom dîn rôter munt?*, "Say, where are thy lips so red?" (§252, ll. 28-29 and l. 27; vol. 1, p. 143). Noticing that Parzival is now wearing the magic sword (made by an ingenious smith, the famous Trebuchet) that Anfortas had given him, Sigune asks again whether Parzival asked *the* question, *niemen ist sô riche, / der gein dir koste mege hân, / hâstu vrâge ir reht getân*, "The crown of blessings fair / Uplifted o'er all earth's noblest henceforward thine head shall bear. / And thine is desire's fulfilment, and none with thy wealth and might / May measure himself, if the question hath won at thy lips its right!". This time Parzival admits, *ich hân gevrâget niht*, "Nay, I asked no question," to which Sigune responds in dismay, *ôwê daz iuch mîn ouge siht* […] *sît ir vrâgens sît verzagt!*, "Alas! […] That ever mine eyes have seen thee, who to question wast sore afraid!" (§254, l.28-§255, l.4; vol. 1, p. 144). Sigune curses Parzival, *gûnerter lîp, vervluochtet man!*, "Alas! wherefore hast thou sought me? Dishonoured, accurst art thou / Who bearest wolf's fang empoisoned!" and she forcefully rejects his expression of regret, *ir lebt, und sît an saelden tôt* […] *ir sult wandels sîn erlân*, "Now thou livest, and yet I tell thee to bliss are thou henceforth dead! […] Little good may repentance do thee" (§255, ll. 20 and 24; p. 145). Sigune refuses to say another word, and Parzival rides off.

Parzival's identity is thus intimately bound up with the Grail itself: One might say that *his quest for the Grail is the quest for his identity*. Now Parzival is struck with remorse: "That his lips were so slow to question when he sat by the mournful king, / To the heart of the gallant hero must surrow and rueing bring," and his self-accusation and the heat of the day have him covered in sweat. And then — something happens: *er kom ûf eine niuwe slâ*, "Then he saw a fresh track" (§256, ll. 5-6 and 11; vol. 1, p. 145). Throughout his quest, Parzival's journey is full of signs and pointers, none more famous than in Book 6 when Parzival is in search of King Arthur's camp and sees three drops of blood on the white snow (§282). Unbeknownst to him, Parzival had been following the path of King Arthur's falcon (§282, ll. 11-12), and the falcon had earlier attacked a goose: "In its flight from the wounds there brake / Three blood-drops, all glowing crimson, and fell on the spotless snow, / As Parzival's eyes beheld them, swift sorrow his heart must know!" (§282, ll. 10-12; vol. 1, p. 160). The sorrow this sight brings him is because it reminds him of his beloved wife, Condwiramurs: *wer hât sînen vlîz / gewant an dise varwe clâr? / Cundwîer âmûrs*, "Say what hand hath painted these colours that here I see? / Kondwiramur, I think well, these tints sure shall liken thee!" (282, ll. 26-29; vol. 1, p. 161).

The motif of drops of blood on snow as a symbol of white skin and rosy cheeks (and hence as an image of feminine beauty) is well known,[45] and Parzival himself interprets this sight as follows:

> "[…] — in this snow that so spotless lies,
> 'Gainst the blood-drops, that ruddy-gleaming, glow crimson beneath mine eyes,
> I find ever thy face so gracious, my lady, Kondwiramur,
> Red as blood-drops and white as the snowdrift, it rejoiceth me evermore!"
>
> (§283, ll. 4-9; vol. 1, p. 161)

Yet the motif of blood also links in with the other themes and symbols of the work: the theme of blood relations (in the world of *Parzival*, almost everybody is related to everybody else); the blood dripping from the spear in the first Grail scene; and, of course, the redeeming blood of Christ. The impact of the sight on Parzival is significant, *sus begrunde er sich verdenken*, "Little recked he of aught around, / But wrapped in love and longing, saw naught but the blood-stained ground," and he falls into a kind of catatonic

[45] DKV, vol. 2, p. 604-605.

state: *sus hielt er als er sliefe*, "So held he him still, as sleeping" (§283, ll. 16-17 and 23; vol. 1, p. 161).

Precisely at this moment, a squire runs by, observes Parzival sitting on his horse, fully clothed for battle with a lance in his hand ("And a knight there abode in armour, and his lance he aloft did bear / As one who here patient waited the joust that he fain would ride"), and runs back to Arthur's camp (and to Cunneware, the sister of Orilus, the Duke of Lalant, whom Parzival had earlier, in Book 5, both fought in battle and reconciled with his wife, Jeschute of Karnant). Back at the camp, the squire raises the alarm, warning that a knight is waiting to do battle! One of King Arthur's knights, Segramors — *der ie nâch strîte ranc*, "ever his heart did long / To be in the midst of conflict" — rushes off to oblige. Segramors challenges Parzival, who remains lost in his thoughts of love: *unversunnen hielt dâ Parzivâl*, "There held fast by threefold might, / And the power of red blood-drops threefold stood ever the stranger knight" (§287, ll. 9-10; vol. 1, p. 163).

Here as elsewhere, Wolfram personifies Love as an allegorical figure, *vrou Minne*:

> Frau Minne with force constrained him, as here on his
> wife he thought,
> And by magic of colours mystic, a spell on his senses
> wrought.
>
> (§283, ll. 18-22; vol. 1, p. 161)

(and see §291-§293, §532-§534, and §585-§587). Wolfram's narrator develops the personification of *minne*, confessing that he, too, has succumbed to her power: "Yea, well I myself have known this, how Frau Minne with power may hold, / And holding, the senses scatter, and with passion of grief untold / Shall fill the heart to o'erflowing" (§287, ll. 11-13; vol. 1, p. 163).[46]

---

[46] This personification of Love, or *Minne,* as an allegorical figure is a convention of the time, found also in Eilhart von Oberge (see *Tristrant*, ll. 2505 and 2464) and in

Overwhelmed by the power of love personified by *vrou Minne*, Parzival remains unaware of the danger, until Segramors turns his horse around and prepares to attack. In response, Parzival's own horse turns round, and suddenly Parzival wakes up: "Round wheeled him the war-horse good / On whose back the gallant hero yet sate in mystic mood, / And ever he gazed on the blood-drops; as his charger turned him round / Awhile from his eyes they vanished, and fame in their stead he found!" and as Lady Reason (*vrou Witze*) replaces Lady Love (*vrou Minne*), Parzival makes ready for battle: "For swift as the blood-drops crimson thus passed from his dazzled sight, / He hearkened the voice of the foeman, and braced him anew for fight" (§288, ll. 7-10 and 11-12; vol. 1, p. 164).

Parzival defeats Segramors; then "brave" Keie, lord high steward and seneschal at Arthur's court (and, in Wolfram's narrator's view, a much-maligned man…) has a go — and he loses, too.[47] After the battle, Parzival returns to gaze at the blood drops on the snow:

> Thus he who know naught of falsehood was guided of
> truth to know
> His message in blood-drops threefold, on the white of
> the drifted snow.
> 'Twas tear-drops, not blood, that he saw there, and
> well might his senses fail,
> And the thoughts of his heart wax heavy, as he mused
> on the wondrous Grail,

Hartmann von Aue (see *Erec*, l. 3718; and frequently in *Iwein*), and it is a common device in the lyric work of Walther von Vogelweide. Wolfram innovates, however, by introducing the figures of *frou Witze* (§288, l. 14) and *frou Liebe* (§291, l. 17). See DKV, vol. 2, p. 606.

[47] The narrator's view of Keie is surprising, given the negative way he is depicted elsewhere; and likewise in Hartmann von Aue's *Erec* (ll. 4636-4664) and *Iwein* (ll. 2565-74), Keie is a problematic figure. It seems that Wolfram, in the figure of the belligerent seneschal, is trying to reconcile two irreconcilables: Keie's rôle as a figure of discontent within the plot, and the supposedly ideal nature of the Arthurian court (DKV, vol. 2, p. 610).

And sorely the semblance grieved him that spake of
his wife and queen
(§296, ll. 1-8; vol. 1, p. 168)

— that is, of course, Condwiramurs. In fact, it is not until Gawan — who becomes the hero of the subsidiary, complementary action of the work — rides out to Parzival that the spell of Lady Love is broken. When Gawan finds Parzival in the forest, the latter is still lost in contemplation again:

Fair spake Gawain the stranger, to greeting deaf was he,
Frau Minne yet held him captive, how other might it
be?
True son of Herzeleide, to this lot was he born,
To lose himself for love's sake; such passion as had torn
The hearts of these his parents, afresh in his heart awoke,
And but little his ear might hearken what the mouth of
Gawain spoke.
(§300, ll. 11-22; vol. 1, p. 171)

Because he, too, has once also been caught in the binds of love (in his case, with queen Inguse de Bahtarliez — the episode itself has been lost in the tradition of Arthurian romance), Gawan realizes what the problem might be:

"It may be Frau Minne dealeth so with this
goodly man,
As she dealt with me of old time, so claspeth him in
the ban
Of her magic spells fair-woven, that his spirit within
the snare
She holdeth fast entangled"
(§301, ll. 22-25; vol. 1, p. 171).

And so he also realizes what the solution is, and quickly covers up the drops of blood in the snow:

— Then his eyes on the snow-flakes fair
He cast, and he knew the token, and swift from the
spell-bound sight
With cloth of fair silk and sendal, he covered the
blood-drops bright.
(§301, ll. 26-30; vol. 1, p. 171)

Gawan's intervention brings Parzival back to his senses; or, as Wolfram's narrator puts it, the Queen of Belrepeire, that is, Condwiramurs — as if embodying Frau Minne — allows him to return to his senses. (By contrast, in Chrétien de Troyes's version, the magical power of love melts as the snow melts in the sun.)[48]

Thus restored to the world, Parzival is escorted by Gawan back to Arthur's camp, where he is welcomed by Cunneware for avenging the wrong that Keie had done to her. Whereas previously Parzival had been dressed like a fool, he now appears resplendent:

And robed was the gallant hero, and so bright and so
fair was he,
That all men who there beheld him, they sware he for
sure must be
The flower and the crown of manhood, a knight
without shame or fear;
And they looked upon him, and they praised him and
his colour waxed bright and clear [...].
(§306, ll. 20-29; p. 174)[49]

---

[48] See Chrétien de Troyes, *Perceval* (ll. 4413-4456). Gawan's intervention can be read as a "rationalistic" device on Wolfram's part, as opposed to Chrétien's more "natural" account (see DKV, vol. 2, p. 613).

[49] The theme of wounded masculinity in *Parzival* has been discussed in various online essays by Richard A. Sanderson, including "Wounded Masculinity: Parsifal and the Fisher King Wound," available HTTP http://howellgroup.org/parsifal.html

Indeed, he is not only the "flower of all men," but it is said that he *looks like an angel*:

> And so fair was the knight and radiant, that all men
> beheld his face
> As an angel from heaven, that wingless, abideth on
> earth a space.
>
> (§308, ll. 1-3; p. 175)

Thus attired, Parzival is introduced to King Arthur, and he becomes a knight of the Round Table (§308-§309). Arthur's wife, Queen Ginover, forgives Parzival for having killed Ither of Gaheviez, or the "Red Knight," whose death has "wrought sorrow unto many a woman dear" (§311, l. 3; vol. 1, p. 177).

Precisely at this moment of resolution and integration, however, Cundrie the sorceress arrives, riding on a mule. Wolfram's narrator describes her unflatteringly as having long, dark hair, as soft as boar's bristles; a nose like a dog; a pair of tusks; braided eyebrows; ears like a bear; in short, "never the eye might trace / A shy glance of love, or longing, I ween in that wondrous face" (§313, l. 30-§314, l. 1; vol. 1, p. 178). In fact, she is described as being *trûrens urhap, vröuden twinc* ("a source of sadness, a grave of happiness") (§314, l. 12), and she rides up to Arthur and laments the current reputation — thanks to Parzival and his killing of the "Red Knight" — of the Round Table. Then she rides up to Parzival himself and curses him for not asking the question, thus allowing Anfortas's suffering to continue. "Oh! thou false and faithless guest [*vil ungetriwer gast*]," she says, "For hadst thou had pity on him, his anguish had gotten rest," calling him "Thou hook in fair feathers hidden, bright serpent with poisoned fang," and chastising him for

(accessed 30 September 2013); and HTTP https://www.camilogallardo.com/index.php/resources/wounded-masculinity (accessed 19 February 2024) his silence: "The goal of thy sins, this thy silence, of Hell's horde art thou now the sport, / And dishonour upon thy body, Sir Parzival, has thou wrought. / Saw'st thou not how they bare before the Grail, and the bleeding spear, / And sharp silver? Thy joy's destruction, and thy shelter from grief were here!" (§316, ll. 2-3, 20, 24-28; vol. 1, pp. 179-180). Her final words are a bitter lament: "Ah! woe unto thee, Monsalväsch, thou dwelling and goal of grief, / Since no man hath pity on three, or bringeth thy woe relief!" (§318, ll. 29-30; vol. 1, p. 181).

At the same time, Cundrie issues a challenge. What has happened, she asks, to the courtly ideals: "Is there here a knight / Who yearneth for love's rewarding, and for honour and fame would fight?" (§318, ll. 13-15; vol. 1, p. 181). And she tells the assembled company about the four queens and 400 maidens who are being held captive at Schastel merveile (or the Castle of Wonders), awaiting rescue. To rescue them would be, says Cundrie, a real adventure, *al âventiure ist ein wint, / wan die man dâ bezalen mac*, "and like to the empty air / Shall be all knightly ventures to the venture that Burg within" (§318, ll. 20-21; vol. 1, p. 181), thereby evoking the key concept of courtly literature — the medieval concept of *âventiure* as found in the Arthurian epics, where it refers a *Bewährungsprobe* or test which the hero has successfully to pass. Or, as Ingrid Kasten puts it, "the *âventiure* is no longer an arbitrary fate that befalls the hero, but a dangerous test of his worth that he seeks out on his own initiative and is destined for him alone through a wondrous stroke of good fortune" (*die âventiure [...] ist nicht mehr willkürliches Geschick, das dem Helden zustößt, sondern eine von ihm aus eigenem Antrieb gesuchte und durch wunderbare Fügung für ihn allein bestimmte gefahrvolle Bewährungsprobe*).[50] The *âventiure* thus demonstrates many of the structural principles of the hero's

[50] Ingrid Kasten and Volker Merstens, "Aventure (âventiure)," in *Lexikon des Mittelalters* (LexMA), vol. 1 (Munich and Zurich: Artemis & Winkler, 1980), cols. 1289-1290.

journey and its archetypal framework of typical situations and figures.

And thus, the next set of episodes is set in motion. As Cundrie leaves, the figure of Kingrimursel, the landgrave and burgrave of Schanpfanzun, rides up to challenge Gawan for having killed his uncle, Kingrisin. One of Gawan's brothers, Beaucurs, offers himself as surety for the fight between Gawan and Kingrimursel, and Gawan prepares to depart for his fight with Kingrimursel before the King of Asculan in Schanpfanzun. At this point, the narrative bifurcates, following alternately Gawan and Parzival on their respective journeys. For his part, Parzival, lamenting his failure to help Anfortas by asking the question, resolves to seek the Grail: "No joy shall my portion be," he says, "Or long or short my wanderings, till the Grail once again I see!" (§329, ll. 25-30; vol. 1, p. 187). At the same time, he now questions the advice he had been given by Gurnemanz (or advice that he has incorrectly interpreted?): "If a courteous and knightly bearing but bringeth rewarding still / In shame, and in this world's mocking, then methinks I was counselled ill: / For 'twas Gurnemanz who bade me of questions rash beware, / And from words and ways unfitting a courteous knight forbear" (§330, ll. 1-6; vol. 1, p. 187).

As he sets off, Gawan wishes that God will bring him good luck, "God guide thee upon thy way" (§331, l. 27), which reminds Parzival of his original question to his mother, *wê waz ist got*, "Woe is me! Who is He, this mighty God?" and in an astonishing passage, for which there is no equivalent whatsoever in previous versions of the story, Parzival renounces God:

> "Woe is me! Who is He, this mighty God?
> Had He power, methinks our portion had ne'er been
> this shame abhorred!
> Small power shall be His! I served Him from the day
> I first knew His grace,

Henceforth I renounce His service; doth He hate me,
His hate I'll face!
And, friend, in thine hour of peril, as thy shield may a
wife's love stand,
Dost thou know her for pure and holy, then the thought
of her guide thine hand,
And her love from all evil guard thee, — as I wish,
may it be to thee,
For little I wot of the future, if thy face I again may
see!"

(§332, ll. 1-16; vol. 1, p. 188)

What is at stake here is not so much the *existence* of God — we are a long way off from Nietzsche's cry that God is dead — as His *nature*, that is to say, whether He is like a feudal lord who displays *triuwe* to his vassals, failing which the vassals are allowed to revoke the relationship and refuse further obedience. Previously seen by earlier critics as *the* great sin on the part of Parzival, his renunciation of God is now usually related to the motif of *zwîvel* in the prologue and the question of how to respond to a world in which certainty is not possible. (In his conversation with Parzival in Book 9, Trevrizent suggests there may be various sins for which Parzival should atone, not just this *sünde*.)[51] Instead of protection from God, Parzival thus urges Gawan to seek protection from an earthly source — the love of a virtuous woman. At this point, all now go their separate ways: Gawan goes off to Asculan (§335, ll. 1-3), Arthur's court sets out to find the Castle of Wonders (§334, ll. 1-7), and Parzival sets out in search of the Grail (§333, ll. 27-30).

[51] Cf. DKV, vol. 2, pp. 622-623.

Book 9

We next meet Parzival in Book 9, which opens with an apostrophe by Wolfram's narrator to *vrou Âventiure* or Lady Adventure (§433). We learn that Parzival has traveled widely across land (by horse) and sea (by boat), engaging in knightly combat. Although the sword given to him by Anfortas once shattered in a duel, it was repaired thanks to the restorative powers of a spring near Karnant known as Lac (§434, ll. 25-29). One day, riding through a forest, Parzival encounters Sigune for a third time. She is now living as an anchoress above the tomb of her dead lover, Schionatulander, whose death she laments: "All her life was a prayer," we are told, "and her lips, erst so red and glowing, had faded as life-joys fade" (§435, ll. 25 and 26-27; vol. 1, p. 252). Yet again, they fail to recognize each other, and in response to his questions (is Parzival beginning to learn his lesson …?), Sigune tells him how she receives food from the Grail, brought to her once a week by Cundry the sorceress. This can only mean one thing: that Munsalvaesche is close by!

Finally, Parzival and Sigune do recognize each other, and Parzival expresses his deep regret at not having asked the question and his desire to rediscover the Grail:

> "Alas! For my joy is fled,
> And the Grail hath but wrought me sorrow, and mischance in fair fortune's stead.
> For the land that as king had crowned me must I leave, and yet more, I ween,
> The fairest of wives, and the sweetest, that ever a man hath seen.
> For no lovelier form I think me on earth of mankind was born,
> And I yearn for her tender greeting, and full sore for her love I mourn!
> And yet know I a deeper sorrow and I strive for a higher prize,

For the day when the Burg of Monsalväsch, and the
Grail shall rejoice my eyes!
[…]"

(§441, ll. 4-14; vol. 1, p. 255)

Sigune confirms the gravity of the consequences of Parzival's error, as she tells him:

"From henceforth, my cousin, mine anger will
I forswear,
For too much of thy joy lieth forfeit since the question
thou didst forbear!
And I would not too sorely grieve thee — Alas! that
thou didst withhold
The word that had brought thee honour, and the tale of
his griefs had told
Who sat there as thine host beside thee — nor thine
host alone was he,
Anfortas, for joy and blessing his presence had
brought to thee!
And thy question great bliss had brought thee, and thy
silence had wrought thee woe,
And thy spirit shall fail, and heart-sorrow as thy
comrade thou well shalt know.
[…]"

(§441, ll. 18-28; vol. 1, p. 255)

This line, *dîn herze sorge hât gezemt*, announces a great theme in German literature — one that reaches from Wolfram von Eschenbach to Johann Wolfgang Goethe's *Faust* and beyond to the existentialism of Martin Heidegger (1889-1976) and to C.G. Jung: namely, the theme of *Sorge*. Sometimes, as here or as in Goethe's *Faust*, *Sorge* is presented as an allegorical personification. In *Being and Time* (1927), Heidegger offers extensive phenomenological analysis of *Sorge* (care), along with *das Gerede* (idle talk), *die Neugier* (curiosity), *die Zweideutigkeit* (ambiguity), *das Verfallen* and *die Geworfenheit* (falling and thrownness), and *Angst* (anxiety).[52] What happens to us in "everydayness," in "the press of things"? We "lose" ourselves, we "forget" ourselves, Heidegger says (106).

In Goethe's *Faust II*, Sorge is one of the four gray women who emerge from the ashes of Philemon's and Baucis's burned cottage, respectively identified as Want, Debt, Care, and Need. Of these four, Sorge is the most intimidating, as she tells Faust: "In an ever-changing guise / Cruel power I exercise" (*In verwandelter Gestalt / Üb' ich grimmige Gewalt*) (ll. 11426-27), and the question that she asks Faust, "Hast thou not Care already known?" (*Hast du die Sorge nie gekannt?*) is one that might be asked of us all.[53]

Sigune advises Parzival to follow the tracks left by Cundrie that might lead him to Munsalvaesche, but — not for the first time — the tracks disappear, and he loses his way:

> But farewell did he bid to the maiden; and he followed the woodland way,
> And fresh were the tracks before him, but such pathway the mule must choose
> Thro' the depths of the dusky thicket that its traces he soon must lose.
> As the Grail he had lost of aforetime, so he lost It again to-day,

[52] See §35, §36, §37, §40, and §41, in Heidegger, *Being and Time*, trans. John Macquarrie and Edward Robinson (Oxford: Blackwell, 1962), pp. 211-224, 228-235, 235-241. For further discussion of *Gerede*, see Jesús Adrián Escudero, "Heidegger on Discourse and Idle Talk: The Role of Aristotelian Rhetoric," *Gatherings: The Heidegger Circle Annual*, 3 (2013), 1-17.

[53] For further discussion, see Konrad Burdach, "Faust und die Sorge," *Deutsche Vierteljahrsschrift für Literaturwissenschaft und Geistesgeschichte*, 1 (1923), 1-60; and Margarita Kranz, "Sorge," in *Historisches Wörterbuch der Philosophie*, ed. Joachim Ritter and Karlfried Gründer, vol. 9 (Basel: Schwabe, 1995), cols. 1086-1090.

And joy and delight fled with It — Yea, had he but found the way,
And reached once again Monsalväsch, far better than erst of old
Had he known how to ask the question — thus in sooth is the venture told.
(§442, l. 26-§443, l. 4; vol. 1, p. 256)

But Parzival then encounters a knight of the Grail, defending its territory; the knight's warning to Parzival is discouraging, to say the least:

"Begone! or receive such token thou shalt wish thyself far from here!
Monsalväsch doth never brook it that men ride thus its walls anear,
And here must thou strive in battle, and win here a victor's fame,
Or such penance be thine, as without there, in the open, men *Death* shall name!"
(§443, ll. 16-20; vol. 1, p. 256)

So Parzival jousts with the knight, defeating him — but, in the process, losing his own horse when it falls into a deep gulley, so he takes the knight's horse and rides off:

Onward he rode, yet wandering, nor further befell mischance,
Nor strife, from the knights of Monsalväsch, yet one grief must vex his soul,
He found not the Grail — Ever further he rode, further fled the goal!
(§445, ll. 27-30; vol. 1, p. 258)

(What sort of knights are the Grail knights — might they belong to the Knights Templar? Otherwise known as the Order of Solomon's Temple, the Templars were founded in 1119 after Hughes de Payens had approached King Baldwin II of Jerusalem and sought permission for a religious order with the military purpose of protecting pilgrims traveling in the Holy Land.[54] After all, Wolfram calls the knight here *der templeis* [§444, l. 23; cf. §468, l. 28], which sounds similar, and both Grail knights and Templars have much in common as chivalric orders, pledged to chastity and with specific objectives.[55] In terms of the reception of the Grail legend, the accusations of heresy made against the Templars, the suppression of the order by Pope Clement V in 1312, and the burning at the stake of its Grand Master, Jacques de Molay, all contributed to lending the Grail a more esoteric significance.) Many weeks later, it is a snowy Good Friday (perhaps in March), and Parzival is riding through a wood.[56]

[54] For further discussion, see Malcolm Barber, *The New Knighthood: A History of the Order of the Temple* (Cambridge: Cambridge University Press, 1994); Malcolm Barber and Keith Bate (eds), *The Templars: Selected Sources* (Manchester: Manchester University Press, 2002); and Malcolm Barber, *The Trial of the Templars*, 2nd edn (Cambridge: Cambridge University Press, 2006). For an anthroposophical approach, see Willem Frederik Veltman, *The Temple and the Grail: The Mysteries of the Order of the Templars and the Grail and their Significance for Our Time* [^{2}1992], trans. Philip Mees (Forest Row: Temple Lodge Publishing, 2021).

[55] See DHV, vol. 2, pp. 660-661. At the same time, there are important differences: There are virgins of the Grail as well, and the Grail coat of arms — the turtle dove — differs from the red cross on the white background of the Templars; and as Giles Morgan and other historians have noted, the Templars were not a particularly well-known or established order in Germany at the time when Wolfram was writing (*The Holy Grail* (Harpenden: Pocket Essentials, 2005), p. 91).

[56] On the question of the relation between events narrated in *Parzival* and the liturgical calendar, see Hermann J. Weigand, "Die epischen Zeitverhältnisse in den Graldichtungen Chrestiens und Wolframs," *Publications of the Modern Language Association of America*, 54 (1938), 917-950; Arthur B. Groos, "Time Reference and the Liturgical Calendar in Wolfram von Eschenbach's *Parzival*," *Deutsche Vierteljahrsschrift für Literaturwissenschaft und Geistesgeschichte*, 49 (1975), 43-65; Harald Haferland, "Parzivals Pfingsten: Heilsgeschichte im *Parzival* Wolframs von Eschenbach," *Euphorion: Zeitschrift für Literaturgeschichte*, 88 (1994), 263-301; and Alfred Büchler, "Psalter und Zeitrechnung in Wolframs *Parzival*," *Amsterdamer Beiträge zur älteren Germanistik*, 50 (1998), 95-109.

This time he encounters an aged gray knight (Gabenis), accompanied by his gray-haired wife and his two daughters, also dressed in gray. All four are barefoot, a sign of penitence. In response to Parzival's question (so it seems he really *is* learning!), the gray knight gives a friendly reply, but gently chides Parzval for not riding unarmed or walking barefoot in observance of the religious day. In his reply, Parzival confesses that he does not know what day it is and expresses his sense of bitterness at having been abandoned by God:

> "Nay, I know not what the time of the year may be,
> Or how men the tale may reckon of the weeks as they swiftly flee,
> How the days shall be named I know not, long have I forgot such lore!
> Of old time I served a master, and *God* was the name He bore.
> But He bare unto me no favor, and for guerdon He mocking gave,
> Tho' ne'er had my heart turned from Him — Men said, 'If from God ye crave
> For succour, He sure will give it'; but I deem well they spake a lie,
> For He who they said would help me, did help unto me deny!"
>
> (§447, ll. 19-30; vol. 1, p. 259)

In response to this outburst, the gray knight patiently explains that today is Good Friday, and he expounds the religious meaning of the day (and its theological and liturgical significance):

> "For to-day all men call Good Friday, and the world it rejoiceth still

O'er the day that her chains were riven; tho' she mourneth her Saviour's pain.
Speak, knowest thou of faith more faithful than the faith God hath kept with men,
Since He hung in the cross for men's sake? Such woe as He bare for three,
Sir Knight, sure must work thee sorrow, since baptized thou shalt surely be!
For *our* sin His life was forfeit, or else had mankind been lost,
And Hell as his prey had held us, and Hell's torments had paid sin's cost.
Sir Knight, if thou be not heathen, thou shalt honour this Holy Day — […]."
(§448, ll. 7-20; vol. 1, p. 259)

He encourages Parzival, *rîtet vürbaz ûf unser spor*, "ride on along our tracks," and he advises Parzival to seek penance from Trevrizent, the holy hermit.

At Fontane la Salvaesche, Parzival finds the austere figure of Trevrizent, who will inform Parzival in further detail about the Grail. But before he does so, Wolfram's narrator addresses the reader directly with more information about the Grail from his alleged source, the mysterious figure of Kyot Laschantiure, alias "the Provençal."[57] In turn, Kyot is said to have had his own

[57] **A brief footnote on Kyot:** Wolfram claims that Kyot was a Provençal poet who had served as a source for his work. Although Wolfram may have been referring to the northern French poet or trouvère Guiot (or Guyot) de Provins, from the town of Provins in the Champagne area, there is no evidence that Guiot wrote anything about the Grail. Was the figure of Kyot, then, an invention by Wolfram, a narrative device to signal his distance from his main source, Chrétien de Troyes' *Perceval*? According to Joachim Bumke, four points stand in favor of Kyot as a historical source and against the interpretation that he is no more than a narrative device: (a) Wolfram's reverence for the House of Anjou; (b) the allusions to the Knights Templar, known for their hostility towards the Germans; (c) the demonstrable

source of information about the Grail, a Muslim astronomer (and a descendant of Solomon) called Flegetanis,[58] according to whom the Grail is linked to astrology:

knowledge of French literature on Wolfram's part; (d) the points of agreement between Wolfram and the French Grail tradition *after* Chrétien. According to A.T. Hatto, however, these obstacles may be resolved as follows: (a) the House of Anjou had widespread connections across England, France, Italy, and had lands in Styria; (b) the admirable nobility of the Knights Templar, thanks to their role as guardians of the Holy Sepulcher; (c) Wolfram demonstrates remarkable knowledgeability about numerous subjects (falconry, precious tones, the planets, etc.) — Adrian Stevens talks about Wolfram's "extraordinary eclecticism, the sheer breadth and diversity of his knowledge" ("Fiction, Plot and Discourse: Wolfram's *Parzival* and its Narrative Sources," in Will Hasty (ed.), *A Companion to Wolfram's "Parzival"* (Rochester, NY, and Woodbridge: Camden House, 1999), pp. 99-123 [p. 109]) — not just about French literature; (d) the points of contact between Wolfram and the post-Chrétien tradition occur at different points, rather than constituting a discrete narrative strand ("An Introduction to a Second Reading," in *Parzival* (Harmondsworth: Penguin, 1980), pp. 412-438 [pp. 428-429]). That the figure of Kyot, and Wolfram's claim at the end of the work that "if Chretien of Troyes, the master, hath done to this tale a wrong, / Then Kiot may well be wrathful, for he taught us aright the song [*diu rehten maere*]" (§827, ll. 1-4), represents a real *Stein des Anstoßes* for literary critics is demonstrated by the following remarks with which Hatto prefaces his discussion of this putative independent source: "Ideally and for the most part in practice," he writes, "scholarship is conducted according to the convention that all other scholars are of the highest possible intelligence and perspicacity" and "thus if any wish to take Wolfram's statements on Kyot at their face value they are free to do so, even if these statements are utterly lacking in external support and even if they ironize, not to say mock themselves." "I myself," he adds, inserting the knife, "respect this convention for its optimism and courtesy, and because most scholars out of touch with reality are innocuous and self-supporting," and then he gives the knife a twist: "Nevertheless, it is my hope that one day a far more learned, formidable, and above all blunt scholar than I will arise to bury the 'Kyot controversy' for ever" (p. 427)! Why, one wonders, such anger? Even if the critical consensus is that Kyot and his Grail story "constitute an elaborate literary hoax" (Stevens, p. 110), its function is to highlight the literary, textual embellishment of the ultimate source of the Grail story, *diu âventiure* (personified by Wolfram as *frou âventiure* — *âventiure* understood here in an archetypal sense. Thus the relationship between "Kyot," Chrétien, and the archetypal basis of the story could be summarized in simple diagrammatic form. (This diagram is available online on the site *MediaeWiki - Das Wiki für Inhalte der Mediävistik*, where it is in the public realm at this address HTTP http://mediaewiki.de/w/images/7/70/Quellensystematik.png). In other words, using the terms used by Chrétien, Wolfram brings a *bele conjunture* (verse 14) to a *conte d'aventure* (verse 13), i.e., a literary treatment of an archetypal experience (see Stevens, p. 101).

[58] According to the art historian Hermann Goetz (1898-1976), the name Flegetanis has two possible sources: first, the Kabbalah of Spanish-Arabian Jews and its notion of the *Falak-ath-Thani* (or "second heaven") as speculating on the throne of Jehovah

And the heathen, Flegetanis, could read in the heavens high
How the stars roll on their courses, how they circle the silent sky,
And the time when their wandering endeth — and the life and the lot of men
He read in the stars, and strange secrets he saw, and he spake again
Low, with beated breath and fearful, of the thing that is called the Grail [*ez hiez ein dinc der grâl*],
In a cluster of stars was it written, the name, nor their lore shall fail.
And he quoth thus, "A host of angels this marvel to earth once bore,
But too pure for earth's sin and sorrow the heaven they sought once more,
And the sons of baptized men hold It, and guard It with humble heart,
And the best of mankind shall those knights be who have in such service part."

(§454, ll. 9-30; vol. 1, p. 262)

(These angels will later be described by Trevrizent as "neutral" angels who, in the struggle between Lucifer and the divine Trinity,

in the vision of Ezekiel; and second, a legendary Islamic magician and astrologer called *Aflaton*, whose reputation was influenced by translations — made from the Greek during the Abbasid Caliphate — of pseudo-Hermetic literature on astrology, alchemy, and magic as well as Neoplatonic editions of Plato's writings, and whose name could have been parodied as an apotropaic gesture or as an insult by associating it with *Phlegethon*, one of the five rivers in Hades and described in the *Phaedo* as a "stream of fire" (112b) ("Der Orient der Kreuzzüge in Wolframs Parzival," *Archiv für Kulturforschung*, vol. 2, no. 1 (1967), 1-42 [p. 3]); cf. Joseph Campbell, *The Masks of God*, vol. 4, *Creative Mythology* (New York: Viking Penguin, 1968), p. 430. See also DKV, vol. 2, p. 666-667.

did not take sides, and so were banished to the earth and assigned the role of protecting the Grail [§471, ll. 15-21].)

After discovering the document ascribed to Flegetanis written in Arabic in Toledo, Kyot embarked on extensive research, consulting works written in Latin and chronicles of Britain, France, and Ireland, and establishing that the house of Anjou had been chosen as a line to protect the Grail, and that Titurel and his son, Frimuntel, had bequeathed the Grail to Anfortas. Herzeloyde, Anfortas's sister, had given birth to a son by Gahmuret — none other, of course, than Parzival; thc same Parzival who, even now, is riding along the fresh tracks left by the gray knight …

Parzival approaches Trevrizent explicitly as a penitent, "I am one who hath sinned, and rede at thy lips I crave!" (§456, ll. 29-30). On the altar in Trevrizent's cave, Parzival recognizes a reliquary as one on which, in an earlier episode, he had sworn an oath that had turned Jeschute of Karnant's suffering (*leit*) to joy (*liebe*) by exonerating her, and Trevrizent uses his knowledge of the liturgical calendar to calculate (with amazing precision) that it is four-and-a-half years and three days since Parzival had found (and taken) a painted lance next to the reliquary. Yet this sense of temporal order stands in stark contrast to Parzival's sense of psychological disorder. In a remarkable speech, Parzival confesses his hatred for God, laments his joyless life, and expresses his sense of abandonment:

> "Now first do I learn them, the days that I aimless stray,
> And the weeks and the years that have vanished, since my joy hath been reft away.
> […] Now indeed me-seemeth that my bliss it was but a dream,
> For heavy the load of sorrow that so long hath my portion been!

And, Sir Host, I yet more would tell thee, where cloister or church shall be
And men unto God give honour, there no eye hath looked on me,
And naught but strife have I sought me, tho' the time as thou sayst be long,
For I against God bear hatred, and my wrath ever waxeth strong.
For my sorrow and shame hath He cherished, and He watched them greater grow
Till too high they waxed, and my gladness, yet living, He buried low!
And I think were God fain to help me other anchor my joy had found
Than this, which so deep hath sunk it, and with sorrow hath closed it round.
A man's heart is mine, and sore wounded, it acheth, and acheth still,
Yet once was it glad and joyous, and free from all thought of ill!
Ere sorrow her crown of sorrow, thorn-woven, with stern hand pressed
On the honour my hand had won me o'er many a foeman's crest!
And I do well to lay it on Him, the burden of this my shame,
Who can help if He will, nor withholdeth the aid that men fain would claim.
But *me* alone, hath He helped not, whate'er men of Him may speak,
But ever He turneth from me, and His wrath on my head doth wreak!"

(§461, ll. 1-26; vol. 1, p. 266)

Parzival's confession will later find its counterpart in Faust's confession in the "Midnight" scene in Act 5 of Part 2 when, in conversation with the figure of Care, he realizes: "Athwart the world I have but flown, / Grasped by the hair whatever I did covet, / Loosed it, had I no pleasure of it, / Did it elude me, made no moan. / I did but wish, achieve, and then again / Did wish, and thus I stormed through life amain, / First vehemently, with majestic passion, / But shrewdly now I tread, in heedful fashion" (ll. 11433-11440; p. 317); and, in *The Red Book*, in those passages where Jung confesses, "I had achieved everything that I had wished for myself. I had achieved honour, power, wealth, knowledge, and every human happiness. Then my desire for the increase of trappings ceased, the desire ebbed from me and horror came over me" (RB, 127); when he realizes, "I had become aware that I had lost my soul" (RB, 129); and when he admits, "I wandered for many years, so long that I forgot that I possessed a soul" (RB, 131).

Trevrizent advises Parzival to put his faith in God, and he goes on to expound a strange, Neo-Gnostic cosmogony revolving around the fall of Lucifer (and related in greater length in *Willehalm*, §308, ll. 1-30).[59] The purpose of the myth is to warn against *wanc* ("playing God false") and against *haz* ("hate") (§462, l. 30 and §46, l. 2), and the fate of Lucifer, together with Astiroth and Belcimon, Belet and Radamant (§463, ll. 10-11), serves as just such a warning. Trevrizent tells of how God created Adam from the dust of the earth and Eve from the ribs of Adam, of how Cain murdered Abel, and of how Cain robbed Mother Earth (Cain's grandmother) of her virginity (the latter a favorite Patristic theme).[60] Trevrizent urges Parzival to do penance,

[59] DKV, vol. 2, p. 673. See toward the end of Book 6 in Wolfram von Eschenbach, *Willehalm*, trans. Marion E. Gibbs and Sidney M. Johnson (Harmondsworth: Penguin, 1984), p. 156.

[60] DKV, vol. 2, p. 675. See, for example, Tertullian's *De carne Christi*, §17, 1-5 [PL 2, 827-28], cited in Luigi Gambero, *Mary and the Fathers of the Church: The Blessed Virgin Mary in Patristic Thought* [1991], trans. Thomas Buffer (San Francisco:

"No longer be wroth with thy Maker! If thou wouldst
not thy soul were lost —
And here for thy sin do penance, nor longer thus
rashly boast,
For he who, with words untamèd, is fain to avenge
his wrong,
His own mouth shall, I ween, speak his judgment ere
ever the time be long."
(§465, ll. 11-18; vol. 1, p. 268);

recounts how Plato and the Sybils had foretold how redemption was to come (another Patristic theme);

"For Plato alike and the Sibyls in their day spake
words so true,
And long years ere the time had ripened His coming
they did foretell
Who made for our sin's Atonement, and drew us from
depths of Hell."
(§465, ll. 21-27; vol. 1, p. 268);

and emphasizes the theme of God as light, *der ist ein durchliuhtec lieht*, "For He is a Light all-lightening, and never His faith doth cease" (§466, l. 3) (cf. §119, l. 19; cf. 1 John 1: 5). In fact, Trevrizent significantly develops this theme of God as light at length, emphasizing God's purity as penetrating the darkness itself:

Ignatius, 1999), pp. 67-68: "And this is the new birth: that man is born in God when God is born in man, having assumed the flesh of the old seed, but without using this seed, in order to reform the flesh through a new seed, a spiritual seed, and to purify the flesh after having eliminated all its ancient stains. But, as it happened, this whole new manner of birth was prefigured in the ancient wise design that depended upon a virgin. When man was created by God's action, the earth was still virgin, not yet pressed down by man's toil, not having been sown. We know that, from this virgin earth, God created man as a living soul" (p. 67).

> "From the shrine of his heart, who shall keep Him?
> Tho' hidden the thought within,
> And secret, and thro' its darkness no sunbeam its way may win,
> (For thought is a secret chamber, fast locked, tho' no lock it bear),
> Yet, tho' against man it be closèd, God's light ever shineth there.
> He pierceth the wall of darkness, and silent and swift His spring,
> As no sound betrayed His coming, as no footstep was heard to ring,
> So silent His way He goeth [...]."
> (§466, ll. 16-24; vol. 1, p. 269)

In response to Trevrizent, Parzival now declares his twofold ambition to find the Grail and to return to Condwiramurs, and it now appears that there might be some kind of a link between these two ambitions: "Of my sorrows the chiefest is for the Grail, / And then for my wife — none fairer e'er hung on a mother's breast, / For the twain is my heart yet yearning, with desire that ne'er findeth rest," *nâch den beiden sent sich mîn gelust* (§467, ll. 26-30; vol. 1, p. 269). A philological or allegorical link between them is not hard to find, inasmuch as Condwiramur's very name (*conduire amours* or "to guide love") embodies the quest for love, and the Grail itself is an embodiment of the grace of divine love.

Responding in turn, Trevrizent tells Parzival that no one can find the Grail unless called by it, "But if for the *Grail* thou grievest, then much must I mourn thy woe, / O! foolish man, since fruitless thy labours, for thou shalt know / That none win the Grail save those only whose names are in Heaven known, / They who to the Grail do service, they are chosen of God alone" (§468, ll. 10-14; vol. 1, p. 270). Although described by Trevrizent as a *tumber man*, that is, a fool, Parzival is by now not so foolish as to admit that he has already seen the Grail, while at the same time eliciting from Trevrizent the information that he himself, too, has seen it.

Trevrizent goes on to tell Parzival how the Grail provides sustenance to the knights of Munsalvaesche, how it is called *lapsit exillis* (see below), and how it has marvelous powers to preserve the youthfulness of anyone who looks at it. Indeed, in the Grail Castle Parzival had witnessed the power of the Grail, which was described in Book 5 as "the crown of blessing, the fulness of earth's delight, / And Its joys I right well may liken to the glories of Heaven's height" (§238, ll. 21-24; vol. 1, p. 136), possessing the power to provide those who dwell in the Castle with the food and drink of their choice. Furthermore, Trevrizent explains, the Grail can bestow youthfulness and immortality, and however ill one might be, from the day when one sees the Grail, one cannot die for that week or lose one's youthful freshness (§469, ll. 14-24). In the tragic case of Anfortas, however, the power of the Grail serves only to prolong his agony and his sufferings. The vital power of the Grail is expressed through the symbolic image of the phoenix, for the same restorative powers of the Grail enable the phoenix to burn to ashes from which it then re-emerges:

> "[…] Men call it *Lapis Exilis* — by its magic the wondrous bird,
> The Phœnix, becometh ashes, and yet doth such virtue flow
> From the stone, that afresh it riseth renewed from the ashes glow,
> And the plumes that erewhile it moulted spring forth yet more fair and bright —
> […]."
>
> (§469, ll. 8-13; vol. 1, p. 270)

The symbol of the Grail is clearly of such central importance to Wolfram's *Parzival* and indeed to the tradition of Arthurian literature as a whole that we must pause for a moment to consider the import of the symbolism, which inevitably caught the attention of Jung himself as well.

The Grail and the Hermetic Vessel

In relation to the central image of the Grail, Jung notes in "Individual Dream Symbolism in Relation to Alchemy" (1936), now part of *Psychology and Alchemy* (CW 12), the close relation between the Grail and the Hermetic vessel, pointing out that Wolfram (through the figure of Trevrizent) calls the stone of the Grail "*lapsit exillis*" — a term whose significance remains a matter of controversy (CW 12 §246, fn; cf. Book 9, §469, l. 7), and we should note the entire context of the passage just quoted from the discourse of Trevrizent:

> "[…] Then know, by a *stone* they live,
> And that stone is both pure and precious — Its name has thou never heard?
> Men call it *Lapis Exilis* — by its magic the wondrous bird,
> The Phœnix, becometh ashes, and yet doth such virtue flow
> From that stone, that afresh it riseth renewed from the ashes glow,
> And the plumes that erewhile it moulted spring forth yet more fair and bright —
> And tho' faint be the man and feeble, yet the day that his failing sight
> Beholdeth the stone, he dies not, nor can, till eight days be gone,
> Nor his countenance wax less youthful — If one daily behold that stone,

(If a man it shall be, or a maiden 'tis the same,) for a
hundred years,
If they look on its power, their hair groweth not grey,
and their face appears
The same as when first they saw it, nor their flesh not
their bone shall fail
But young they abide for ever — And this stone all
men call the Grail."

(§469, ll. 7-28; vol. 1, p. 270)

A huge variety of explanations for this Latin term for the Grail has been offered by literary scholars, most of which read *lapsit* as meaning *lapis*, or "stone":[61]

- *lapis erilis* = stone of the Lord (San-Marte, the pseudonym for Albert Schulz, 1802-1893)
- *lapis electrix* = the amber stone (Julius Zacher)
- *lapis textilis* = the asbestos stone (J.F.D. Blöte)
- *lapis elixir* = the stone of the wise (Rudolf Palgen, Gottfried Weber)
- *lapis exilis* = the small, unassuming stone (Gustav Ehrismann, Friedrich Ranke); "a thing with no appearance, no show at all, a vile thing" (C.G. Jung)[62]
- *lapis ex celis* = the stone from heaven (Samuel Singer)
- *lapis exiliens* = the stone that flares up (Helen Adolf)

[61] Joachim Bumke, *Wolfram von Eschenbach*, 8th edn (Stuttgart: Metzler; Poescheln, 2004), pp. 139-140; and DKV, vol. 2, pp. 679-680. For further bibliographical references, see Bumke, pp. 139-140; and for an overview of the various manuscript readings, see Eberhard Nellmann, "Lapsit exillis? Jaspis exillix?: Die Lesarten der Handschriften," *Zeitschrift für deutsche Philologie*, vol. 119, no. 3 (2000), 416-420.
[62] C.G. Jung, *Dream Symbols of the Individuation Process: Notes of C.G. Jung's Seminar Wolfgang Pauli's Dreams*, ed. Suzanne Gieser (Princeton and Oxford: Princeton University Press, 2019), p. 285. Jung takes at face value Wolfram's claim in the Apology that he "couldn't even write and [...] didn't understand Latin," and suggests that in writing *lapsit exillis* instead of *lapis exilis* Wolfgang "probably made a mistake."

- *lapis exsulis* = the stone of the banished (Arthur E. Waite, Hermann Goetz)[63]
- *lapis exilii* = the stone of exile (Herbert Kolb)
- *lapis ex silice* = the stone from pebble (Petrus W. Tax)
- *lapis excilis* = the inconspicuous stone, paltry stone (C.G. Jung)[64]

In 1952, Bodo Mergell construed the term as *lapsit exillis*, discerning in its significance a fourfold reference to the stone of Daniel (*lapis abscissus de monte*), the stone of Alexander (*lapis iste exilis*), biblical and liturgical altar stones and portable altars (see above), and the vision of the "throne set in heaven" or the *Sedes Domini* (*similis lapidis iaspidis et sardinis*) in Revelations 4:2.[65] And in 1957, Hans Sperber advanced the ingenious thesis that *lapsit exillis* derived from the Old French *l'absite exilli(é)s*, i.e., the semi-precious stone of the exiled (referring here in this context to the so-called "neutral" angels).[66] As Eberhard Nellmann notes in his commentary, none of these interpretations has succeeded in finding broad acceptance.[67]

For his part, throwing interpretative caution aside, in "Individual Dream Symbolism in Relation to Alchemy" Jung also notes that, in the *Rosarium philosophorum* (1550) attributed to Arnaldus de Villa Nova (c.1240-1311), the *lapis* (i.e., the philosopher's stone) is called the "lapis exilis," that is, the uncomely

[63] According to Hermann Goetz, Wolfram's Grail is an amalgam of the alchemical *lapis exillis*, the *lapis exulis* or the embodied Shekhinah (i.e., the "divine manifestation," "earthly residence," or "dwelling" or presence of God) of the Kabbalah, and the so-called "sacred bowl" in the Cathedral of San Lorenzo in Genoa — a vase in green jasper (Goetz, "Der Orient der Kreuzzüge in Wolframs Parzival," p. 5).

[64] Jung, *Dream Symbols of the Individuation Process*, ed. Gieser, p. 136.

[65] Bodo Mergell, *Der Gral in Wolframs Parzival: Entstehung und Ausbildung der Gralsage im Hochmittelalter* (Halle (Saale): Niemeyer, 1952).

[66] Hans Sperber, "*lapsit exillis* und *sarapandratest*," *Zeitschrift für deutsches Altertum und deutsche Literatur*, vol. 87, no. 4 (1957), 270-275.

[67] DKV, vol. 2, pp. 679-680.

stone (*Artis auriferae*, Basel 1693, vol. 2, pp. 204-384 [p. 210]), suggesting that this description "may be of importance for the interpretation of Wolfram's term" (CW 12 §246, fn. 125).[68] Later in *Mysterium coniunctionis* (1955-1956) Jung speculates whether the English alchemist Sir George Ripley (c. 1415-1490) might have been "acquainted" with the Grail tradition, mentioning the "doubtful" evidence of an etymological link between *lapis exilis* and *lapsit exiliis* (as found in Wolfram) and referring to the parallels between the "mystic vessel of transformation" in alchemical symbolism and the chalice used in the liturgy of the Mass (CW 14 §369).

(In his reading of the symbolism of the Grail in "Individual Dream Symbolism in Relation to Alchemy," Jung compares the philosopher's stone in alchemy to the Grail, seeing it as a representation of "the creative vessel, the *elixir vitae*," depicted in one of the dreams he analyzes in this paper as "surrounded by a spiral, the symbol of indirect approach by means of the *circumambulatio*" (CW 12 §245, fn. 124). More generally, it is depicted in dreams, visions, and in artistic traditions in the East and West alike using the symbolism of the mandala. In alchemical terms, the *vas* is said to be often understood as "the uterus where the 'child' is gestated," and this image finds parallels in the calyx of the Indian lotus, the "seat and birthplace of the gods" which is called the *padma* and has "a feminine significance"; in the Litany of Loreto, where the Blessed Virgin is acclaimed three times as the "vas" (viz., "vas spirituale," "vas honorabile," and "vas insigne devotionis"), and in medieval poetry where she is described as the "flower of the sea," sheltering the Christ; and more generally in mandala symbolism as the center of the mandala (§246, fn. 125). Nothing speaks more eloquently to the idea that the Grail, like the mandala, is a symbol of totality than the inclusion of a picture, taken from a 15th-cenury Parisian manuscript, of the vision of the Grail in the *Roman de Lancelot du*

[68] See *Artis auriferae*, Basel 1693, vol. 2, pp. 204-384 [p. 210]).

Lac [fig. 88]. As Perceval, Parzival is included in this picture, an example of the ongoing development of the Grail legend after its treatment by Chrétien de Troyes and by Wolfram.)

The origin of the word "grail" has been traced by some scholars back to the ancient Greek word κρατήρ or *kratēr*,[69] literally a "mixing vessel" as used in ancient Greece to dilute wine with water. Jung might have shared this view, as he argues at one point in his seminar on Nietzsche's *Zarathustra* that "in the pagan Hermetic philosophy [...] the *kratēr*, the mixing jar, the famous vase of Hermes that was made by God after the creation [...] is the origin probably of the Grail" (SNZ, vol. 2, p. 936).[70] When he rehearses this argument a year later in his lectures given in 1937 on "Psychology and Religion," Jung notes that, in the tradition of philosophical alchemy, a "spirit" is imprisoned in the earth as a "white dove," comparable to the *nous* in the *kratēr* of Hermes (CW 11 §150), but also a parallel to the white dove which, every Good Friday, brings a small white wafer (*ein kleine wîze oblât*) from heaven and places it on the stone: "And the stone from the Host receiveth all good that on earth may be / Of food or of drink, the earth beareth as the fulness of Paradise" (Book 9, §470, ll. 11-14; vol. 1, p. 271). (As we shall see in Chapter 3, the Gnostic and Hermetic origins of the Grail acquire added significance in light of the link between the Grail as *kratēr* and the *kratēr* as Grail).[71]

---

[69] According to Diez, the word *graal* = Provençal *grazal*, < *cratalis*, i.e., *cratus* for *crater*; see Friedrich Diez, *Etymologisches Wörterbuch der romanischen Sprachen* (Bonn: A. Marcus, 1853), p. 648; cited in Peter Kingsley, *Catafalque: Carl Jung and the End of Humanity*, 2 vols (London: Catafalque Press, 2018), vol. 2, p. 602.

[70] For further references to the likely Gnostic and Hermetic origins of the Grail, see Kingsley, *Catafalque*, vol. 2, pp. 601-602. For further discussion, see David Fideler, "The Path Toward the Grail: The Hermetic Sources and Structure of Wolfram von Eschenbach's *Parzival*," *Alexandria: The Journal of the Western Cosmological Traditions*, 1 (1991), 187-227; and Henry and Renée Kahane, with Angelina Pietrangeli, *The Krater and the Grail: Hermetic Sources of the "Parzival"* (Urbana, IL: University of Illinois Press, 1965). For Jung's discussion of the "well-known and widespread symbolism of the vessel" in *Psychological Types*, see CW 6 §396-§406.

[71] Kingsley, *Catafalque*, vol. 2, p. 601.

The curative properties of the Grail are rich in archetypal significance, as is the wound from which Anfortas suffers. Commenting in *Transformations and Symbols of the Libido* (1911-1912) on the figure of Philoctetes, the hero and archer who was the only person on the Trojan expedition who knew the location of the hidden sanctuary of Chryse the nymph, Jung notes that, according to one legend, he was bitten on his foot while approaching the altar by a poisonous serpent, and from then on was ailing. In a footnote, Jung points out the similarity to the Lord of the Grail, who guards the chalice, or in other words the mother symbol (PU §461, fn. 36). (In this extensive footnote, a little masterpiece of scholarship, Jung relates the myth of Philoctetes to the Hercules myth, even detecting a resonance of the mythologem of the journey of the sun to the western sea in Faust's contemplation of suicide in the "Night" scene of Part 1: "And though all Hell its flames assemble / Above the narrow mouth, press boldly through [*Nach jenem Durchgang hinzustreben*]" [ll. 716-717].)

In turn, this detail of having one's foot bitten by a poisonous serpent might remind us of the episode in Nietzsche's *Zarathustra* where Zarathustra has fallen asleep under a fig tree and an adder comes and bites him in the neck. In conversation with the adder, it tells him that its poison is fatal, but Zarathustra only smiles. "When did ever a dragon die of a serpent's poison?" he asks and tells the adder: "But take thy poison back! Thou art not rich enough to present it to me," and the adder falls again on his neck and licks his wound (Z I 19). This episode also looks forward to the vision of the shepherd and the snake in "Of the Vision and the Riddle" (Z III 2 §2), although in his seminar on *Zarathustra* when he discusses this chapter called "Of the Adder's Bite," Jung does not mention this parallel or the possible parallel with Philoctetes, interpreting the episode instead along the lines that Zarathustra, being more or less the *logos* or the mind, needed to link up with the serpent as representing the body or the lower nervous centers or the instinctive world (SNZ, vol. 2, pp. 769-770; cf. SNZ, vol. 1, pp. 748-764).

In the concluding chapter of the "mystic peregrination" (as Jung called it, cf. CW 14 §276) undertaken by the German alchemist Michael Maier (1568-1622) in his *Symbola aureae mensae duodecim nationum* (or *The Symbols of the Golden Table of the Twelve Nations*) (1617), Maier describes his quest for the phoenix.[72] Titled *Allegoria Bella* (and published separately in the *Musaeum Hermeticum* as *A Subtle Allegory concerning the Secrets of Alchemy*),[73] this chapter begins with Maier's account of his decision to go in quest of this fabulous bird. Ever since Clement of Alexandria in his First Letter to the Corinthians, §25,[74] and the fourth-century allegorical bestiary, the *Physiologus*,[75] had come to be a symbol for Christ. Moreover, in the figure of the phoenix, the two great works of God — the Bible and the Book of Nature, i.e., Christ and the "universal medicine" — are jointly signified (217). According to the *Allegoria Bella*, the phoenix is synonymous with νηπενθές (i.e., *nēpenthés*), the mythical cure for sorrow or the "drug of forgetfulness" given by the Queen of Egypt to Helen of Troy who, according to Homer in Book 4 of the *Odyssey*, administered it to Telemachus and Menelaos (Book 4, ll. 219-221) (218).[76]

Leaving his hometown of Holstein on his quest — a quest, not for the Grail, but for the phoenix — on the day "when the Moon

[72] See Hereward Tilton, *The Quest for the Phoenix: Spiritual Alchemy and Rosicrucianism in the Work of Count Michael Maier (1569-1621)* (Berlin and New York: de Gruyter, 2003), pp. 215-232.
[73] See the full title in the translation by Arthur E. Waite in the second volume of *The Hermetic Museum*, viz. *A Subtle Allegory concerning the Secrets of Alchemy, Very Useful to Possess and Pleasant to Read.*
[74] *The Apostolic Fathers*, vol. 1, ed. and trans. Bart D. Ehrman (Cambridge, MA, and London: Harvard University Press, 2003), pp. 81-83.
[75] *Physiologus*, trans. Michael J. Curley [1979] (Chicago and London: University of Chicago Press, 2009), pp. 13-14.
[76] Homer, *The Odyssey*, ed. and trans. Albert Cook (New York and London: Norton, 1993), p. 38.

and Sun were both in the sign of Aries," i.e., the vernal equinox, Maier sets out "with the intention of first travelling through Europe, and to enquire everywhere after the Phœnix."[77] After failing to find the phoenix in Europe (representing the element of earth), Maier travels to America (standing for water), Asia (for air), and Africa (for fire). Not far from the Red Sea lives the Erythræan Sibyl, the prophetess who foretold the coming of Christ, and whose rocky cave Maier visits to inquire about the phoenix. She tells him:

> The object of your search […] is a great and glorious one; doubt is the first stage of knowledge, and you have also come to the right place and the right person. […] Araby the Blest and Egypt have from of old rejoiced in the sole possession of the Phœnix, whose neck is of a golden hue, while the rest of its body is purple, and its head is crowned with a beautiful crest. It is sacred to the Sun, lives 660 years, and when the last hour of its life approaches, it builds a nest of cassia and frankincense, fills it with fragrant spices, kindles it by flapping its wings towards the Sun, and is burnt to ashes with it. From these ashes there is generated a worm, and out of the worm a young bird which takes the nest, with the remains of its parent, and carries it to Heliopolis (or Thebes), the sacred city of the Sun, in Egypt. Now, this whole tale which you find in the books of the Ancients is addressed to the mind rather than to the ear; it is a mystical narrative, and like the hieroglyphics of the Egyptians, should be mystically (not historically) understood. An ancient Egyptian writer tells us that the Phœnix rejoices in the Sun, and that this predilection

[77] *The Hermetic Museum*, trans. Arthur Edward Waite, 2 vols (London: Elliot, 1893), vol. 2, p. 206.

> is its chief reason for coming to Egypt. He also relates that his Countrymen were in the habit of embalming the Phœnix if it died before its time. If you therefore regard this tale as an allegory, you will not be far wrong; and you know that the flesh and feathers of this bird were of old used in Heliopolis as a remedy for anger and grief.[78]

(The ancient Egyptian writer in question is Horapollo, or Horus Apollo, an Egyptian priest who was the author of a treatise on Egyptian hieroglyphics.) On the advice of the Sibyl, Maier journeys to the seven mouths of the Nile, the dwelling place of Mercury himself, who has been granted "authority to shew you this bird, and its Medicine." (In his "Concerning Virtue and its Interpretation," Zosimos of Panopolis had said, "Go to the waters of the Nile; there you will find a stone which has a spirit; take it, cut it in two; put your hand in its interior and draw out the heart: because its soul is in its heart.")[79]

Yet when Maier arrives at the ancient Egyptian city of Canopus (near modern-day Abu Qir, in the Nile Delta), he discovers that when he asks about the whereabouts of Mercury, some people were "hopelessly puzzled" by his questions, although others tell him that because, "according to Hermes, Egypt exhibits an image of the heavens, and the seven mouths of the Nile (of which the Canopic is the most considerable) correspond to the seven planets; the Canopic mouth they called the habitation of Saturn, the grandfather of Mercury," Mercury was "to be found domiciled in some other mouth of the river."[80] (On the basis of a correspondence between the planets and the metals, this advice can be read as an

[78] *The Hermetic Museum*, trans. Waite, vol. 2, pp. 218-219.

[79] Marcellin Berthelot (ed.), *Collection des anciens alchimistes grecs*, vols 2-3 (Paris: Steinheil, 1888), pp. 127-139 (p. 129); cited Tilton, *The Quest for the Phoenix*, p. 229; and cf. Jung, CW 12 §405.

[80] *The Hermetic Museum*, trans. Waite, vol. 2, pp. 220-221.

allusion to the progress of metallic development in the womb of the earth, beginning with Saturn or lead — the "first gate to the arcana," according to Abū Bakr al-Rāzī, known as al-Razi or Rhazes.)[81]

Yet searching the Canopic, Bolbitic, Sebennitic, Pelusian, Tanitic, Phanitic, and Mendesian mouths of the Nile yields no results: at the sixth (i.e., Phanitic) mouth, Mercury had once lived but had "long since migrated somewhere else," while at the seventh (i.e., Mendesian) mouth, "nothing whatever was known about him." Retracing his steps to the Canopic mouth, however, Maier finally succeeds in finding Mercury in one of the mouths, where "the people had at first appeared to know nothing about him." (Could this have been the fifth or Tanitic mouth, corresponding to the fourth planet from Saturn, that is, Mercury?) Mercury instructs Maier about where he must look for the phoenix and "obtain possession" of it; yet a further disappointment arises when, on reaching the place to which Mercury had directed him, it turns out that the phoenix has "temporarily deserted it," for it has been "chosen umpire between the owl and other birds which pursue it, of which battle we have treated otherwise" — an allusion to Maier's *Jocus Severus* and its account of a court of judgment held by various birds to judge the owl (a bird sacred to Pallas Athene, an embodiment of *chemia* as the highest science, and a symbol of Rosicrucianism).[82]

On the one hand, this quest looks as if it has ended in defeat: as Jung observed in "Religious Ideas in Alchemy," there is a tragic dimension to Maier's quest: "at the end of his chef-d'œuvre he confesses that in the course of his grand peregrinatio he found neither Mercurius nor the phoenix, but only a feather — his pen!" (CW 12 §515). Analogously, the Arabic alchemist Baqsam had declared that "when a man thinks he has done and has the world" and the seeker believes the Art is perfected, "he shall find nothing

[81] Tilton, *The Quest for the Phoenix*, p. 230, cf. p. 42.
[82] *The Hermetic Museum*, vol. 2, p. 221; see Tilton, *The Quest for the Phoenix*, p. 231, cf. pp. 132-133.

in his hands."[83] On the other, however, Maier turns this defeat into a victory, precisely through his quill pen, by composing a series of epigrams "in honour of the Sibyl, Mercury, the Phœnix, and the Medicine." As Hereward Tilton has shrewdly observed, Maier has "found the phoenix in the face of its very absence," inasmuch as the Sibyl emphasizes that the tale of the phoenix is "addressed to the mind rather than to the ear," is a "mystical narrative," and should be "mystically (not historically) understood"; [84] what Horapollo says is "an allegory," and it is in this light that one should read his statements about the ancient: first, that "when they would denote a soul continuing a long time here, or an inundation, they depict the PHŒNIX the bird: and they denote the soul by it, because this is the longest lived of all creatures in the world; and an inundation, because the Phœnix is a symbol of the sun, than which nothing is greater in the universe. For the sun passes over all and scrutinises all" (Book 1, §34; pp. 54-55); and second, that "to denote a man returning home after a long time from a foreign land they again delineate the PHŒNIX the bird: for this creature, after an interval of 580 years, when the time of death is about to overtake him, returns to Egypt, and as soon as he pays the debt of nature in Egypt, he is mystically served with funeral rites; and whatever rites the Egyptians pay to the rest of the sacred animals, the same are due to the Phœnix" (Book 1, §35; pp. 55-56).

Elsewhere in his *Hieroglyphics*, Horapollo explains that "when they [i.e., the Egyptians] would denote the great cyclical

[83] Tilton, *The Quest for the Phoenix*, pp. 214 and 231; cf. *The Turba Philosophorum or Assembly of the Sages*, trans. Arthur Edward Waite (London: Redway, 1896), dictum 39 (pp. 127-131 [p. 129]; cited in H.M.E. de Jong (ed.), *Michael Meier's Atalanta Fugiens: Sources of an Alchemical Book of Emblems* [1969] (York Beach, ME: Nicolas-Hays, 2002), emblem 27 (pp. 201-206 [p. 203]).

[84] Tilton, *The Quest for the Phoenix*, p. 231; *A Subtle Allegory concerning the Secrets of Alchemy*, p. 219; and Alexander Turner Cory, *The Hieroglyphics of Horapollo Nilous* (London: Pickering, 1840). For an alternative translation, see *The Hieroglyphics of Horapollo*, trans. George Boas [1950] (Princeton, NJ: Princeton University Press, 1993).

renovation, they portray the bird PHŒNIX": "For when he is produced a renovation of things takes place, and he is produced in this manner. When the Phœnix is about to die, he casts himself vehemently upon the ground, and is wounded by the blow, and from the ichor, which flows from the wound, another phœnix is produced; which as soon as it is fledged, goes with his father to the city of the sun in Egypt; who when he is come thither, dies in that place at the rising of the sun. And after the death of his father, the young one departs again to his own country; and the priests of Egypt bury the phœnix that is dead" (Book 2, §57; pp. 121-122). Thus these passages — *not quoted by Maier in the "Allegoria Bella"* — inscribe the phoenix within the tradition of cyclical return: both the procession of all things from God (to whom they must return) or the movement of the *spiritus* through the sun to gold and the human heart (before it returns to its source); and the "return to the monad," as it is called in *Atalanta Fugiens* — "make a circle out of a man and a woman, derive from it a square, and from the square a triangle: make a circle again and you will have the Philosophers' Stone" (232).[85]

So perhaps another clue to its meaning of the Grail (or to one of its meanings) can be found in this archetypal image of the phoenix, to the idea of whose power both Nietzsche and Jung in their turn equally have recourse.[86] In the chapter on *Thus Spoke Zarathustra* in *Ecce Homo*, Nietzsche relates how "the fundamental idea" of that work, namely, "the Eternal Recurrence of all things — this highest of all possible formulae of a Yea-saying philosophy," first occurred to Nietzsche in August 1881, when he was "wandering through the woods alongside of the lake of Silvaplana, and [...]

[85] For further discussion, see Chapter 3 below.

[86] For further discussion of the phoenix in relation to the Grail, see Werner Wolf, "Der Vogel Phönix und der Gral," in Richard Kienast (ed.), *Studien zur deutschen Philologie des Mittelalters: Friedrich Panzer zum 80. Geburtstag* (Heidelberg: Winter, 1950), pp. 730-795.

halted beside a huge, pyramidal and towering rock not far from Surlei" — and was then "struck" by the thought. This episode had, however, been anticipated two months earlier by "an omen of its coming in the form of a sudden and decisive alteration" in his musical tastes: "It would even be possible to consider all 'Zarathustra' as a musical composition. At all events, a very necessary condition in its production was a renaissance in myself of the art of hearing. In a small mountain resort (Recoaro) near Vicenza, where I spent the spring of 1881, I and my friend and Maestro, Peter Gast — also one who had been born again — discovered that the phoenix music that hovered over us, wore lighter and brighter plumes than it had done theretofore" (*Ecce Homo*, "Thus Spoke Zarathustra," §1).

(In his seminar on Nietzsche's *Zarathustra*, Jung interpreted a line from "Of Joys and Passions," "But that bird built its nest beside me: therefore, I love and cherish it — now sitteth it beside me on its golden eggs" (Z I 5), with reference to the haṁsa, a gooselike or swanlike bird, used in Indian and Southeast Asian culture as a Hindu symbol of the *vāhana* (i.e., vehicle) of Brahmā, Gāyatrī, Sarasvatī, and Viśvakarmā.[87] Jung explained the haṁsa as "a sort of phoenix, because the wise old man" — in this case, Zarathustra — "knows of the elixir of life" and can "give himself rebirth" and "always rise again from his ashes," adding: "We could say that this bird is quality, virtue — made visible in the figure of Zarathustra, the greater one in Nietzsche" (SNZ, vol. 1, p. 430). A line in "Of the Way of the Creator," "Ready must thou be to burn thyself in thine own flame; how couldst thou become new if thou have not first become ashes!" (Z I 17), was interpreted by Jung in terms of the phoenix myth, remarking that "when a man is on the way to himself, he will see his other side, and there will be a tremendous conflict; it will be a conflagration, a flame in which

---

[87] See the entry for "haṁsa" in Margaret and James Stutley, *A Dictionary of Hinduism: Its Mythology, Folklore and Development, 1500 B.C.-A.D. 1500* (London and Henley: Routledge & Kegan Paul, 1977), p. 108.

he is burned up" (SNZ, vol. 1, p. 722). The injunction from "Of the Gift-Giving Virtue," "Therefore shall ye be creators!" (Z I 22), was read by him in relation to the principle that "nothing can be created without destruction"; to the Latin sentence, *Creatio unius est corruptio alterius* (i.e., "the creation of the one is the corruption of the other");[88] and to the myth of the phoenix as "burn[ing] itself up — that is destruction — and then it comes back recreated" (SNZ, vol. 2, p. 818). And he glossed the beginning of a line from "Of the Rabble," "On the tree of the future we build our nest; [...]" (Z II 6), as another way for Nietzsche of saying that he had wings, he was a bird, he made his nest on the marvelous Yoga tree, that is, the tree of knowledge, the *arbor philosophorum* (or "the philosophical tree [...] the tree with immortal fruits — a Hermetic symbol"), the world tree in the Edda, the tree Yggdrasil, and hence assimilable to the phoenix, the symbol of renewal and rebirth [SNZ, vol. 2, p. 1072].)

Even though Goethe himself did not use the image of the phoenix in *Faust*, it did not escape an early (and perspicacious) reader of the second part of this work, the German philosopher and pedagogue Johann Karl Friedrich Rosenkranz (1805-1879), that precisely the dynamic of the phoenix underpins the dynamic of the opening scene in *Faust*, Part Two (and, one might add, the drama of *Faust* as a whole): "In a delightful spot, lying upon the flowery sward, we see Faust alone, tormented by deep pangs, seeking rest and slumber. Out of pure pity, indifferent whether the unfortunate

[88] See Peter of Tarentaise (c. 1225-1276), *Commentary on the Sentences*, II, D. I, Q. 2, art. 3, 6 and ad 6 (cited in Ann Giletti, "Early Witness: Thomas Aquinas, Albert the Great and Peter of Tarentaise in Ramon Martí's *Pugio fidei* (c. 1278)," in Görge K. Hasselhoff and Alexander Fidora (eds), *Ramon Martí's "Pugio fidei": Studies and Texts* (Santa Coloma de Queralt: Obrador Edèndum, 2017), pp. 121-156 [p. 133]). For an analogous idea, see Lucretius, *De rerum natura*, book 1, ll. 670-671: "For whatever by being changed passes outside its own boundaries, at once this is the death of that which was before" (Lucretius, *De rerum natura*, trans. W.H.D. Rouse, revised Martin Ferguson Smith (Cambridge, MA; London: Harvard University Press, 1992), pp. 55-57).

man is holy or wicked, elves hover around him and fan him to sleep, in order that the past may be sunk into the Lethe of forgetfulness; [...]. The secret of renewing ourselves perpetually consists in this, that we can destroy ourselves within ourselves, and, as a veritable Phœnix, be resurrected from the ashes of self-immolation."[89]

And in his *Red Book*, Jung has brief recourse to the imagery of the phoenix (and far deeper recourse to its notions of regeneration and renewal) when, in "Death" in *Liber Secundus*, he writes: "When I comprehended my darkness, a truly magnificent night came over me and my dream plunged me into the depths of the millennia, and from it my phoenix ascended" (RB, 265). This image of the ascending phoenix with its flaming wings is, of course, cognate with the central imagery in *The Red Book* of the rising sun. (As a heraldic aside: in *Memories, Dreams, Reflections,* we are told that the Jung family originally had a phoenix for its coat of arms, until Jung's grandfather — the one who was, allegedly, a natural son of Goethe (MDR, 52) and who was a keen Freemason and a Grand Master of the Swiss Lodge — changed them. This change, Jung suggests, was made "probably out of a spirit of resistance towards his father" (i.e., to Goethe?), and Jung retained this change, but adding Masonic or Rosicrucian symbols of "heavenly" and "chthonic" elements, i.e., a cross azure and a blue bunch of grapes in a field d'or, separated by a golden star as a uniting symbol equivalent to the *aurum philosophorum* or the alchemical philosopher's gold (MDR, 259). In this way, the same elements of "young," "youth," and "rejuvenation" represented by the phoenix are expressed using a different symbolism.)

[89] Rosenkrantz, trans. D.J. Snider, "Second Part of Goethe's Faust," *The Journal of Speculative Philosophy*, vol. 1, no. 2 (1867), 65-79 (pp. 68-69).

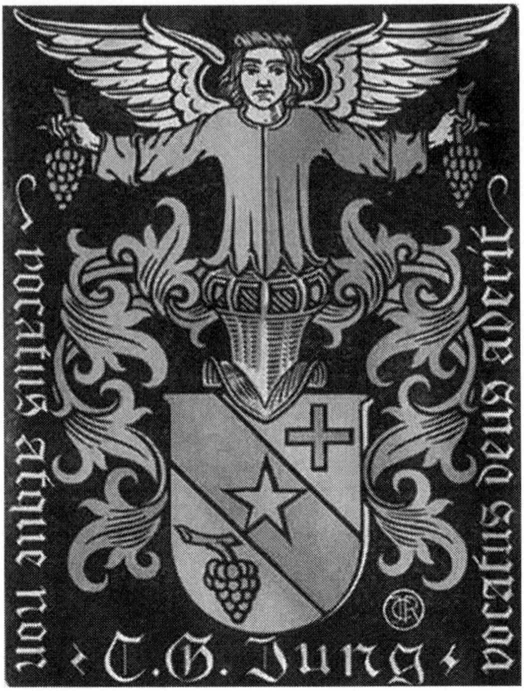

Figure 2. Jung's heraldic coat of arms as an *ex libris*. Image in public domain

Just as these symbols are anchored in classical and other non-Christian traditions, so the Grail in Wolfram is bound up with Christian theology. In Book 9, Trevrizent's account of the Grail now turns to the events that happened on Good Friday — the very day, of course, on which he and Parzival are having this conversation (as the gray knight, Gabenis, had reminded Parzival during their meeting in the snowy wood). Nowadays, Good Friday is for most people just a bank holiday, but within the Christian calendar, it is a day of immense significance. It is the day that commemorates the death of Christ by crucifixion on Calvary, and liturgically it forms part of the Paschal Triduum, that is: Maundy Thursday (commemorating the institution of the Eucharist), Good Friday (the Crucifixion), and the Holy Saturday vigil. Theologically, it is bound up with the events of Easter and the Resurrection, and this theological background informs in one way or another all four works under discussion here.

For example, Faust is about to kill himself when he hears the bells ringing out and announcing the Resurrection Easter Day; the great motif of Good Friday, the "death of God," informs Nietzsche's *Zarathustra*; and the iconography of the Crucifixion is central to Jung's *Red Book*. (Nietzsche was by no means the first to speak about the "death of God," for the second stanza of an old German hymn, *O Traurigkeit, o Herzeleid*, attributed to the Jesuit Friedrich Spee (1591-1635), adapted for Protestant use by Johann Rist (1607-1667), and turned into a chorale prelude and fugue by Johannes Brahms (1883-1897), contains the line, "God Himself is dead" (*Gott selbst liegt tot*); at the end of Part 3 of *Zarathustra*, his Roundelay appears to allude to it in its eighth line, "Joy: deeper than heart's agony" (*Lust — tiefer noch als Herzeleid*). Indeed, G.W.F. Hegel in his *Lectures on the Philosophy of Religion* (1827) explicitly cites this hymn, reading the line "God Himself is dead" as expressing "an awareness that the human, the finite, the fragile, the weak, the negative are themselves a moment of the divine" and that, if "death is a stripping away of the human, the negative," then "God himself is involved in this.")[90] At the same time, no one could describe these four books as religious works *per se*; rather, the cultural significance of Christianity is taken for granted, although the theological significance of the motif is plainly more significant in Wolfram's *Parzival* than it is in Goethe, Nietzsche, or Jung.

Each year on Good Friday, we learn, a brilliant white dove descends, bringing to the Grail a wafer that imparts its life-sustaining powers. (The dove is a bird associated with the baptism of Jesus by John the Baptist (cf. Matthew 3:16-17; Mark 1:9-11; Luke 3:21-22), and its role here is reminiscent of the ravens who bring food to Elijah in the desert (1 King 17:206), reprised in the case of

[90] Part 3 ("The Consummate Religion"), B ("The Second Element: Representation, Appearance") §2 ("Reconciliation"), §c ("The Death of Christ and the Transition to Spiritual Presence"), in G.W.F. Hegel, *Lectures on the Philosophy of Religion: One-Volume Edition: The Lectures of 1827*, ed. Peter C. Hodgson, trans. Robert F. Brown, Peter C. Hodgson, and J. Michael Stewart (Oxford: Clarendon Press, 2006), p. 468.

Daniel in the lion pit who is miraculously supplied by Habakkuk with food (Daniel 14:33-39). Associated with the Eucharist by such writers as the great Benedictine monk and Doctor of the Church, Peter Damian (c. 1007-1072/1073), and the French bishop and historian of the Crusades, Jacques de Vitry (c. 1160/70-1240), the dove as a transporter of a host links the Grail to the Church and its chief liturgical act, the celebration of the Mass.)[91] On the side of the Grail, inscriptions appear, naming those who have been chosen to be the knights of the Grail, lines that disappear again as soon as they have been read. According to Trevrizent, the Grail is intimately bound up with the fate of the so-called "neutral" angels and with the redemption of humankind:

> "They who took no part in the conflict, when Lucifer would fight
> With the Three-in-One, those angels were cast forth from Heaven's height.
> To the earth they came at God's bidding, and that wondrous stone did tend,
> Not was It less pure for their service, yet their task found at last an end.
> I know not if God forgave them, or if they yet deeper fell,
> This one thing I know of a surety, what God doeth, He doeth well!
> But ever since then to this service nor maiden nor knight shall fail,
> For God calleth them all as shall please Him! — and so standeth it with the Grail!"
>
> (§471, ll. 15-29; vol. 1, p. 271)

[91] DKV, vol. 2, pp. 681-682. For further discussion, see Arthur C.L. Brown, "Did Chrétien Identify the Grail with the Mass?", *Modern Language Notes*, vol. 41, no. 4 (April, 1926), 226-233.

While cautioning Parzival against excessive pride and urging him to practice modesty, Trevrizent relates how Anfortas was wounded while jousting, "For his youth and worldly riches they led him an evil road, / And he sought for Frau Minne's favour in paths where no peace abode" (§472, ll. 27-30) (the woman in question, it turns out, was Orgeluse; cf. Book 12, §616, ll. 11-§617, l. 3). Consequently, the knights of the Grail must remain chaste. Only one person, Trevrizent adds, has come unbidden to Munsalvaesche, "Yet *one*, uncalled, rode thither and evil did then befall, / For foolish he was, and witless, and sin-laden from thence did fare, / Since he asked not his host of his sorrow and the woe that he saw him bear" (§473, ll. 12-16; vol. 1, p. 272), and because he failed to ask about Anfortas's suffering, that man must atone for his sin.

Now Trevrizent asks Parzival who he is, recognizing the turtledove emblem designed by Anfortas on Parzival's horse's saddle and wondering if he is Lähelin (brother of Orilus and Cunneware), who had fought a Grail knight (§473, ll. 22-29; cf. §340, ll. 1-6). Parzival declares himself as the son of Gahmuret and admits to having killed Ither of Gaheviez (i.e., the Red Knight) and to despoiling his corpse. Trevrizent now recognizes Parzival as his nephew, that is, as the son of his sister, Herzeloyde; and he takes Parzival to task for having killed his kinsman, Ither. As the various narrative threads start to be pulled together, Trevrizent now tells Parzival of how Herzeloyde died of grief after he departed from her. In the sections that follow, further details about how various figures in the story are related to each other are explained, and Trevrizent goes into further detail about Anfortas's jousting prowess, how he received the wound through his testicles from a spear thrown by a heathen,[92] and how — while the Grail prevented Anfortas from

[92] Is this spear — "in a joust was he wounded sore / With a poisoned spear, so that healing may be wrought on him nevermore. / For thine uncle, the King Anfortas, he was smitten thro' the thigh / By a heathen who with him battled" (§479, ll. 8-12) — identical with the bleeding spear witnessed by Parzival in the Grail scene (§231, ll.

dying — the wound continues to fester. Nothing, says Trevrizent, has been found that can help Anfortas, not even the golden bough that the Sibyl gave to Aeneas for his journey to the underworld, nor the blood of the pelican, nor the heart of the unicorn, nor trachante (dragon-wort).[93]

Again, let us pause to consider some of these symbols: first, the physical position of the Grail and the imagery of ascent and descent within the work. In his seminar on Nietzsche's *Zarathustra*, Jung links Zarathustra's journey into the underworld (in "Of Great Events") with the legend of the Grail, and he does so through noting the motif of flying or suspension. (Jung associates Zarathustra's ability in that chapter to fly to the figure of the *haṁsa* or heavenly swan in Hindu mythology [see above], which is said because of its pure, sunlight-white color to represent the "universal soul or supreme spirit.")[94] According to one version of the Grail legend, the Grail itself as a physical object is held in a state of suspension, since it is held suspended by angels between heaven and earth (SNZ, vol. 1, 186-187). The motif of suspension has significance in a further context, being an aspect of crucifixion or what Jung terms "the unconscious aspect of transfiguration" (or transformation). As it undergoes this process, the "subtle body" (as it is known in a variety of religious and esoteric traditions) is said to undergo a kind of "martyrdom," itself appearing in a "sort of crucifixion" or a "state of suspension," which "precedes birth or creation." At this point, Jung recalls a passage from the *Runenkunde* of the Edda,

17-22)? For an overview of critical opinion for and against this reading, see DKV, vol. 2, p. 576.

[93] For discussion of the alchemical aspects of these attempts to cure Anfortas, see Joachim Reichert, "'Slaying the Dragon': Der letzte Heilversuch an Anfortas im 'Parzival' Wolframs von Eschenbach (483, 6-18)," *Mediaevistik*, 14 (2001), 149-178.

[94] See the entry for हंस (Hamsa), in Monier Monier-Williams, *A Sanskrit-English Dictionary: Etymologically and Philologically arranged with special reference to Cognate Indo-European Languages* (Oxford: Clarendon Press, 1899), p. 1286.

I know that I hung on the windswept tree
Nine nights through,
Wounded by a spear, dedicated to Odin
I myself to myself,

a passage which he also quoted in *Transformations and Symbols of the Libido* (PU §400) and to which he alludes in *The Red Book* when he finds himself "hang[ing] above the ground on the swaying branch of the divine tree [...] my hands are bound and I am completely helpless" (RB, 443). (Only a few pages later he cries out to Philemon, "damned charlatan, you aped the mysteries for me, you lay the mantle of the stars on me, you played a Christ-fool's comedy with me, carefully and ludicrously, in the tree just like Odin" [RB, 449].)

Almost two years later, we find the motifs of (a) Odin/Wotan, (b) his spear, (c) the Grail, and (d) the unconscious constellated again by Jung when he discusses these lines from "The Child with the Mirror": "And when I want to mount my wildest horse, then doth my spear always help me up best: it is my foot's ever ready servant:— / The spear which I hurl at mine enemies! How grateful am I to mine enemies that I may at last hurl it!" (Z II 1). For Jung, the spear is "a symbol for the intellect on account of its piercing, discriminating, dissecting character," and this symbolism connects with the earlier line where Zarathustra declares, "Wounded am I by my happiness" (SNZ, vol. 2, p. 865). Jung goes on to argue that "th[is] happiness is the consequence of his identification with the spirit [...] by way of the intellect, so by that *détour* it is of course the spear by which he is wounded," a motif that he associates with "the Amfortas problem" and with "the idea of the suffering god" (866). On Jung's somewhat unusual reading of the story of the Crucifixion (which sheds a good deal of light on the use of this motif in *The Red Book*), Christ is said to represent "the human being that was wounded by the overwhelming fact of the spirit, which carried him away and killed his humanity" (866). ("Of course we worship that fact," Jung adds, "but not all of us worship it.") Although this experience of the spirit has "a very marvellous side," inasmuch as it is "really very wonderful to be like a wild river rushing into the wide plains inundating everything and enjoying the play," its corollary is that "on the other side there is any amount of destruction linked up with it" (867). Precisely this ambivalence can be seen, Jung believes, in the case of Nietzsche here: "It is a very wonderful experience to be identical with the spirit, in spite of all sorts of indications that it is not such a particularly happy event," as is reflected in Zarathustra's words that he is *wounded by his own happiness*, that he *hurls a spear against his enemies*, and that he is *grateful that he has enemies*, someone upon whom he can inflict the wound again (867). So, if the spirit manifests itself as "a one-sided thing," then the unconscious mind foresees "some compensating truth" — something shown, Jung believes, "in the symbolism of the Grail and in similar symbolism of the unconscious" (867).

Another couple of years later in his discussion of "The Bedwarfing Virtue," Jung returned to this point, emphasizing how Nietzsche "often liked to think of himself as a religious reformer" and that "not in vain did he take the name of Zarathustra to express his historical role" (SNZ, vol. 2, p. 1364). Thus Nietzsche presented Zarathustra as "a Saoshyant, a new savior," who has "come back in order to heal the wound he caused" (1364). Consequently, Nietzsche's idea of an *Übermensch* would be "the man who was beyond that wound, who had healed that wound," and here lies for Jung the link to the Grail mystery — for "the suffering king who is to be cured by a saviour" is really "the Christian man who carries that moral wound," similar to how "the Persian man was rent asunder" by (the historical) Zoroaster's teaching about good and evil as "moral opposites" (1364).

According to Jung, Nietzsche believed that "his task in the history of the world was to cure [humankind] of that incurable wound he has suffered from hitherto"; or in other words, Nietzsche saw himself as a kind of Parzival-figure! Jung insists that Nietzsche had not been "simply playing" with this idea, but that it was "a deep-rooted conviction in him amounting to a sort of mystical experience" — hence the quasi-reality of the figure of Zarathustra as "more than a speech metaphor" (1364-1365). This background explains, Jung added, why it was precisely the opera *Parsifal* that had caused "the bitterest estrangement" between the two former friends, Nietzsche and Wagner (as we shall discuss further in Chapter 3).

Second, in his comparative, cross-cultural analysis of the figure of the unicorn in Chapter 6, titled "Alchemical Symbolism in the History of Religion," in "Religious Ideas in Alchemy" (1937) included in *Psychology and Alchemy*, Jung shows how the symbolism of Mercurius came to become intermingled with the traditions of pagan Gnosticism and of the Church (CW 12 §518). Here Jung defines the unconscious as the "matrix of symbols" and chooses as a paradigm the symbol of the unicorn. His analysis encompasses the unicorn in alchemy; in ecclesiastical allegory; in Gnosticism; in those great religious texts of ancient India, the Vedas; the creation myth of Zoroastrianism, the Bundahishn; in the Jewish tradition in the Talmud and various examples of midrash; and in Chinese traditions, before turning to the symbol of the unicorn cup (in the context of which he mentions Wolfram's *Parzival*). These assorted unicorn symbolisms, Jung argues, provide us with but a sample of what he calls the "extremely intricate and tangled connections" between pagan and natural philosophy, Gnosticism, alchemy, and ecclesiastical tradition: connections which, in turn, exercised a "deep and lasting influence on the world of medieval alchemy" — and beyond. For Jung's attempt to uncover "just how far alchemy was a religious-philosophical or 'mystical' movement" goes so far as to suggest that the alchemical tradition may well have "reached its peak" in Goethe's "religious *Weltanschauung*, as this is presented for us in *Faust*" (§554).

As just mentioned, in this discussion Jung includes the example of the unicorn cup. In his meeting with Trevrizent the hermit in Book 9, Parzival learns that nothing could be found to help Anfortas (not the Sibyl's bough, the pelican's blood, the unicorn's heart, nor trachonte or dragon-wort). The figure of the unicorn is described by Trevrizent as follows:

> "A strange beast, the Unicorn, liveth, and it doth in such honour keep
> The heart of a spotless maiden that it oft at her knee will sleep.
> And the heart of that beast we took us, and we took us the red-fire stone
> That lies 'neath its horn,[95] if the king's wound might its healing virtue own.
> And we laid on the wound the carbuncle, and we put it the wound within,
> Yet still was the sore empoisoned nor aid from the stone might win!"
>
> (§482, ll. 23-§483, l. 1; vol. 1, p. 277)

As an emblem of "vigour and strength," Jung remarks, the horn has a "masculine character," but at the same time, it is a cup which, according to the German Indologist Isidor Scheftelowitz (1875-1934), "as a receptacle, is feminine" (§553). Leaving aside those gender stereotypes (which may nevertheless not have been so problematic for Wolfram), let us note that what matters for Jung is that "the secret of the cup is also the secret of the horn, which in its turn contains the essence of the unicorn as bestower of strength, health, and life" (§552). Precisely these qualities are attributed

[95] Does a confusion between *cor* (i.e., horn) and *cœur* (i.e., heart) underlie Wolfram's description of the curative properties of the unicorn's heart and his location of the "carbuncle" (or *karfunkelstein*) beneath its horn (see DK, vol. 2, p. 690)?

by the alchemists to the philosopher's stone or "carbuncle" (*karfunkelstein*, cf. §482, l. 29); and it is to the legend that this stone may be found under the horn of the unicorn that Wolfram is here referring (§552). In so doing, Jung argues, Wolfram is making use of a "uniting symbol" (*vereinigendes Symbol*), that is, a symbol that expresses the bipolarity of the archetype (§553). As we shall see, in *Psychological Types* this notion of the "uniting symbol" is explicitly discussed by Jung with reference not to Wolfram's *Parzival* but to Wagner's *Parsifal* and to Goethe's *Faust*.

So, neither the golden bough nor the pelican's blood nor the unicorn's heart nor dragon-wort can help cure Anfortas. Only one remedy, it seems, remained, as described by the mysteriously appearing inscriptions on the side of the Grail itself:

> "Ye shall mark this, forewarning shall bring but ill,
> And in the first night of his coming must the healer his task fulfil,
> Or the question shall lose its virtue; but if at the chosen hour
> He shall speak, *his* shall be the kingdom, and the evil hath lost its power.
> So the hand of the Highest sendeth to Anfortas the end of woe,
> Yet *King* shall he be no longer tho' healing and bliss he know."
>
> (§483, l. 29-§484, l. 8; vol. 1, p. 278)

Yet while this knight had indeed come, he had failed to ask the question!

Everything, then, turns on this one question, whether formulated as "*hêrre, wie stêt iuwer nôt?*" (i.e., "Sire, what ails you?") or as "*oeheim, waz wirret dir?*" (i.e., "Uncle, what ails you?")

(§484, l. 27, cf. §795, l. 29). (Similarly, the plot of *Faust* turns on the wager between Faust and Mephistopheles, formulated with slight variation; while textual precision is important, it is equally important not to get caught up in semantics.) When Parzival finally confesses that *he* is the knight in question, Trevrizent is aghast:

> "Alas! my nephew, thou speakest the words of woe,
> Vanished our joy, and sorrow henceforth must we grasp and know,
> Since folly of bliss betrayed thee: senses five did God give to thee,
> And methinks, in the hour of thy testing, their counsel should better be.
> Why guarded they not thine honour, and thy love as a man to men,
> In the hour that thou satst by Anfortas? Of a truth hadst thou spoken then!"
>
> (§488, ll. 21-30; vol. 1, p. 280)

This passage underscores how Parzival's *tumpheit* (§488, l. 15) does not consist in a failure to be privy to some esoteric knowledge but in a failure to make use of his five senses; one might say, to use his common sense(s). In fact, even when he was being warned not to ask too many questions, Parzival was specifically told by Gurnemanz to make use of his senses, "Thou canst hear and see, I wot well full five shalt thy senses be, / An thou use them aright, then wisdom it draweth anear to thee" (§171, ll. 22-24; vol. 1, p. 96). The message of *Parzival* is thus not about fleeing this world but about positioning ourselves correctly in it, trusting to our senses without allowing ourselves to be deceived by them; and this same message can be found in *Faust*, *Zarathustra*, and *The Red Book*, namely: that the coordination of our various faculties, including the intellect and the senses (especially sight and touch, or the hand and the eye), or the rational and the irrational, or ultimately consciousness and the unconscious, is the precondition for salvation; indeed, in a sense it *is* salvation itself.

Within the economy of the narrative of Wolfram's *Parzival*, this salvation is represented by Trevrizent himself, who tells Parzival, "Mourn not for thy fault too sore, / Thou shalt, in a fitting measure, bewail thee, and grief give o'er. / For strange are the ways, and fitful, of mankind," *dui menschheit hât an witze vart* (§489, ll. 2-5; vol. 1, p. 280), and reassures him: "God thee, as His knight, shall claim! / Thro' my mouth would God teach thee wisdom," *ich bin von gote dîn râtes wer* (§489, ll. 20-21; vol. 1, p. 281). After further discussion (from Trevrizent) about the use of the spear to soothe Anfortas's wound and his habit of bathing in the lake Brumbane, and (from Parzival) about the 25 maidens who care for the Grail, Trevrizent explains how a knight who wishes to serve the Grail must renounce the love of women, "He who would to the Grail do service, he shall women's love forswear: / A wife shall none have save the Grail king, and his wife a pure heart must bear" (§495, ll. 7-10) — a pledge that Trevrizent himself had violated in the past. In conclusion, Trevrizent summarizes Parzival's two grave sins as (a) having slain Ither, the "Red Knight"; and (b) having to lament his mother's death:

> "Yet God *He* hath not forgotten, and thy deed shall He count for sin,
> And I wot thou shalt first to penance ere thou to His peace shalt win.
> And, weeping, this truth I tell thee, two mortal sins shall lie
> On thine heart, thou hast slain thy kinsman, and thy mother, thro' thee, must die."
>
> (§499, ll. 15-22; vol. 1, p. 286)

Parzival stays with Trevrizent for another 15 days, and before he leaves, Trevrizent gives Parzival a final piece of advice — never to mistreat women or priests:

> "An thou wouldst that thy life be adornèd with true worth as thy crown of fame,
> Then ne'er mayst thou hate a woman, but shall honour, as knight, her name,
> For women and priests, thou knowest, unarmèd shall be their hand,
> Yet the blessing of God watcheth o'er them, and as shield round the priest doth stand; [...]."
>
> (§502, ll. 4-9; vol. 1, p. 287)

This encomium of the priesthood marks an important difference between the medieval, theocentric world of *Parzival* and the modern, post-Christian world of Goethe, Nietzsche, and Jung. In the case of Goethe, for instance, there is the skepticism shown toward the clergy (one thinks, for example, of Mephisto's horror at the way Gretchen's mother gives the box of jewels intended to seduce Gretchen to the local priest or the figure of the Archbishop in Act 4 of *Faust*, Part Two); and in the case of Nietzsche, there is the sharp rejection of the priests by Zarathustra (in "Of the Priests"), whom he describes as his "enemies," even while recognizing a certain kinship or affinity with them, not to mention the figure of the Last Pope. For his part, Jung frequently reminded the audience at his seminar on *Zarathustra* that Nietzsche, like him, was the son of a parson, adding: "I know what *that* means" (SNZ, vol. 1, p. 31; cf. pp. 69, 261, 429, 576; vol. 2, pp. 961, 1095)! By contrast, Trevrizent sees the office of the priest as being one without equal, given his power to celebrate Mass and to forgive sins, "And his hand hath been blest for the holding of the pledge on the altar laid, /

To assure us of sin's forgiveness, and the price for our pardon paid" (§502, ll. 17-19; vol. 1, p. 288).

And implicitly, this encomium raises the interesting question of the relation of the Grail to the Church: Is it a supplementary conduit of salvation alongside the Church or is it an entirely separate source of salvation? Do its institutions (its knights, its servants, etc.) stand in parallel — or in a subordinate position, or even in a superior position — to ecclesiastical authority? This question is never explored by Wolfram (nor, indeed, is it by Chrétien de Troyes), and yet it has huge implications: To cast the question in the terms of St. Cyprian of Carthage, is it true that *extra Ecclesiam nulla salus* (i.e., "outside the Church there is no salvation")? For now, perhaps it is sufficient to note how the Grail legend, in ways explored above, forms a bridge between Christian theology and the pagan traditions underpinning the Arthurian tradition.

Books 10 to 16

In Book 10, the narrative pivots back to Gawan, with whom it remains in Books 11, 12, and 13. It certainly narrates *wilden maeren*, "strange adventures" (§503, l. 1)! In Book 10, Gawan meets the haughty Orgeluse (previously loved by Anfortas) and fights Lischois Gwelljus, the knight who serves her; in Book 11, he enters the magical Castle of Wonders (Schastel marveile), survives his adventures there (including the marvelous bed), and breaks its magic spell; and in Book 12, he encounters Gramoflanz (an enemy of King Arthur, and the owner of the territory on which stands a tree, from which Orgeluse asks him to break off a twig, thus issuing a territorial challenge), and finally (thanks to the help of a magical pillar that allows him to see into the distance) he rides after Orgeluse and, this time, wins her love. In Book 13, Gawan becomes lord of the Castle of Wonders, and he learns from Arnive (one of the women he had earlier liberated, and who turns out to be Arthur's mother, and hence Gawan's grandmother) the story of Clinschor the magician. (As a castrated sorcerer who is descended from Virgil, Clinschor's history forms a kind of pagan parallel to the story of Anfortas.) Toward the end of Book 13, the two narrative arcs begin to converge, as Gawan prepares for his joust with Gramoflanz at Joflanze, and encounters a knight by the river. It is Parzival — but Gawan does not recognize him.

Thus, Book 14 opens with a description of the fierce joust that takes place between Gawan and Parzival, until some of Arthur's pages cry out Gawan's name, and Parzival throws down his sword and declares his identity. Back in Arthur's camp, Parzival asks Gawan to allow him to fight Gramoflanz in his stead, but Gawan refuses. But when Gramoflanz comes looking for his fight the next day, Parzival secretly goes out to engage him, and their joust begins. Once again, Parzival is on the verge of victory, but some of Arthur's knights interrupt the battle-weary pair, and the end of the joust is postponed. Romantic love intrigues and family concerns lead to Arthur's intervention to resolve the various disputes, leading to reconciliation between Gawan and Granoflanz, who marries Gawan's youngest sister, Itonje; Lischois, the duke in the service of Orgeluse, marries Gawan's other sister, Cundrie (not to be confused with Cundrie the sorceress); and Lischois's companion in the service of Orgeluse, Florant of Itolac, marries Sangive (the former wife of Lot, Arthur's sister, and Gawan's mother).[96] While this reconciliation and marital union is celebrated by a sumptuous marriage feast, Parzival recalls his love for Condwiramurs that has not faded during his quest for the Grail:

> "Since to Love I wakened but ill hath Love dealt with me,
> Of Love was I born, how comes it that I must from her presence flee?

[96] For further discussion, see Siegfried Christoph, "Conflict Resolution and the Concept of Honor in Wolfram's 'Parzival,'" *Colloquia Germanica*, vol. 15, no. 1/2 (1982), 32-45.

Tho' my hand for the Grail be seeking yet desire it
doth rend my heart,
And I yearn for her sweet embraces; ah, too long have
we dwelt apart!
Shall I look with mine eyes on rejoicing while my
heart seeth naught but woe?
The twain fit but ill together, and no man thereby shall
know
High courage, a knight befitting — Now Good Fortune
direct my way,
And show me what best beseemeth!"

(§732, ll. 15-29; vol. 2, p. 130)

Once again, however, Parzival laments his lot, "Since this sorrow must be my portion I care not else my lot, / Little reck I what shall befall me, since my joy Heaven willeth not!", *got wil mîner vröude niht* (§733, ll. 6-8; vol. 2, p. 131), and while wishing those celebrating well, he renounces his own happiness, "May God give to this folk rejoicing! But I from their joy must flee, / And wend lonely as of aforetime, since gladness is not for me!" (733, ll. 19-20; vol. 2, p. 131). And so he rides off at dawn.

Here (as elsewhere in *Parzival* and across the epic tradition) we have a clear narrative structure of crisis and resolution; for no sooner is one crisis is resolved (here, the enmity between Gawan and Giroflanz, and a series of minor romantic love intrigues), then another one begins (here, the final stages of Parzival's quest to rediscover the Grail). As we shall see, this structure informs not just *Parzival* but *Faust*, *Zarathustra*, and *The Red Book*: indeed, it is arguably *the* archetypal narrative structure of the epic. Not for nothing does this structure of crisis and resolution map onto the structure of the so-called monomyth as proposed by Joseph Campbell; in fact, it underpins it.

The action of Book 15 takes Parzival decisively closer to attaining his goal — that of rediscovering the Grail. Going through the forest, Parzival comes across an unknown knight; so, of course, he fights him (for this is how things work in Wolfram's world). This knight is described as "a prince of battles who dauntless to strife doth ride, / And unbaptized was the foeman who rode here in his heathen pride," and he is richly clad, "His blazoned coat was costly, and naught but the truth I say, / Ruby and Chalcedony, ye had held them not fair that day. / And bright as the sun was his vesture, on the mount of Agremontein, / In the glowing fires, Salamanders had welded that garment's shine" (§735, ll. 2-4 and ll. 20-27; vol. 2, p. 135). Like most knights, he is in search of love and fame, "His desire was for love's rewarding, and the winning of high renown" (§736, ll. 1-2), and on his helmet is depicted as a sign of his great deeds a curious animal — an ecidemon, "As reward for his deeds of knighthood on his helmet a beast he bare, / Ecidemon, all poisonous serpents they must of its power beware" (§736, ll. 9-11; cf. §739, l.16 and §741, ll. 15-20).[97]

Parzival does not recognize the knight; so, of course, he must be related to him (for this is also how things work in Wolfram's world). The sword that Gaheviez has given Parzival shatters when he smashes it down on his opponent's helmet, and the joust is paused; in the ensuing conversation, the knight turns out to be none other than Parzival's infidel half-brother, Feirefiz. Parzival knows that Feirefiz is meant to be *als ein geschriben permint, / swarz und blanc her unde dâ*, "As written parchment, both black and white is he" (§747, ll. 26-27; vol. 2, p. 142), and removing his helment, Feirefiz confirms that it is he, "For straightway he knew the other, (as a magpie, I ween, his face,) / And hatred and wrath were slain here in a brotherly embrace" (§748, ll. 6-9; vol. 2, p. 142). In his

[97] For further discussion of this strange, weasel-like animal that can kill poisonous snakes, see Johannes Siebert, "*Ecidemôn*," *Journal for German Philology*, 62 (1937), 248-264.

joy, the so-called pagan Feirefiz cries out and expresses polytheistic thanks to his *gote unt gotinne*, "gods and goddesses," especially Juno and Jupiter. (Obviously, this is a grotesque misrepresentation of the monotheism of Islam, and it is unclear whether Feirefiz is meant to be a Muslim or a pagan; whatever his religious beliefs, he falls into the category of non-Christian Other.)

Parzival persuades Feirefiz to return with him to Arthur's camp, where he introduces him to Gawan. Jofreit, son of Idœl, announces plans for a great feast at Joflanze, which Clinschor's knights and ladies attend. Feirefiz tells Arthur of his knightly ambitions, after which Arthur tells him of Parzival's high ambition to find the Grail, *er suochet einen hôhen vunt, / nâch dem grâle wirbet er*, "For he seeketh a lofty guerdon, and he rideth to find the Grail" (§769, ll. 24-25; vol. 2, p. 153). The feast begins; and, for a second time, Cundrie the sorceress turns up. This time, however, she is splendidly dressed in garments decorated with the Grail emblem of the flock of turtledoves. (Together with the laughing lion, a flock of doves is the sign awaited by Zarathustra; a sign which, in the closing chapter, "cometh," and which indicates, as the doves whisk over the nose of the lion, making it shake its head and wonder and laugh, that, in Zarathustra's words, "My children are nigh, my children" [Z IV 20].)

And this time Cundrie greets Parzival with great warmth, hailing him as Gahmuret's son and as *du crône menschlichen heiles*, "the crown of all earthly blessings" (§781, l. 14), and she brings him a message from the Grail itself:

> "For read is the mystic writing — The Grail, It doth
> hail thee king,
> And Kondwiramur, thy true wife, thou shalt to thy
> kingdom bring,
> For the Grail, It hath called her thither — Yea, and
> Lohengrin, thy son,

For e'en as thou left her kingdom twin babes thou by
her hadst won.
And Kardeiss, he shall have in that kingdom a heritage
rich I trow!
And were no other bliss thy portion than that which I
tell thee now —
That with true lips and pure, thou shalt greet him,
Anfortas the king, again,
And thy mouth thro' the mystic question shall rid him
of all his pain,
For sorrow hath been his portion — If joy's light thro'
thy deed shall shine
On his life, then of all earth's children whose bliss
shall be like to thine?"
(§781, ll. 15-30; vol. 2, p. 159)

Cundrie concludes by pointing to the favorable astrological constellation observable in the skies, using Arabic names for the planets in a way that is comprehensible to Feirefiz, *der vor ir saz swarz unde wîz*, "who sat there, both black and white" (§782, l. 4), and she closes her speech by telling Parzival that he has overcome *sorge* and discovered *des lîbes vröude* or "bodily joy": "For thou hast thy soul's rest won, / And in grief thou o'er-long hast waited for the joy that is now begun" (§782, ll. 27-30; vol. 2, p. 160). Thus, the quest for the Grail turns out to be not just a quest for identity but also a quest for joy (*vröude*). Parzival chooses Feirefiz to be his companion for this final adventure, and together with Cundrie they ride off — to the Grail.

Wolfram's artful narrative has already begun to bring together a number of storylines, such as the adventures of Gawan and the adventures of Parzival as well as diverse romantic love intrigues, at the same time as opening up new lines of narrative development. These include the two sons born by Condwiramurs from Parzival, Kardeiz and his twin brother Loherangrin, the subject of another strand of Arthurian legend — and another Wagner opera, of course.[98] (The figure of Prester John is another new narrative opening.) So in the final book of *Parzival*, what remains is to bring the narrative arc of the Grail and the sufferings of Anfortas to a conclusion and to narrate how Parzival becomes lord of the Grail. And this Book 16 does, which means that Wolfram's *Parzival* is complete in a way that Goethe's *Faust*, Nietzsche's *Zarathustra*, and Jung's *Red Book* are not. For in the second part of *Faust*, the scene of Faust's descent to Persephone in the Classical Walpurgisnacht of Act 2 remained unwritten; Nietzsche had plans for a part 5 and a part 6 of *Zarathustra*, which were never brought to fruition; and Jung's *Red Book* lacks a proper conclusion, and breaks off *in media res*. Curiously, then, this medieval work enjoys a completeness missing in its Weimar classical (or German Romantic), modernist, and postmodern counterparts.

Book 16 opens with a reminder of Anfortas's lamentable sufferings. It is a grim scene: Anfortas is screaming in pain, and the stench of his wound means that his room has to be kept well ventilated. In the hope that relief is at hand in the form of the return of Parzival, the Grail knights are reluctant to put him out of his suffering and turn instead to a bizarre series of "alternative therapies," including the use of no fewer than 58 gemstones. Guided by Cundrie, Parzival and his brother arrive at Terre salvaesche and are spotted by a knight who cries, *unser sorge ein ende hât*, "Now an end hath it found, our grief" (§792, l. 28; vol. 2, p. 168) — more precisely, an end to *sorge* (or "Care"). His group of knights welcomes Parzival and accompany his party to Munsalvaesche and its great hall. As Anfortas begs him to let him die, Parzival asks the crucial question, *oeheim, waz wirret dir?*, "*What aileth*

[98] For further discussion, see Alastair Matthews, *The Medieval German "Lohengrin": Narrative Poetics in the Story of the Swan Knight* (Rochester, NY: Camden House, 2016).

thee here, mine uncle?" (§795, l. 29; vol. 2, p. 169). These words unlock God's healing powers, just as Pope St. Silvester is said to have brought a bull back to life (see the *Kaiserchronik* or *Imperial Chronicle*, ll.10030-336) and Jesus brought Lazarus back from the grave (John 12:1-11). Significantly, Anfortas is returned not just to good health but to blossoming, flourishing *beauty*:

> [...] and all men beheld the king,
> And what French folk shall know as "*Florie*" it shone on his face so fair,
> And Parzival's manly beauty was but as the empty air!
> Yea, Vergulacht, Askalon's monarch, and Absalom, David's son,
> And all who the dower of beauty as their birthright shall e'er have won —
> E'en Gamuret, as men saw him draw near unto Kanvoleis,
> So wondrous fair to look on — they were naught unto all men's eyes
> When matched with the radiant beauty that forth from his bitter woe
> He bare, the King Anfortas — such skill God doth surely know!
>
> (§796, ll. 2-16; vol. 2, p. 170)

Thus, the redemption around which *Parzival* revolves is ultimately not just a biological or a spiritual one, but an *aesthetic* one. And as if to drive home the point, Wolfram's narrator says that neither the proverbial beauty of Absalom, "But in all Israel there was not a man so comely, and so exceedingly beautiful, as Absalom: from the sole of the foot to the crown of his head there was no blemish in him" (2 Samuel 14:25), nor the beauty of Parzival's cousin Vergulaht of Ascalun, nor of Parzival's father, Gahmuret, nor of Parzival himself could rival the beauty of the transformed Anfortas. As Wolfram's narrator puts it, *got noch künste kan genuoc*, i.e., God has his "powers" (*künste*), and the highest expression of these powers is expressed in beauty, so that Hatto is surely right to translate this line as follows, "God's power to apply his artistry is undiminished today" (395).

His task now finally achieved, Parzival is declared king and the new lord of the Grail. As Condwiramurs, guided by Kyot (her paternal uncle) and others, rides out toward Munsalvaesche, Parzival rides away to Trevrizent, who hails his achievement, "Greater marvel I ne'er may see / Than that thou by thy wrath has won blessing, and th' Eternal trinity / Hath given thee thy desiring!" (§798, ll.2-5; vol. 2, p. 171): in other words, Parzival's achievement is less a case of fulfilling a divine plan and more a case of a triumph of his individual will (*willen*). (In this brief scene, there is the intriguing suggestion that, in their earlier encounter, Trevrizent had deliberately misled Parzival, "Yet aforetime in sooth I lied, / For I thought from the Grail to bring thee, and the truth I from thee would hide" (§798, ll. 6-7; vol. 2, p. 171), a remark usually explained in relation to what he had said about the "neutral" angels (cf. §454, ll. 24-216 and §471, ll. 15-21), but the passage remains highly problematic.)[99]

Taking his leave from Trevrizent, Parzival rides through the night to meet Condwiramurs, arriving to find her asleep in a bed with their two sons, Loherangrin and Kardeiz. Embracing Parzival and (so Wolfram's narrator coyly remarks) apparently kissing him, Condwiramurs cries, *mir hât gelücke dich / gesenet, herzen vröude mîn*, "The joy of my heart! Good Fortune hath sent thee again to me" (§801, ll. 6-7), and she adds: "Now in sooth I should wrathful be, / Yet have I no heart for anger! Ah! Blest be the dawn and the day / That this dear embrace hath brought me, which all sorrow

[99] DKV, vol. 2, p. 776.

must drive away. / For now at last have I found thee, whom my heart hath desired so long, / And grief in my heart is vanquished, and sighing is turned to song," *ich hân nu des mîn herze gert: / sorge ist an mir vil ungewert* (§801, ll. 9-14; vol. 2, p. 172). Once again, *sorge* has been replaced by *vröude*, that is, worry or anxiety or care is replaced by joy.

Once again, Wolfram's narrator insists on the physicality of that *vröude*, contrasting the moment in Book 6, when Parzival had been held in unconscious fascination by the drops of blood on the snow, with the physical pleasures of *minne* enjoyed by Parzival, who has remained true to his wife: "I ween that in bliss he lay, / And converse sweet, till morning drew night to middle day" (§802, ll. 9-10; vol. 2, p. 173). Not just the physical world, but also the social one is deeply implicated in this outcome, as we see in the remaining lines of the epic. (Here lies perhaps a significant major difference between our modern age of the individual, so often bewildered about the way the world works, and a much older view that regards suffering and salvation as essentially collective matters.)[100] Kardeiz is crowned king of Parzival's secular realms (i.e., Brobarz, Anjou, Waleis, and Norgals), and as they eat a late breakfast on the banks of the river Plimizoel, Parzival asks about the hermitage where Sigune was living. Riding to the site, Sigune is found to be dead, and Parzival

[100] Compare with Jung's remark in *Psychological Types* (1921): "What we understand by the concept 'individual' is a relatively recent acquisition in the history of the human mind and human culture," in contrast to "the earlier all-powerful collective attitude" (CW 6 §12). Tatsuhiro Nakajima suggests that Wolfram's *Parzival* plays a pivotal rôle in the history of the West, inasmuch as, "in the context of Aristotelian psychology, *Parzival* is a dramatization of the passage from not knowing to knowing, the soul's movement from the passive intellect, without asking any question at all, to the active intellect through imagination," adding that "it was soon after *Parzival* was written that *principium individuationis* become a subject matter of [the] medieval philosophy of Duns Scotus" and noting that, "already in *Parzival*, an increased emphasis on the role of the individual can be found" (Tatsuhiro Nakajima, "Psychology of the 12th Century Renaissance in Wolfram von Eschenbach's *Parzival*," *Studia Hermetica Journal*, vol. 8, no. 1 ("Hermetism and the Underworld") (2018), 23-40 [p. 34]). For further discussion, see David Blamires, *Characterization and Individuality in Wolfram's "Parzival"* (Cambridge: Cambridge University Press), 1966.

orders that she be buried next to her beloved Schionatulander in the same coffin. And they return to Munsalvaesche.

When Loherangrin is taken to his uncle Feirefiz, he is afraid of him, *dô der was swarz unde wîz*, "who was black and white": "And so the babe turned aside nor would kiss him — as children oft do from fright!" (§805, l. 30-§806, ll.1-2). In response (and thankfully, perhaps), Feirefiz simply laughs. Now the figure of Feirefiz — mottled, or black and white, so neither black *nor* white, and moreover heathen (or at least, non-Christian) — has somehow to be integrated into the world of the Grail, that is, into its symbolic universe of light. The figure by which this is achieved is Repanse de Schoye (whose name contains the "joy," or *joie*, that is so important in this work). For it is she who brings forth the Grail, because of her radiant beauty, "And the Grail, so men have told me, might be borne by her hands alone; / Pure was her heart, and radiant as sunlight her fair face shone," *ir vel des blickes flôrî* (or as Hatto translates this passage, "the flesh without was a blossoming of all brightness") (§809, ll. 10-14; vol. 2, p. 176). But significantly, *Fierefiz cannot see the Grail*, only a green achmardi (i.e., a green- and gold-brocaded silk cloth). He can, however, see Repanse, who displaces Secundille (queen of Tribalibot in India) in his erotic affections, and with whom he now falls in love. Anfortas's grandfather (and Parzival's great-grandfather), Titurel, explains that the Grail cannot be seen by a heathen, "If he be a heathen" — *ein heidensch man* — "then such thought shall he put away / As that eyes unbaptized may win them power to behold the Grail! / Such barriers are built around It, his sight to the task shall fail" (§813, ll. 17-22; vol. 2, pp. 178-179). If it will help him in love, however, Feirefiz is willing to be baptized, and he agrees to renounce both Jupiter (as his god) and queen Secundille (as his partner or spouse).

The baptism offered to Feirefiz does, however, seem to be of a special kind, given the restorative, even magical, properties of the water involved:

"In water was He baptizèd, in Whose likeness was
Adam made,
And each tree from the water draweth its sap, and its
leafy shade.
By water all flesh is nourished, and all that on earth
doth live,
And the eyes of man are quickened, such virtue doth
water give;
And many a soul it cleanseth, till it shineth so pure
and white
That the angels themselves in heaven methinks shall
be scarce so bright!"
(§8117, ll. 23-30; vol. 2, p. 181)

(This water sounds, as Julius Evola has suggested, less like the water of Christian baptism and more like "a real enlightenment, the water having here more or less the same meaning of the 'divine water' or of Hermeticism's 'philosophical water.'")[101] After his baptism, Feirefiz can immediately see the Grail, and a new set of inscriptions appears on the Grail, with the following instructions about any Templar knights who undertake missionary work in another country:

"The Templar whom God henceforward to a strange
folk should send as head,
Must forbid all word or question of his country, or
name, or race,
If they willed he aright should help them, and they
would in his sight find grace.
For the day that they ask the question that folk must
he leave straightway" —
(§818, l. 26-§819, l. 2; vol. 2, p. 182)

[101] Julius Evola, *The Mystery of the Grail: Initiation and Magic in the Quest of the Spirit*, trans. by Guido Stucco (Rochester, VT: Inner Traditions, 1997), p. 105.

This curious reinstallation of the *Frageverbot* or the proscription of asking questions opens the way to integrate the story of Loherangrin into the story of Parzival (and into its narrative logic).

And in fact, the final stanzas of Book 16 both close the story of Parzival and open up wider perspectives. Feirefiz invites Anfortas to sail away with him and return to his court, but Anfortas firmly declines, pledging to serve only the Grail and renouncing the love of women. After 11 days Feirefiz leaves with Repanse de Schoye as his new wife, and Anfortas rides with them as an escort of honor through the forest of Læprisin on his journey back to Joflanze, and thence to India. We learn that, in India, Repanse will give birth to a son called "Prester John," a legendary Christian priest-king in India (later said to have ruled over a Christian nation in the East).[102]

Now Wolfram's narrator briefly recounts the story of Loherangrin — of how he was sent from Munsalvaesche to be a husband for Elsa, princess of Brabant, and arrives at Antwerp in a boat pulled by a swan. He pledges to marry her and serve as lord of Brabant, but on one condition: namely, *gevrâget nimmer wer ich sî*, "ask thou never who I may be" (§825, l. 19; vol. 2, p. 185). But of course, she does — and Loherangrin departs again, pulled by the swan; but this is another literary work (be it in the form of the late 13th-century Middle High German epic *Lohengrin*, attributed to Nouhusius; the Middle High German verse romance by Konrad von Würzburg, *Der Schwanritter*; or the 16th-century adaptation in the form of a Meisterlied called *Lorengel*) and, of course, another Wagnerian operatic work (1850).

That there is a specific literary theme here in Arthurian romance in the form of the proscription of questions is illustrated by Wolfram's narrator's brief reference to Hartmann von Aue's *Erec*,

[102] For further discussion of this legendary figure, see Charles F. Beckingham and Bernard Hamilton (eds), *Prester John, the Mongols and the Ten Lost Tribes* (Aldershot: Variorum, 1996); and Nicholas Jubber, *The Prester Quest* (London: Doubleday, 2005).

"Here Herr Erec should speak, for, I think me, he knoweth the tale to tell / Of revenging for broken pledges, and the fate that such speech befell!" (§826, ll. 29-30; vol. 2, p. 186). (In Hartmann's epic, Erec, a knight at Arthur's court, wins the hand of the beautiful Enite, but out of devotion to his wife, he begins to neglect his knightly duties as a ruler. He sets out from the court looking for adventure, accompanied by Enite, whom he forbids to speak to him. In a series of adventures, Enite breaks Erec's command and speaks, but only to warn him of danger and to save his life. The final adventure is known as the *Joie de la Curt* ["joy of the court"].) Sometimes it is a mistake to ask a question, sometimes it is a mistake *not* to ask; what makes the hero a hero is knowing *when* to ask and *when not*.

It is Wolfram's genius to have taken this motif — and, indeed, all his source materials — and to have transformed those sources into such a fascinating, rich, and complex work, which puzzles, perplexes, and delights right to its very last lines. In the end, in a final self-reflexive move, Wolfram's narrator expresses the same kind of joy (albeit in a more modest form) at having told his tale that Parzival experienced in realizing his destiny as the lord of the Grail, "And if good and gracious women shall think I be worthy praise, / Since I tell to its end my story, then joyful shall be my days. / And since for the love of a woman I have sung it, this song of old, / I would that, in sweet words gentle, my guerdon by her be told!" (§827, ll. 25-30; vol. 2, p. 186) — or, as Hatto translates these lines, "If I have any well-wishers among good women of discernment I shall be valued the more for my having told this tale to its end. And if it was done to please one in particular, she must own I have said some agreeable things" (411).

Whatever the Grail in Wolfram's *Parzival* might be (whether a stone or a portable altar or anything else), what is evident is its *transformative* effect. Not only does it enable Anfortas to be cured of his wound, it enables Parzival to become the lord of the Grail and thus the true hero he was meant to be. In the end, Parzival succeeds in his quest: in his quest for identity, in his quest for joy, and — insofar as this is possible — in his quest to answer the question "what is God?" If this transformation takes place outside the usual channels of grace, that is, the Church, it is nevertheless situated against a firm theological background: even if the world is full of radical uncertainty, there *is* a God, and it *is* possible to know something about him. In the works that follow on *Parzival* in the German epic tradition, the level of that uncertainty increases and the possibility of knowing anything about God recedes. (In *Faust*, the theological background itself is questioned as it is inverted in the course of the work; in *Zarathustra*, God is declared to be "dead," and the transformation that concerns Nietzsche's prophetic hero is the transformative "self-overcoming" of the human individual into the *Übermensch*; while in *The Red Book*, Jung's god Izdubar becomes "squeezed [...] into the size of an egg" and placed in Jung's pocket — how practical is that? — while it becomes increasingly clear that it is not humankind that needs salvation, but God Himself: a salvation that is found by "precisely what one would actually consider fatal, namely by declaring him a figment of the imagination," which stops Him from "pass[ing] away" by instead "becom[ing] a living fantasy" [RB, 295].) Although Jung only discusses Wolfram's *Parzival* directly on a couple of occasions, the Grail legend nevertheless formed a significant part of his historico-cultural outlook, as we shall explore in the following chapter.

Chapter 3

Jung and the Grail Myth: Analytical Psychology as a New Form of Quest for Transformation

As a child Jung is said to have had an "absolute craving" to "read every scrap of printed matter" that fell into his hands (MDR, 46). At school his Latin teacher would allow him to skip classes and to fetch books for him from the University of Basel library, and his reading came to include Homer's *Odyssey*, Virgil's *Aeneid*, the *Eclogues*, and Horace.[1] In addition, he read the stories of the Grail, stories which he described as having been "of the great importance" to him since he read them for the first time at the age of 15 (MDR, 189). This account is confirmed by a recently published conversation with Aniela Jaffé in 1957, when Jung claimed that two books had made the great impression on him when he was a child.

The first was the legend of the Grail, which he described as his "favourite book when he was a child," as "something quite wonderful" (*etwas ganz Wunderbares*), and as a work which he immediately "read through twice."[2] Thanks to reading this work,

---

[1] Sonu Shamdasani, *C.G. Jung: A Biography in Books* (New York and London: Norton 2012), p. 11.

[2] Aniela Jaffé, *Streiflichter zu Leben und Denken C.G. Jungs* (Einsiedeln: Daimon Verlag, 2021), p. 37. The catalog to Jung's library reveals the extent of his interest in the Grail legend, and it includes the seminal study by Adolf Birch-Hirschfeld (1849-1917), *Die Sage vom Graal: Ihre Entwicklung und dichterische Ausbildung in Frankreich und Deutschland, im 12. und 13. Jahrhundert: Eine literarhistorische Untersuchung* (Leipzig: F.C.W. Vogel, 1877), as well as a compilation of various short works published between 1855 and 1872 in German, French, English, or Latin (including one titled "Die Sage von Parcival und vom Gral"), bound together as a

Jung noted that the figures in the Grail story were familiar to him and exercised an "uncanny fascination" on him. Yet he explained that he only mentioned them rarely in his writings, because his wife, Emma Jung, had begun writing about the Grail legend. In fact, on another occasion in 1958, Jung told Jaffé of a dream he had had about his wife after her death, when he dreamed they had spent a day in Provence while she worked on her studies of the Grail.[3] (The second book that had influenced him, it should be added, was Goethe's *Faust.*) Emma Jung's work on the Grail was presented at the Psychological Club in Zurich in 1944 and greatly interested the theoretical physicist Wolfgang Pauli (1900-1958), who corresponded with her about it.[4]

In 1920 and again in 1923, Jung gave a seminar in Cornwall (at Sennen Cove and Polzeath, respectively), and during these stays he took the opportunity to visit nearby megalithic monuments:[5] Tintagel Castle (known as the birthplace of King Arthur) and Glastonbury (where Joseph of Arimathea is said to have brought the Grail). And in 1938, during a visit to India, Jung had a vivid dream about the Grail, the significance of which we shall explore

---

book and with an ex libris bearing the name Karl Vollmüller and the date 1887. This book was part of Emma's library, and the pencil marks in the book suggest that it may have been acquired secondhand, possibly by Emma herself. (For information about this work, I am grateful to Dr. Carl C. Jung of the Stiftung der Werke von C.G. Jung).

[3] Jaffé, *Streiflichter zu Leben und Denken C.G. Jungs*, p. 187. In the introduction to their study of the Grail legend published in 1960 as *Die Graalslegende in psychologischer Sicht*, Marie-Louise von Franz noted that Emma Jung had been researching the Grail for some 30 years before her work was cut short by her death in 1955 — work which it then fell to von Franz to complete and bring to publication (Emma Jung and Marie-Louise von Franz, *The Grail Legend* (Boston, MA: Sigo Press, 1986), p. 7).

[4] See Pauli's letter to Emma Jung of 16 November 1950, in *Atom and Archetype: The Pauli/Jung Letters, 1932-1958*, ed. C.A. Meier, trans. David Roscoe (Princeton, NJ, and Oxford: Princeton University Press, 2001), pp. 49-53. Pauli observed that "although the solution in Wolfram's version emerges as the more psychological one, [...] in the French versions the story ends tragically with the disappearance of the Grail" (p. 49).

[5] William McGuire, "Firm Affinities: Jung's Relation with Britain and the United States," *Journal of Analytical Psychology*, 40 (1995), 301-326 (pp. 313 and 316).

below. The key tenets of Jungian psychology — the collective unconscious, the archetypes, the importance of the symbol — offered a unique toolkit with which to analyze the Arthurian stories and the Grail myths, and it is no disrespect to the work of Emma Jung and Marie-Louise von Franz to describe their joint study on the Grail as an example of "applied Jungianism." On their account, the main characters of the Grail legend fall neatly into their (archetypal) place: Parzival is the "holy fool," about to embark on a journey; Gurnemanz is the "wise old man," who gives him the advice he needs; and the adventure on which Parzival is embarking is nothing less than the process of individuation. Thus, the quest for the Grail is the search for higher, spiritual understanding — for the attainment, in other words, of the Self. As we saw in Chapter 2, Jung noted the proximities and parallels between the Grail quest and alchemy; first, inasmuch as alchemy was a kind of subterranean tradition beneath a dominant Christianity, compensating for the lacunae left by the tension of opposites within Christianity;[6] and second, inasmuch as in both the Grail quest and in alchemy what is central is the experience of transformation.

There can be no doubt of the significance that Jung attached to the medieval period, the age when the Grail legend flourished.[7] In *Psychological Types* (1921), Jung draws attention to the "medieval background" of Goethe's *Faust*, arguing that the special significance of this background lies in the fact that "there actually was a medieval element that stood at the cradle of modern individualism" (CW 6 §376). For modern individualism began, or so Jung explains, with the worship of women (or *Frauendienst*, a notion in the tradition of courtly love), as a consequence of which "the soul of the man became considerably strengthened as a psychological factor"

[6] Jung and von Franz, *The Grail Legend*, p. 34; cf. CW 12 §25-§27.
[7] For an overview of the Grail legend and its various versions, see Richard Barber, *The Holy Grail: Imagination and Belief* (London: Allen Lane, 2004); and the literature discussed in the Preface.

(§376). This is so, Jung declares, because the worship of woman really meant the worship of the soul (*Seelendienst*).

Further consideration of this point leads Jung to discuss Dante's *Divine Comedy*, especially Canto XXXIII of the *Paradiso* (see CW 6 §377), in which the fact that Dante speaks here through the mouth of St. Bernard is seen by Jung as an "indication of the transformation [*Umgestaltung*] and exaltation [*Erhöhung*] of his own being" (§378). Corresponding to Dante's transformation as a "spiritual knight" is, of course, the transformation of the figure of his lady: Her image is exalted (*erhöht*) into the "otherworldly, mystical figure of the Mother of God — a figure that has detached itself from the object and turned into the personification of a purely psychological affair, namely: those unconscious contents whose personification I have termed the soul [*Seele*]" (§377).

And then there is — tellingly — the legend of the Grail. According to Jung, there exist significant psychological relations between the worship of woman (*Frauendienst*) and the legend of the Grail that he regards as being so "peculiarly characteristic" of the early Middle Ages (CW 6 §401). One of the greatest versions of the Grail legend was, of course, Wolfram's *Parzival*, and although Jung does not specifically mention Wolfram here, his remarks are nevertheless pertinent for our understanding of that work. Now Jung reminds us that the "central religious idea" in the numerous variants of this legend is the sacred vessel (or, in the case of Wolfram, a sacred stone), an image that Jung describes as being "obvious to everyone" as "thoroughly un-Christian," and whose origin must surely lie in extra-canonical sources (§401). In fact, in a footnote Jung mentions the thesis that the pagan roots of this vessel symbolism are found in the "magic cauldron" (*Zaubertopf*) of Celtic mythology. In this tradition, the Dagda is a god, described as a large, bearded man or giant in a hooded cloak who owns a magic staff or club (the *lorg mór* or *lorg anfaid*) which kills with one end and brings to life with the other, a magic harp (*uaithne*) which can control human emotions and change the seasons, and a cauldron (the *coire ansic*) which never runs empty and can supply all with the food they need. Likewise, the Celtic god Bran is said to possess a vessel of renewal (and it has been suggested that the name "Brons" — one of the figures in the Grail legend, who in the *Joseph of Arimathea* attributed to Robert de Boron catches a wonderful fish used later to distinguish the righteous from the sinners and who becomes known as the "Rich Fisher" (verse 3348) — is in fact derived from Bran). Jung mentions the view of Alfred Nutt (1856-1910), the British folklorist and Celticologist, that the figures of "Bran" as lord of the cauldron and "Brons" represent stages in the transformation of the Celtic saga of Peredur into the quest of the Holy Grail, suggesting that the source of the Grail motifs is to be found in Celtic mythology.[8]

Yet rather than pursue these Celtic connections, Jung turns to the tradition of Gnosticism, whose symbolism of the vessel he has just been examining (see CW 6 §396-§398). The Grail vessel is, he suspects, a "genuine piece" of Gnosticism (*ein echtes Stück Gnosis*), a relic that has, thanks to a secret tradition, survived the extermination of heresies, or owes its revival to "an unconscious reaction against the official rule of Christianity" (§401). This unconscious revivification of the symbol of the vessel is an indication of "a strengthening of the feminine principle in the masculine psychology of that time"; but, if this all sounds a bit too Freudian, Jung is quick to add that "its symbolization in an enigmatic image signifies a spiritualization of the eroticism that the worship of woman had stimulated" (§401). On Jung's account,

[8] As the source of this information, Jung acknowledges the Scottish psychiatrist and author Maurice Nicoll (1884-1953), a noted Fourth Way teacher who is known for his collection of talks published as *Psychological Commentaries on the Teaching of Gurdjieff and Ouspensky*. For further discussion of Nicoll's friendship with Jung (and Jung's skepticism about Gurdjieff), see McGuire, "Firm Affinities," p. 316 (and L2, 180).

this spiritualization (*Vergeistigung*) involves holding back a certain amount of libido which would otherwise be directly enjoyed as sexuality, with the result that part of this libido flows into the "spiritualized expression" while the remainder sinks into the unconscious. Here it activates corresponding images that express themselves in the symbol of the vessel which, living through the restraint imposed on certain forms of libido, in turn brings about the restraint of those libidinal forms. As a magical or redeeming symbol, it possesses an unassailable nature and serves as the "best possible expression of the prevailing world-view [*Weltanschauung*]" (§401). Indeed, it cannot in its essence be overcome, for so far removed from comprehension does it stand that the critical intellect lacks all means to be able to dissolve it, and in its aesthetic form it appeals so convincingly to our feeling that no emotional arguments can be raised against it. In Jung's view, such was the function of the symbol of the Grail: "for a certain time it filled these demands and owed its vital effect to this fact," as the example of Richard Wagner shows (§401). For, thanks to Wagner, whose *Parsifal* was in part a revival of Wolfram's *Parzival*, we can see how its vitality is even today still not exhausted, "even if our age and our psychology constantly strive for its dissolution," he adds (§401).

Further on, Jung writes that the fascination of early medieval psychology for "three of the greatest minds of Germany" (CW 6 §408) offered proof of the lasting influence exercised by the medieval period. These great minds are, of course, Goethe (who parodies Dante in the concluding scene of *Faust II*), Nietzsche (whose notion of a "master caste" with a "master morality" Jung sees as embodied in the "many blond-haired heroic and knightly figures" of the Middle Ages),[9] and Wagner (who uses the Grail

[9] Jung might also have been thinking of Nietzsche's explicit reference in *Beyond Good and Evil* to the troubadours, "the Provençal knight-poets, those magnificent and inventive human beings of the '*gai saber*'" (§260), and his allusion in the title of *The Gay Science* to "the Provençal concept of *gaya scienza* — that unity of *singer, knight,*

legend in *Parsifal*) (§408; trans. modified). Or as Jung had put it in his *Red Book*, "I must catch up with a piece of the Middle Ages — within myself. We have only finished the Middle Ages — of others. I must begin early; in that period when the hermits died out" (RB, 330). On Jung's account, what inspired such knightly orders of the Middle Ages as, for instance, the Templars, was "that strange something" (*jenes fremdartige Etwas*) which found expression in the legend of the Grail: in short, "the germ or the bud of a new possibility of orientation" or, in other words, "a new symbol" (§409; trans. modified). What is this strange or mysterious thing? In this chapter, I consider Jung's reception of the Grail myth and relate some key Jungian concepts to Wolfram von Eschenbach's *Parzival*.

Whom Does the Grail Serve?

According to Chrétien de Troyes' version of the story of Perceval/Parzival/Parsifal, the magical question that has to be asked is "Whom does the Grail serve?"[10] For Wolfram von Eschenbach, the question is, "What ails thee?"[11] For Jung, however, the decisive question in life itself was: "Are you related to something infinite or not?" (MDR, 356). Yet perhaps these different questions are ways of articulating the same thing, inasmuch as "the Grail legend speaks very plainly about the one crucial question that has to be asked — just like Jung's question about whether each individual is related

and *free spirit* which distinguishes the wonderful early culture of the Provençals from all equivocal cultures" (*Ecce Homo*, "The Gay Science" (Friedrich Nietzsche, *Basic Writings*, ed. and trans. Walter Kaufmann (New York: Modern Library, 1968), pp. 398 and 750).

[10] *Perceval, ou le conte du Graal*, in Chrétien de Troyes, *Œuvres complètes*, ed. Daniel Poirion (Paris: Gallimard, 1994), ll. 3552-3555, 3568-3571, and 3583-3592 (pp. 773-774) and ll. 6413-6414 (p. 843); cf. p. 1352.

[11] Whether formulated as "*hêrre, wie stêt iuwer nôt?*" (i.e., "Sire, what ails you?") or as "*oeheim, waz wirret dir?*", (i.e., "Uncle, what ails you?") (§484, l. 27, cf. §795, l. 29).

to something infinite, or not — before the Grail itself can be won," and "until then the whole earth remains desolate; wasted; dead."[12] In his recent work, *Catafalque* (2018), Peter Kingsley has drawn attention to the importance for Jung of the Grail legend (or, perhaps, it would be more accurate to say the Grail *myth*).[13] "You might suppose," Kingsley dramatically warns his readers, "you know the general direction in which the Grail is to be found," and "you may be ever so confident you have it in your grasp," but "without that one question being asked, then answered, it's not just that all your own accomplished efforts are ultimately useless — all your strivings for personal individuation utterly useless": no, "even the world around you is going to be lifeless."[14] And so, "for the real life to come back, nothing is more important than to know that magical question which has to be asked": Whom does the Grail serve? Or: What ails us? Or: Are we related to something infinite — or not?

Kingsley points to a passage in the Jaffé Protocols, Aniela Jaffé's original transcript of the material she noted in her interviews with Jung between 1956 and 1958, where Jung offers an extended commentary on two dreams about the search for Grail, in which he "explains that this dream figure of the knight represents his own ancient forefather or ancestor; describes how the Grail is a reward for living the life of a true knight and how one can only set off in quest of the Grail after inwardly being accepted as abiding by the rules for becoming a knight; and emphasizes in no uncertain terms that the mysterious gift of the Grail received by a knight is the deepest secret possible for a human, which is the true secret, or mystery, of individuation."[15] These Protocols have not (yet) been

[12] Peter Kingsley, *Catafalque: Carl Jung and the End of Humanity*, 2 vols (London: Catafalque Press, 2018), vol. 1, p. 123.
[13] Mythology, that is, in the sense used by the Roman historian Sallust in *On the Gods and the World*, §4, "Now these things never happened, but always are" (in Gilbert Murray, *Five Stages of Greek Religion* [31955] (Mineola, NY: Dover, 2002), p. 195).
[14] Kingsley, *Catafalque*, vol. 1, p. 123.
[15] Kingsley, *Catafalque*, vol. 2, pp. 526-527.

published, but the dream image of a knight is mentioned twice in the published version of Jung's biography which we know as *Memories, Dreams, Reflections* (1961).

The first of those dreams is mentioned in the context of Jung's work on *Transformations and Symbols of the Libido* (1911-1912) and is said to presage his imminent break with Freud (MDR, 186). As it is told in *Memories, Dreams, Reflections*, this dream had two parts: In the first, set toward evening in a mountainous region of the Swiss-Austrian border, Jung sees the ghost of an elderly Imperial Austrian customs official, described by someone else in the dream as "one of those who still couldn't properly die" (MDR, 186-187).[16] And in the second, set in the fierce light of midday in an Italian city that bore a curious resemblance to Basel, Jung is suddenly approached by a medieval Knight Templar dressed in a helmet, chain armor, and a white tunic into which was woven a large red cross. An unidentifiable voice tells Jung, "Yes, this is a regular apparition. The knight always passes by here between twelve and one o'clock, and has been doing so for a very long time" — apparently, for centuries — "and everyone knows about it" (MDR, 188-190).

How should we interpret these dreams? Jung has some suggestions: He points out a conceptual connection between *Zoll* ("customs") and *Zensur* ("censorship"), inasmuch as both relate to the order of a border, be this the border between consciousness and the unconscious, or between Freud's psychology and his own. Intriguingly, Jung proposes that an analysis is like a border control: The embarrassment of having to open one's suitcases and have them checked for contraband is, he suggests, similar to the discovery of

[16] In his *Black Books*, this dream is recorded in the entry for 26 November 1913, where Jung interprets the customs guard as representing Freud and the knight as representing himself, while hinting that the dream speaks of larger issues, inasmuch as a voice in Jung's head calls out, "It is all empty and disgusting" (see BB 2, 160-161; cited in RB, "Introduction," 16).

unconscious assumptions and repressed desires. In that case, there is no doubt whom the sour-faced customs official represents: Freud himself! What about the second dream? Here Jung highlights the contrast between the figures of the customs official and the knight: the former "shadowy," someone who "still couldn't die properly," a "fading apparition," whereas the knight was "full of life" (*lebensvoll*) and "completely real" (*völlig wirklich*) (MDR, 187 and 189). Similarly, the scene on the Swiss-Austrian border was "dull" (*nüchtern*) and "not very impressive [*eindrucksvoll*]," whereas the second scene was "numinous in a high degree" (*in hohem Maße numinos*) (MDR, 189). Clearly, the second dream held a greater significance for Jung than the first — but what?

In the period following these dreams, i.e., in the years following 1911-1912 (which is, of course, the period during which work on *The Black Books*, then *The Red Book* began), Jung gave (or so we learn from *Memories, Dreams, Reflections*) a good deal of thought to the mysterious figure of the knight. After extensive meditation on the dream, Jung began to discern what its meaning might be. After all, the knight belonged to the 12th century, and the 12th century was the period when alchemy was beginning. But it was also the period of the quest for the Holy Grail, as Jung observes. The stories of the Grail had, as we have seen, been of "the greatest importance" to Jung, ever since he first read them at the age of 15 — a reading which is described as "an unforgettable experience" (*ein unverlierbares Erlebnis*) and as something that left "an impression that has never let go" of him (*ein Eindruck, der mich nie mehr losgelassen hat*) (ETG, 169). For Jung had the intuitive feeling that "a great secret" (*ein Geheimnis*) lay hidden in those stories (ETG, 189). Hence it seemed, we are told, quite natural that the dream should conjure up the world of the Grail Knights and their quest — as a symbol of Jung's sense of meaning and purpose in the world that had nothing whatsoever to do with Freud. "My whole being," we read, was "seeking for something still unknown which *might confer meaning upon the banality of life*" (ETG, 189).

This was one aspect of the Grail: the quest for "something still unknown" (*ein noch Unbekanntes*). A later chapter records how the quest for the Grail King and the image of the Fisher King had often come to his mind while working on his treatise called *Aion* (1951) and its discussion of the symbol of the *ikhthýs* (or ἰχθύς), the first-century Christian symbol composed of two intersecting arcs, the ends of the right side extending beyond the point of intersection to resemble the profile of a fish. Had it not been for the reluctance on Jung's part to intrude on the research of his wife, Emma Jung, who had been working on a study of the Grail legend which after her death was completed by Marie-Louise von Franz,[17] he would unquestionably have included the Grail legend in his studies of alchemy, we are told (MDR, 241). (Perhaps Emma Jung might have also appreciated it if Jung had been more reluctant to spend so much time with Toni Wolff?)

Another aspect was more personal: Jung's memory of his own father, Johann Paul Achilles Jung (1842-1896), as a kind of "Fisher King," as someone suffering from a sort of Anfortas wound — a wound that would not heal and a wound that is presented as "the Christian suffering for which the alchemists sought the panacea" (MDR, 241-242). (The circumlocutory remarks in *Memories, Dreams, Reflections* do not necessarily make it clear to readers what exactly Jung's father was suffering from, nor do we need to know… Suffice it to say that it seems to have involved a crisis of faith, a crisis of sexuality, and a crisis of intellect as well.) If his

[17] Emma Jung and Marie-Louise von Franz, *Die Graalslegende in psychologischer Sicht* (Zurich: Publications of the C.G. Jung Institute, 1960). In 1944, Emma Jung gave four lectures at the Psychological Club in Zurich titled *Die Graalssage: "Le Conte del Graal" von Chretien de Troyes: Psychologische Kommentare*, followed by a series of three lectures (held on 16 and 18 November and 2 December 1944) titled *Die Graalssage II: Le roman de l'estoire dou Graal von Robert de Boron*. This work fed into the study as revised and completed by von Franz.

father was Anfortas, this means that Jung himself was Parzival — *ein »thumber« Parzival*, a "dumb" Parzival who witnessed his father's sickness and yet never asked about it.

A later Grail dream is recorded in *Memories, Dreams, Reflections* that can be dated to 1938, the year when Jung accepted an invitation from the British Government in India to participate in celebrations of the 25th anniversary of the University of Calcutta (as it was then known). This was a journey on which Jung, despite or because of his knowledge of Indian philosophy and religious history, took with him the first volume of the *Theatrum Chemicum* (1602), which contains the principal writings of Gerhard Dorn (c. 1530-1584); during the voyage, Jung studied these writings from beginning to end. On the one hand, this choice of reading material reflects the intensive study of alchemical philosophy on which Jung was, at that time, engaged, and in which the trip to India formed a kind of intermezzo. On the other, it reflects his conviction of the value of "Oriental wisdom," as well as his belief that both European and Indian thought had emerged from "primordial psychic experiences of the unconscious" (*aus den seelischen Urerfahrungen des Unbewußten*) (ETG, 278) and had therefore produced "the same, similar, or at last comparable insights" (MDR, 304). Jung's impressions of "a foreign mentality and culture" (*eines fremden Kulturgeistes*) thus served, in an entirely uncolonial way, as "a point of constant contact" (*konstante Berührung*)[18] with "fundamently European intellectual traditions" (*ureuropäisches Gedankengut*) (ETG, 278).

Jung's trip took him to Allahabad, Benares, and Calcutta (or as we would call them today: Prayagraj, Varanasi, and Kolkata), in each of which he was honoured with a doctorate. (Jung's gratitude was expressed after his return to Zurich in the form of two articles

[18] The German phrase is thus precisely the opposite of the translation offered by Richard and Clara Winston, who translate it in terms of "constant counter[pointing]" (MDR, 304).

published in the magazine *Asia*, "The Dreamlike World of India" [January 1939] and "What India Can Teach Us" [February, 1939].) In Kolkata, Jung fell ill with dysentery and had to go into hospital, an experience which Jung cheerfully describes as offering a place where he could contemplate — using a Chinese phrase which reflects the principle of infinite creativity — "the ten thousand things."[19] On his return, in better health, to his hotel, Jung had another dream about the Grail.

In this dream, Jung found himself with many of his friends from Zurich on a small, unknown island off the coast of southern England. This island is described as a narrow strip of land running from north to south with a medieval castle situated on the rocky coast of its southern end. Like a group of tourists, Jung and his friends stand in its courtyard, looking up at its imposing keep, through the gate of which a wide stone staircase is visible, leading to columned hall, lit by candles. And Jung suddenly understands where he is: They are standing in front of the castle of — the Grail. That very evening, the Grail ceremony — or as it is expressed in the dream, "a celebration of the Grail" (*der Gral* [*werde*] *gefeiert*) — is going to take place (MDR, 311). Among the friends with Jung is an old German professor, described as being strikingly reminiscent of Mommsen, that is, Theodor Mommsen (1817-1903), the great German classical scholar. Jung is impressed with this figure's scholarly learning and sparkling intelligence, but he is bothered by one thing. Although this professor can talk learnedly about the relationship of the British to the French sources of the Grail story and has lots to say about a dead past, *he knows nothing about the*

[19] The expression "the ten thousand things" is an allusion to a line attributed by Aldous Huxley in *The Perennial Philosophy* to Sengcan, known as the Third Chinese Patriarch of Chán after Bodhidharma and 30th Patriarch after Siddhārtha Gautama Buddha, whose poem *Xinxin Ming* (i.e., "Inscription of Faith in Mind") includes the line, "When the Ten Thousand things are viewed in their oneness, we return to the Origin and remain where we have always been" (*The Perennial Philosophy* (London: Chatto & Windus, 1947), p. 21).

meaning of the legend and its living present (MDR, 311). For his part, however, Jung is "intensely" aware of both.

And so the professor continues on and on, as if he were in the lecture hall, *but he cannot see the staircase or the festive glow in the hall*, however much Jung tries to draw them to his attention. Looking around him, Jung realizes that he is standing next to the castle wall, and he notices an interesting detail: The lower part of the wall is decorated with a kind of trellis, made not of wood but of black iron, skillfully formed into a grapevine with leaves, tendrils, and grapes; on the horizontal branches of this grapevine are little iron houses. Then suddenly, something moves, and in the foliage, Jung sees a tiny, iron hooded gnome, a *cucullatus* (or "hooded" figure), scurrying from one house to the next. "Now, will you look at that ...," Jung says in astonishment to the professor, and the dream changes.

The same group of friends, minus the professor, is now standing *outside* the castle in a rocky landscape without trees. Jung senses that something had to happen, because the Grail is not yet in the castle, but the ceremony was due to take place that very evening. The Grail, it seems, has been hidden in a small, abandoned house in the northern part of the island, and Jung realizes that it falls to him and his friends to go and bring the Grail to the castle. And so six of them set out and begin their journey to the north. After several hours of strenuous walking, they reach the narrowest part of the island, divided into two halves by an inlet of the sea. By now, the sun has set, and night is descending, and Jung and his friends make camp for the night on the ground, overlooking the hundred yards or so of water that forms the narrowest part of the inlet. The landscape is bleak and desolate; only grass and rocks, no trees and no shrubs; and it is cold. One after the other, Jung's friends fall asleep, until only he is awake, wondering what to do. Until he concludes that he alone must swim across the water *and fetch the Grail*. And as in the dream he undresses — Jung suddenly awoke.

There is so much to say about this dream, which is relatively little discussed compared with Jung's childhood visions of the subterranean phallus or God defecating onto the roof of Basel Cathedral, or the dream of the two-story house with a cellar (MDR, 182-183). First, it is obviously a critique of academia: The Mommsen-like professor knows everything there is to know about the Grail legend, but he has no actual understanding of it. In terms of the hermeneutic distinction made by Wilhelm Dilthey (1833-1911), the professor can *erklären* ("explain"), but he cannot *verstehen* ("understand"). Jung, by contrast, is able to do both, and he is said to be alert to the "meaning" (*Sinn*) of the legend as well as its "living present" (*lebendige Gegenwart*). Second, in the trelliswork on the castle wall there is the symbolism of the grapes, recalling the dream from 1914 of a leaf-bearing tree (described as the "tree of life"), whose leaves are transformed by the effects of frost into sweet grapes, full of healing juices, which Jung plucks and gives to a large, waiting crowd (MDR, 200),[20] as well as the symbolism of Jung's coat of arms, with its blue cross in the upper right and blue grapes in a field of gold in the lower left, separated by a blue bar with a gold star, which is said to be Masonic or Rosicrucian in its symbolism of "heavenly" and "chthonic" elements (MDR, 259).

Third, there is the little, gnomelike hooded figure of the *cucullatus*, equivalent to the *kabir* figures of the manikin carved by Jung as a child which he kept in a pencil case in the loft (MDR, 36-39), the homunculus or Telesphorus of Asklepios that Jung carved in stone at his Tower in Bollingen (MDR, 253-254), or the Cabiri — derived from F.W.J. Schelling via Goethe — that feature in *The Red Book* (RB, 425-429). These enigmatic, chthonic deities were worshipped as part of the mystery cult associated with Hephaestus

[20] For further discussion of this dream, see Peter Homans, *Jung in Context: Modernity and the Making of a Psychology* (Chicago and London: University of Chicago Press, 1979), pp. 79-80; citing John E. Gedo, *Magna est vis veritatis tuae et praevalebit: Comments on the Freud-Jung Correspondence* (unpublished MS).

found on Lemnos and Samothrace, and the figure of the *kabir* is linked by Jung with "the creative impulse," "a supply of life-force," and ultimately "the breath of life" (MDR, 39). At the same time, in the context of Jung's visit to India, the *cucullatus* is a kind of external equivalent to the homunculus in the alchemical retort — a figure which Jung uses as a way to describe how, during in his trip, he "remained within himself" (MDR, 304). In fact, Jung remained so within himself during this journey that when, on the way back, the ship docked at Bombay (or Mumbai), he decided not to go ashore and visit the city but "buried himself in his Latin alchemical texts" (MDR, 314)!

Finally, there is Jung's own interpretation of this dream. For Jung, it represents "a quintessentially European dream" (*dieser ureuropäische Traum*), and it is significant that it emerged while Jung was working his way through the overwhelming variety of his impressions from India (MDR, 312). Ten years earlier, we are told, Jung had apparently discovered that the myth of the Grail was alive and well in England and that, "despite all the scholarship that has accumulated around this tradition," *der Traum vom Gral noch nicht ausgeträumt ist* — a sentence one might paraphrase as "the dream of the Grail shall never die!" (MDR, 312). Jung had been struck by the "concordance" or "agreement" (*Übereinstimmung*) between, on the one hand, the "poetic myth" (*poetischer Mythus*) of the Grail legend and, on the other, the tradition of alchemy with its *unum vas* ("the one vessel"), the *una medicina* ("the one medicine"), and the *unus lapis* ("the one stone") (MDR, 312). At this juncture, Jung makes a programmatic statement about his entire approach to culture:

> Myths which day has forgotten continue to be told by night, and powerful figures which consciousness has reduced to banality and ridiculous triviality are recognized again by poets and prophetically revived;

> therefore they can also be recognized "in changed form" [*in veränderter Gestalt*] by the thoughtful person. The great ones of the past have not died, as we like to think; they have merely changed their names. "Small and slight, but great in might," the veiled *kabir* enters a new house. (MDR, 312)

The fundamental thesis of this proposition is clear enough, but it also supports the argument that there is a fundamental continuity with the German tradition as expressed in the four works studied in this series. For in this statement Jung has artfully woven in two allusions to Goethe's *Faust*: "in changed form" (*in veränderter Gestalt*) echoes the words of the figure of Sorge in Part Two (*in verwandelter Gestalt / Üb'ich grimmige Gewalt*) (ll. 11426-11427), while "Small and slight, but great in might" (*Klein von Gestalt, / Groß von Gewalt*) is obviously a reference to the "Cabiri Scene" in the Classical Walpurgisnacht (ll. 8174-8175).[21]

So this dream is said to have wiped away all the intensive impressions of India and to have returned Jung to "the all-too-long-neglected concerns of the Occident" which had formerly been expressed in the quest for the Holy Grail as well as in the search for the "philosophers' stone" (MDR, 312-313). Thus seen, Jung's visit to India had served to remind him that his real goal was nothing to do with the East and everything to do with the West:[22] It urged him to seek for himself and for those like him "the healing vessel, the

[21] For Jung's use of this second phrase in the context of occult phenomena and externalized psychic energy in general and of UFOs in particular, see Jaffé, *Streiflichter zu Leben und Denken C.G. Jungs*, p. 122.

[22] Jung's statement that "India was not my task [*nicht meine Aufgabe*], but only a part of the way [*ein Stück des Weges*] — admittedly a significant one —which should carry me closer to my goal [*meinem Ziel annähern*]" (MDR, 313), is reminiscent of that passage in *Ecce Homo* where Nietzsche says that "even the *blunders* of life — the temporary sidepaths and wrong turnings, the delays, the "modesties," the seriousness squandered on tasks [*Aufgaben*] which lie outside *the* task [*jenseits* der *Aufgabe*] — have their own meaning and value" (EH Why I am So Clever §9).

servator/salvator mundi [i.e., the servant or saviour of the world], which you urgently need" (MDR, 313).[23] On Jung's account, this task is especially urgent, because we are "in imminent danger of destroying everything that centuries have built up" (MDR, 313).

Yet Jung did not regard himself as being an entirely solitary figure in this task. For, in his seminar on Nietzsche's *Zarathustra*, Jung related the Grail legend to the task that Nietzsche had undertaken in this work. On 26 October 1938, Jung reminded his audience how Nietzsche had chosen the figure of Zarathustra because the historical Zoroaster had been the originator of the moral opposites of good and evil. (In *Ecce Homo*, Nietzsche writes that because Zarathustra was "the first to see in the struggle between good and evil the actual wheel in the working of things" and "*created* this most fateful of errors, morality," "consequently he must also be the first to *recognize* it" [EH Why I am a Destiny §3].) Or as Jung put it, if the historical Zoroaster had "caused that great split in humanity of the moral problem," Nietzsche's Zarathustra has to be understood as "a Saoshyant, a new savior," who "has to come back in order to heal the wound he caused," and as a result Nietzsche conceived the *Übermensch* as "the man who was beyond that wound, who had healed that wound" (SNZ, vol. 2, p. 364).[24]

And it is this idea, Jung adds, that one finds in the Grail mystery embodied in the figure of Anfortas, that is, in "the suffering

---

[23] MDR corrects ETG's *salvator mundi* to *servator mundi* (MDR, 313; cf. ETG, 286). On this expression, see Peter Kingsley's comment: "*Servator mundi* is an older form of *salvator mundi* and means preserver or saviour of the world. In ancient and then medieval texts they were both standard ways of referring to Jesus Christ. Inside the Latin alchemical literature Jung was so familiar with, it's exactly the same story. […] But by using this particular expression — *servator mundi*, cosmic protector or preserver — he was making a link that binds Christ to the central essence of his own work and duty and labour far tighter, stronger, closer" (*Catafalque*, vol. 1, pp. 132-133). For a scholarly gloss on both terms, see *Catafalque*, vol. 2, pp. 550-551.

[24] For the relation of the Saoshyant figure to the Grail legend, see the anthroposophical (as well as astrosophical) study by Arthur Schult (1893-1969) titled *Die Weltsendung des Heiligen Gral im Parzival des Wolfram von Eschenbach* (Bietigheim-Bissingen: Turm-Verlag, 1975).

king who is to be cured by a savior [...] the Christian man who carries that mortal wound, as the Persian man was rent asunder by Zarathustra's teaching" (SNZ, vol. 2, p. 1364). On this account, Nietzsche saw his task in the history of the world as being "to cure man of that incurable wound he has suffered from hithero," and Jung adds that Nietzsche "was not simply playing with this idea"; rather, it was "a deep-rooted conviction in him amounting to a sort of mystical experience" (1364). For Jung, Nietzsche's little poem, "Sils-Maria," with its famous lines, *Da, plötzlich, Freundin! wurde Eins zu Zwei — / — Und Zarathustra gieng an mir vorbei* ("Then, suddenly, friend, one turned into two — / — And Zarathustra walked into my view"),[25] expresses "the visionary living nature of the Zarathustra experience," meaning that Zarathustra was "always more than a speech metaphor" and was "a more or less real figure" (1365).

And then Jung makes another move, pointing out that Nietzsche was a contemporary of Richard Wagner, and arguing that "it is not without meaning that Wagner occupied himself with *Parsifal*, which contains this very problem" (SNZ, vol. 2, p. 1365) (and Wagner's *Parsifal* is, of course, based largely on Wolfram's *Parzival*).[26] Curiously enough, Jung observes, it was precisely the opera *Parsifal* which caused the final estrangement between Nietzsche and Wagner, alluding to the accusation leveled in *Nietzsche contra Wagner* that in *Parsifal* Wagner "suddenly fell helpless and broken on his knees before the Christian cross ..." (NCW How I Got Rid of Wagner §1). On Jung's account, however, Nietzsche's focus on "the so-called Christian gesture or the Christian sentimentality" of Wagner's *Parsifal* was missing the

[25] Friedrich Nietzsche, *The Gay Science*, ed. and trans. Walter Kaufmann (New York: Vintage Books, 1974), pp. 370-371.

[26] For further discussion, see Mary A. Cicora, "Medievalism and Metaphysics: The Literary Background of *Parsifal*," and James M. McGlathery, "Erotic Love in Chrétien's *Perceval*, Wolfram's *Parzival*, and Wagner's *Parsifal*," in William Kinderman and Katherine R. Syer (eds), *A Companion to Wagner's "Parsifal"* (Rochester, NY, and Woodbridge: Camden House, 2005), pp. 29-53 and 55-79.

point, because "he was not aware of the deeper meaning of that whole fact," by which Jung means "the fact of the occurrence of that idea at that time" (SNZ, vol. 2, p. 1365). In other words, Wagner's *Parsifal* should be understood as "the parallel" of *Zarathustra*, while *Zarathustra* is "the other aspect of the same thing, only expressed in entirely different terms [...] in an unhistorical milieu, in a setting which was beyond history" (1365):[27]

> Zarathustra is in a way historical, but Wagner remained very much more in the tradition, using a legend which was well known and still much appreciated. And he only went back to the Middle Ages, while Nietzsche made a much further regression, going back into the 8th or 9th century BC to fetch his figure or analogy, his myth. But the actual ideas are very much the same — the idea of the cure of the incurable wound. (SNZ, vol. 2, p. 1365).

Thus, Jung explicitly sets up a link between the ancient Persian Zoroaster, the medieval Parzival, and the modern parallel between Nietzsche's *Zarathustra* and Wagner's *Parsifal*.[28]

Now while one can think of plenty of examples of scholars who exemplify the type of professorial pseudo-Mommsen figure in Jung's dream, no one could accuse Peter Kingsley of having no interest in the meaning of the Grail legend or its living presentness. In

[27] See Roger Hollinrake, *Nietzsche, Wagner, and the Philosophy of Pessimism* (London: Allen & Unwin, 1982), which reads *Zarathustra* as an essentially anti-Wagnerian pastiche and polemic.

[28] To this tradition one might add Friedrich Schiller (1759-1805), who declared in his *Aesthetic Education of Humankind* (1794) that "it was civilization [*die Kultur*] which inflicted this wound upon modern man" (Letter 6, §6) and called for us "to restore by means of a higher Art [*eine höhre Kunst*] the totality in our nature which the arts [*die Kunst*] themselves destroyed" (Letter 6, §15) (*On the Aesthetic Education of Humankind*, ed. and trans. Elizabeth M. Wilkinson and L.A. Willoughby (Oxford: Clarendon Press, 1982), pp. 32-33 and 42-43).

Catafalque, Kingsley is insistent precisely on this living significance of the Grail myth, especially in relation to Jung. Referring to the unpublished Jaffé Protocols, Kingsley draws out the link between individuation as a mystery and the mystery of the Grail, arguing that individuation is "a secret that has to remain a total mystery because, in approaching it, even the slightest possibility of human comprehension comes to a very abrupt and sudden end":

> By its very nature, the whole subject is such a secret that it's something no one will ever be able to grasp or understand. And [Jung] explains, in detail, how the mystery of individuation is the mystery of the Grail. [...] The secret of individuation is that the one and only way to discover the Grail is by being it. It will forever remain undiscovered, and undiscoverable, except by simply becoming it. [...] This, as it were, is the quintessential myth behind Jung's psychology: the myth of individuation.[29]

On Kingsley's account, the mystery of individuation as the mystery of the Grail (110 and 140) is the path to an experience of deification or becoming a god, or identifying with "the 'Christ within'" as a symbol of our higher self, of the divine reality hidden inside us (110-117). Yet in the meantime the sacred, the divine or the numinous has been turned into a "therapeutic resource" (121), thereby ignoring the fact that Jung's fundamental concern was the soul of humanity (122).

Drawing on the unpublished Jaffé Protocols, Kingsley points out that Jung's account of this dream of 1939 as described to Aniela Jaffé in one of their interview sessions had included a number of details that are omitted from the version in *Memories, Dreams,*

[29] Kingsley, *Catafalque*, vol. 1, pp. 110-111.

Reflections. First, the friends who were with him on the island were members of the Psychological Club that he had helped found in Zurich. Second, his emphasis on how they arrived at the castle as sightseeing tourists suggests that he was well aware that some of the early Jungians were simply there "for the view" but were only prepared to go so far. And third, on the moment when everyone else arounds him falls asleep, leaving him alone to fetch the Grail, Jung is said to have observed that those friends were like the disciples in the garden of Gethsemane, leaving Christ to pray alone.[30]

With characteristic acuity and shrewdness, Kingsley notes that, in his essay on "The Philosophical Tree" (1945; 1954), Jung had identified the figure of Christ in the garden of Gethsemane as a kind of parallel or prefiguration of "the arcanum" or the (philosopher's) "stone," and hence of "the alchemical *servator cosmi* (preserver of the cosmos), representing the still unconscious idea of the whole and complete individual, who shall bring about what the sacrificial death of Christ has obviously left unfinished, namely the deliverance of the world from evil," and thus anticipating "a future Christ and *salvator microcosmi*" (CW 13 §390). On this account, this late Grail dream ultimately indicates that Jung is "no longer just the brave knight dedicated to rediscovering at all costs the healing vessel of the *servator mundi*," but he has "become the healing vessel himself: Christ the preserver, saviour of the world."[31]

Jung's Letter of 1926

We can read a letter by Jung written (to an unidentified correspondent) in 1926 as addressing Wolfram's Grail question, "what ails thee?" In this letter (not included in his published correspondence) Jung makes the following confession: "[…] I consciously and intentionally made my life miserable, because I wanted God to be

[30] Kingsley, *Catafalque*, vol. 1, pp. 133-134.
[31] Kingsley, *Catafalque*, vol. 1, p. 134.

alive and free from the suffering man has put on him by loving his own reason more than God's secret intentions."[32] In making this remark, Kingsley argues, Jung is "taking his place, very knowingly and deliberately, inside a long tradition of prophecy."[33] For (as Kingsley explains in one of his copious footnotes) this remark about "want[ing] God to be alive and free" echoes Jung's earlier question in "Nox tertia" in *The Red Book*, "Is there a suffering that would be too great to want to undergo for our God?" and his own confession, "For I took my misdeed upon myself so that the God would be healed" (RB, 355-356).

As Kingsley notes, both this question and the confession are steeped in the prophetic language of Isaiah (63:2-6),[34] the biblical prophet whom Jung had cited at the very start of *Liber Primus* (Isaiah 53:1-4; cf. RB, 117).[35] (Isaiah was active in the eighth century B.C.E..) In fact, it is worth noting that Isaiah, especially the prophetic text of Isaiah 9:6, is associated liturgically with the season of Advent, which occupies the period of the year when Jung began working on *The Red Book*;[36] and even Isaiah 53:1-4, from the fourth Song of the Servant, with its theme of suffering which

---

[32] Gerhard Adler, "Aspects of Jung's Personality and Work," *Psychological Perspectives*, vol. 6, no. 1 (1975), 11-12 (p. 12).

[33] Kingsley, *Catafalque*, vol. 1, p. 342; cf. vol. 1, pp. 337-338.

[34] In what the commentary in New Jerusalem Bible (NJB) calls "a fine fragment of apocalyptic poetry," a dialogue between Yahweh and the prophet Isaiah presents Yahweh as a grape-harvester whose clothes are stained with juice (NJB, OT, 1287).

[35] These lines form part of the last of the four "Songs of the Servant of Yahweh," four lyrical passages that depict (in the words of the NJB) "a perfect servant of Yahweh — re-gatherer of his people and light of the nations — one who preaches the true faith, who expiates the people's sins by his own death and is glorified by God" and that "rank among the most closely studied texts in the Old Testament" (NJB, OT, 1169). In the fourth song, the servant takes up the theme of suffering, presenting the persecutions which the servant will very patiently endure and scandalize the spectators as in fact an intercession and an expiation of sins" (NJB, OT, 1273).

[36] In the traditional Divine Office, the use of passages from Isaiah as a source for antiphons and the sequential reading of Isaiah at Matins mark the liturgical season of Advent.

is associated liturgically with Passiontide,[37] is linked by Jung, somewhat surprisingly, in *Psychological Types* with "the birth of the Saviour, the redeeming symbol" as something that occurs "just when one is least expecting it, and in the most improbable of places" (CW 6 §439). Similarly, one of the two quotations from another great biblical prophet, Jeremiah (seventh/sixth centuries B.C.E.), that are placed at the opening of *Liber Secundus* (Jeremiah 23:16 and 25-28; cf. RB, 211) is cited in *Psychological Types* in the context of his account of how Christianity has suppressed fantasy (CW 6 §78-§86).[38] (And in *The Psychology of the Transference* (1946) Jung prefaces his account of the transference phenomena based on the illustrations to the 16th-century alchemical treatise *Rosarium philosophorum* with a quotation from Jeremiah, "The people […] found grace in the desert" [31:2; cf. CW 16 p. 202].)

The fact that both extracts from Jeremiah are taken from a passage described by the New Jerusalem Bible as a tract against false prophets underscores Kingsley's view of the prophetic dimension of *The Red Book*.[39] These correspondences between Jung's letter of 1926 and *The Red Book* should suffice, in Kingsley's words, to "dispose once and for all of the claims sometimes made nowadays that the *Red Book* was little more than a literary exercise or some detached and impersonal experiment in ventriloquism" —[40] and

[37] In the traditional liturgy for Wednesday in Holy Week, Isaiah 62:11; 63:1-7 and Isaiah 53: 1-12 constitute the first and second readings at Mass. For further discussion of this prophetic text and its relevance for the textual origins of Christianity, see Richard E. Averbeck, "Christian Interpretations of Isaiah 43," in Darrell L. Bock and Mitch Glaser (eds), *The Gospel According to Isaiah 53: Encountering the Suffering Servant in Jewish and Christian Theology* (Grand Rapids, MI: Kegel, 2012), pp. 33-60; cited by Kingsley, *Catafalque*, vol. 2, p. 711.

[38] From the Second Sunday of the Passion or Palm Sunday onward, the first readings in the traditional Divine Office at Matins are from the Book of Jeremiah, while in the liturgical service of Tenebrae on the last three days of Holy Week (Maundy Thursday, Good Friday, and Holy Saturday), the lessons of the first Nocturn of Matins are taken from the Book of Lamentations, ascribed to Jeremiah.

[39] Kingsley, *Catafalque*, vol. 2, pp. 667-668.

[40] Kingsley, *Catafalque*, vol. 2, p. 710; cf. *Catafalque*, vol. 1, pp. 339-340: "It's the norm nowadays in our post-modern, post-structural world to note those opening

the same might be said for the correspondences between *The Red Book* and Wolfram's *Parzival*, Goethe's *Faust*, and Nietzsche's *Zarathustra*. (After all, as we shall see in Volumes 2 and 3 in this series, the narrative of Goethe's *Faust* is set against the background of another biblical prophet, namely: Job; and Nietzsche's *Zarathustra* constitutes a veritable kind of "anti-Bible.")

In fact, in his seminar on Nietzsche's *Zarathustra*, Jung defines "the true prophet" as "the man who in his personal life experiences the fate of his people, and who also tries to find the remedy in his personal life for the disease or the misery of his people," citing the case of Hosea, whom Yahweh instructed to marry a whore and get children with a whore, as an example (Hosea 1:2-3; cf. SNZ, vol. 1, p. 496). As the commentary in the NJB points out, while prophets often performed "symbolic actions" (such as Jeremiah's visit to the potter, or the various acts performed by Ezekiel to foretell the siege of Jerusalem), here Hosea's "very life is symbolic of God's mysterious designs."[41] In so acting, Hosea was — according to the earlier commentator, George Leo Haydock (1774-1849) — representing "the Lord's proceedings with his people Israel, who, by spiritual fornication, were continually offending him."[42] While Jung questioned the extent to which Nietzsche's own life could be described as prophetic (we simply "don't know"), he nevertheless characterized Nietzsche as "a dangerous prophet" who "has surely anticipated in words what the unconscious was preparing" and he declared that *Zarathustra* was "certainly […] highly prophetic" (SMZ, vol. 1, p. 496). (As we shall see in Volume 3 in this series, from the outset of his *Zarathustra* seminar Jung compared the figure of Zarathustra to the Saoshyant, an Avestan

quotations from Isaiah for half a second or perhaps even two and rapidly move on to the rest of the text before leaving that behind as well. But […] they are there not only to set the tone for the rest of his 'new book' but, at the same time, to set the tone and serve as model for the rest of his life."

[41] NJB, OT, 1495.

[42] See H, 1112.

expression for an eschatological saviour; cf. SNZ, vol. 1, pp. 12-13 and 24).

On Kingsley's reading of the second part of the sentence from 1926 where Jung talks about humankind "loving his own reason more than God's secret intentions," Jung is suggesting here that "reason has become God's enemy" and that "not just every minute but every moment of our compulsive reasoning, our obsessively reasonable act or word or thought, each tolerably scholarly murder, is a direct offence against the sacred."[43] In this respect, Jung's letter is said to be pointing to "the need deep inside each of us to reach back prophetically to the forgotten logic which has been murdered, which keeps being murdered, by reason itself."[44] Consequently — yet "unnoticed," because there is "such a heavy cost for noticing" — "each statement Jung is making in his letter is the statement of a prophet."[45]

In this letter of 1926, Jung goes on: "Thus I suffered and was miserable, but it seems that life was never wanting and in the blackest night even, and just there, by the grace of God, I could see a Great Light. Somewhere there seems to be great kindness in the abysmal darkness of the deity."[46] In this remarkable passage, Jung echoes several biblical ideas, many of which he took up and discussed in his *Answer to Job* (1952). In Isaiah, Chapter 60, in a passage on the splendor of Jerusalem suffused with imagery of radiance and light, a writer designated as Second Isaiah (or at least one of Isaiah's disciples) calls out, "Arise, be enlightened, O Jerusalem: for thy light is come, and the glory of the Lord is risen upon thee," and declares, "the Lord shall be unto thee for an everlasting light" (Isaiah 60:1 and 19); and (as we saw in Chapter 2) John in his first letter repeats, "God is light, and in him there is

[43] Kinsgley, *Catafalque*, vol. 1, p. 342.
[44] Kingsley, *Catafalque*, vol. 1, p. 343.
[45] Kingsley, *Catafalque*, vol. 1, p. 343.
[46] Adler, "Aspects of Jung's Personality and Work," p. 12.

no darkness" (1 John 1:5). In the First Book of Kings, however, Solomon brings the Ark of the Covenant into the Temple, and, as Yahweh takes possession of his Temple, he declares, "The LORD said that he would dwell in the thick darkness" (1 Kings 8:12, KJV; cf. 2 Chronicles 6:1). This scene echoes the one in the second discourses of Moses in Deuteronomy, where Moses announces the Ten Commandments, adding: "These words the Lord spoke to all the multitude of you in the mountain, out of the midst of the fire and the cloud, and the [thick] darkness, with a loud voice" (Deut. 5: 22), and in Psalm 97 (96), we read, "The Lord hath reigned, let the earth rejoice: [...]. Clouds and [thick] darkness are round about him" (v. 1-2). The choice of thick darkness for the dwelling place of God is often explained in terms of human weakness and our inability to bear the blaze of the divine majesty (see H, 764).

In the episode of Moses on the mountain in Exodus, Chapter 13, Moses asks Yahweh, "Shew me thy glory," a request explained by Haydock with reference to the angel, sent before the Israelites (33:2) and conducting the pillar of cloud by day (and the pillar of fire by night) (cf. Exodus 13:21-22). Either this angel had assumed human form — a form which Moses knew could not fully display the majesty of Yahweh, hence he begged to see His face or His "glory" (cf. vv. 13 and 18), even if Yahweh had declared that this is impossible for any mortal, since the divine effulgence would cause death (cf. v. 20) — or he was robed in darkness, which Moses begged to be removed, a request interpreted by many commentators (such as St. Augustine of Hippo or Philo of Alexandria) as a desire to contemplate the divine essence and by Tertullian as a wish to behold the Messiah (see H, 112). Because Yahweh, via the angel, usually spoke to Moses in the pillar of the cloud, so that Moses, while speaking with Yahweh "face to face, as a man is wont to speak to his friend" (v. 11), could not see His glory, in the vision granted here Moses is allowed to see something of Yahweh in an assumed corporeal form; that is to say, Moses is allowed to look at

Yahweh, not in His face, the rays of which are too bright for mortal eyes to bear, but to view Him as it were from behind, while His face was turned away (see H, 112).

Even in Isaiah, Yahweh declares, "I form the light, and create darkness,"[47] and represents the nations as saying, "Verily, thou art a hidden God, the God of Israel, the Saviour" (Isaiah 45:7 and 15), the source of the doctrine of the *deus absconditus* or the idea of the fundamental unknowability of God. Equally, in another well-known passage from Isaiah, the prophet speaks — after the vision of everlasting peace and the injunction, "O house of Jacob, come ye, and let us walk in the light of the Lord" (2:1-5), the account of the call of Isaiah (Chapter 6), and the story of King Ahaz's request for a sign that elicits the response, "Behold a virgin shall conceive and bear a son" (7:10-17) — of deliverance in terms of a shift from wandering in "anguish, gloom, the confusion of night, swirling darkness" (8:21-23) into joyful luminosity, "The people that walked in darkness, have seen a great light" (9:2).

The biblical tradition on which Jung drew when he spoke about "the abysmal darkness of the deity" and "a Great Light" also informed such later mystics as Pseudo-Dionysius the Areopagite, the late fifth-/early sixth-century theologian and Neoplatonic philosopher who identified himself as the Athenian convert of St. Paul the Apostle, called Dionysius the Areopagite (see Acts 17:34). In his *Divine Names*, Dionysius (let's play along with his self-portrayal) advances what is called a *negative theology* by arguing that "we attribute a lack of reason to [God] because he is above reason, we attribute a lack of perfection to him because he is above and before perfection, and we posit intangible and invisible darkness of that Light which is unapproachable because it so far exceeds the

[47] In relation to the notion of Yahweh as a God of light and darkness, Jung is said to have frequently quoted Isaiah 45:6-7: "I am the Lord, and there is none else. I form the light, and create darkness; I make peace, and create evil; I, the Lord, that do all these things"; see Jaffé, *Streiflichter zu Leben und Denken C.G. Jungs*, p. 217.

visible light."[48] Dionysius tries to explain how "the divine Mind does not acquire knowledge of things from things," but is rather "a single embracing causality which knows and contains all things," and he develops this explanation by taking the example of light: "In itself it has a prior and causal knowledge of darkness. What it knows about darkness it knows not from another, but from the fact of being light. So too the divine Wisdom knows all things by knowing itself."[49]

In the first chapter of *The Mystical Theology*, Dionysius introduces the notion of "the divine darkness," and he opens with an appeal to the Holy Trinity to "lead us up beyond unknowing and light, up to the farthest highest peak of mystic scripture, where the mysteries of God's Word lie simple, absolute and unchangeable in the brilliant darkness of a hidden silence."[50] Citing the authority of the apostle Bartholomew, Dionysius envisages passing "beyond the summit of every holy ascent" and leaving behind "every divine light, every voice, every word from heaven," in order to "plunge into the darkness where, as scripture proclaims, there dwells the One who is beyond all things."[51] In so writing, Dionysius refers to the example of Moses and his experience in Exodus, where Moses "breaks free" of "the heights of those holy places to which the mind at least can rise," and "plunges into the truly mysterious darkness of unknowing" (or in the words of the anonymous English 14th-century treatise, "the cloud of unknowing") and "here, renouncing

[48] Pseudo-Dionysius, *The Complete Works*, trans. Colm Luibheid, ed. Paul Rorem (New York and Mahwah, NJ: Paulist Press, 1987), p. 107; cf. 1 Timothy 6:16, which says of Jesus Christ that he "inhabiteth light inaccessible, whom no man hath seen, nor can see." For further discussion, see Ronald F. Hathaway, *Hierarchy and the Definition of Order in the "Letters" of Pseudo-Dionysius: A Study in the Form and Meaning of the Pseudo-Dionysian Writings* (The Hague: Nijhoff, 1969).
[49] Pseudo-Dionysius, *Complete Works*, p. 108.
[50] Pseudo-Dionysius, *Complete Works*, p. 135.
[51] Pseudo-Dionysius, *Complete Works*, p. 136. See. Exodus 20:21; cf. Exodus 19.

all the mind may conceive, [...] knows beyond the mind by knowing nothing."[52]

In the second chapter, Dionysius prays that we may come to "this darkness so far above light," and that we may "unhiddenly know that unknowing which itself is hidden from all those possessed of knowing amid all beings, so that we may see above being that darkness concealed from all the light among beings."[53] Referring back to his own lost (or, more probably, simply fictitious) treatise titled *The Symbolic Theology*, Dionysius argues that "the more we take flight upward, the more our words are confined to the ideas we are capable of forming; so that now as we plunge into that darkness which is beyond intellect, we shall find ourselves not simply running short of words but actually speechless and unknowing."[54]

Dionysius rehearses the same idea in his correspondence, writing to a monk called Gaius that "darkness disappears in the light, the more so as there is more light" and that "knowing makes unknowing disappear, the more so as there is more knowledge," but adding that one should think of this, not in terms of "deprivation," but in terms of "transcendence": "The unknowing regarding God escapes anyone possessing physical light and knowledge of beings: His transcendent darkness remains hidden from all light and concealed from all knowledge."[55] And in a letter to Dorotheus the deacon, Dionysius declares that "the divine darkness is that 'unapproachable light' where God is said to live" and that "if it is invisible because of a superabundant clarity, if it cannot be

[52] Pseudo-Dionysius, *Complete Works*, p. 137. In his *Life of Moses* (and in §152-§169 in particular), Gregory of Nyssa offered a detailed commentary on the biblical narrative of Moses's ascent (Exodus 19 and 20:18-21) in a way that anticipates many themes found in Dionysius. See Gregory of Nyssa, *The Life of Moses*, ed. and trans. Abraham J. Malherbe and Everett Ferguson (New York and Mahwah, NJ: Paulist Press, 1978), pp. 91-97.
[53] Pseudo-Dionysius, *Complete Works*, p. 138.
[54] Pseudo-Dionysius, *Complete Works*, p. 139.
[55] Pseudo-Dionysius, *Complete Works*, p. 263.

approached because of the outpouring of its transcendent gift of light, yet it is here that is found everyone worthy to know God and to look upon him."[56]

It is into this theological and especially mystical tradition that Jung, by speaking in his letter of 1926 about "the abysmal darkness of the deity" as well as "the Great Light," is inserting himself. In fact, when one looks closely, one can see evidence of him doing so in numerous places: from an inscription on a mural at Bollingen, which includes a line from an alchemical text, *Ego gigno lumen, tenebrae autem naturae meae sunt* ("I give birth to light, even though my nature is darkness"),[57] via his sense as a child of being an initiate into the realms of darkness (as recorded in MDR) and his claims that a dark substance (*dunkle Substanz*) linked him to the alchemists (as reported in the Jaffé Protocols), to his identification with Mercurius as "the primordial light-bringer, who is never himself the light" (CW 13 §300). In *The Red Book*, Jung warned against that "believ[ing] that we can illuminate the darkness with an intention, and in that way aim past the light," and he cautioned: "How can we presume to want to know in advance, from where the light will come to us?" (RB, 144).

Then again, in his chapter on the conjunction in his late, great work, *Mysterium coniunctionis* (1955-1956), Jung remarks the modern individuals cannot even "bring about the *unio mentalis*" — that is, the uniting of spirit and soul, the first of the three stages of the alchemical *coniunctio* as described by Gerhard Dorn in his *De Philosophia meditativa* (*On the Meditative Philosophy*) — which is "required to accomplish the second degree of alchemical conjunction," that is, the *unio corporalis*, or the conjoining of the

[56] Pseudo-Dionysius, *Complete Works*, p. 265; see 1 Timothy 6:16; and cf. Exodus 20:21 and *Mystical Theology*, §1, 1000C 33ff. (*Complete Works*, pp. 136-137).

[57] *Rosarium philosophorum*, in *Artis auriferae*, vol. 2 (Basel 1953), pp. 239-240; cited in Kingsley, *Catafalque*, vol. 1, p. 150 (cf. vol. 2, pp. 563-564). On light and darkness, see *Catafalque*, pp. 150-151 and 548-549.

unity of spirit and soul with the body (CW 14 §752). Like the alchemist apprentice in the past, the modern individual is said to begin with an unseemly *prima materia,* which presents itself "in an unexpected form," perhaps as "a contemptible fantasy" which, like the biblical stone which the builders rejected (Psalm 118:22-23), is "flung into the street" and is so "cheap" that no one even wants to look at it (§752). Yet if we observe this *prima materia* day by day and note its alterations, Jung continues, eventually our eyes shall be opened; or, expressed in alchemical parlance, "until the fish's eyes, or the sparks, shine in the dark solution" (§752).[58]

For the light that gradually dawns on us, if only we allow it to, consists in coming to understand that our fantasy (*Phantasie*) is "a real psychic process" which is happening to us personally (§752). To the extent that we "look on from the outside," we are "impartial"; yet we are *also* an "acting and suffering figure in the drama of the psyche," and it is essential that we realize this — it is an "important advance" (§753). So as long as we simply *look at* the pictures, we are "like the foolish Parsifal [*der törichte Parzival*] who forgot to ask the vital question *because he was not aware of his own participation in the action*" (§753; my italics). We might note here the parallel to (and the contrast with) Faust in the "Hall of Chivalry" scene in *Faust II,* where he conjures up the spirits of Paris and Helena, and gets all too involved, intervening to prevent the rape of Helena and causing an explosion, after which the

[58] On the *scintillae* ("sparks") or *oculi piscium* ("fishes' eyes"), discussed with reference to the alchemists Morienus Romanus (in the 12th century), Sir George Ripley (c. 1415-1490), and Gerhard Dorn (c.15330-1584), see CW 14 §45. In "On the Nature of the Psyche" (1947; 1954), Jung links the "shining eyes, which were yet no eyes" of the serpent in a vision of St. Ignatius of Loyola (1491-1556) with the fish's eyes which crop up in later alchemical authors, and which are said to have the same significance as motif of sparks or *scintillae*, i.e., that the unconscious is a multiple consciousness (CW 8 §394). For discussion of the "little eye of the soul" in the thought of Michael Maier, see Hereward Tilton, *The Quest for the Phoenix: Spiritual Alchemy and Rosicrucianism in the Work of Count Michael Maier (1569-1622)* (Berlin and New York: de Gruyter, 2003), pp. 76, 184-185, and 211.

spirits dissolve in mist (ll. 6549-6563) — all as a result of ignoring Mephistopheles's urgent reminder, *Machst du's doch selbst, das Fratzengeisterspiel!* ("It's your own work, this ghostly mask, you dunce!") (l. 6546). (The contrast resides in the fact that Faust tries to participate in the action; the parallel, in his lack of awareness about what is really happening.)

If we are foolish and act like Parzival, then when the flow of images ceases, "next to nothing has happened," and this will remain the case, even if the process is "repeated a thousand times" (CW 14 §753). But if, however, we *recognize our own involvement*, then we ourselves shall "enter into the process" with our "personal reactions," *just as if we were "one of the fantasy figures"* or, more precisely, "*as if the drama being enacted before your eyes were real*" (CW 14 §753; my italics). On this point, Jung could not possibly be more emphatic: It is a "psychic fact," he insists, that "*this fantasy is happening*" and "*it is as real as you — as a psychic entity — are real*" (§753; my italics). This point about the engagement of the individual in the process of transformation is crucial: without it, "all the changes are left to the flow of images," and we ourselves remain unchanged (§753). Or, in the words of such alchemists as Gerhard Dorn, "you will never make the One unless you have become one yourself" (*Wer aber selber nicht Einer wird, der kann auch das Eine nicht herstellen*) (§753).[59]

That said, Jung recognized there is a danger here, possibly the same danger that is symbolized by Faust's error in identifying with Paris: If one has "a dramatic fantasy," one can "enter the interior world of images [*seine Bilderwelt*] as a *fictitious personality*" and thereby prevent any "real participation"; and, indeed, to do this can even endanger one's consciousness, because there is the risk that one becomes "the victim of one's own fantasy"

[59] For further discussion of the *unarius* (i.e., the "unity of God" or the One), and the *unicus homo* (i.e., the "unitary man") in Dorn, see CW 14 §41 and §493.

and ends up by "succumb[ing] to the powers of the unconscious" — powers whose dangers are only too well known to the analyst (CW 14 §753; CGJ's italics). So what one has to do is this: One has to place oneself "*in the drama as one really is*," which has two effects: first, the drama gains in "actuality" (*Wirklichkeit*); and second, by this "criticism" of the fantasy, one creates "an effective counterbalance" to its tendency to "get out of hand" (§753). And it does so, because something important is now happening: The "decisive rapprochement with the unconscious" is taking place, a moment when "insight, the *unio mentalis*, begins to become real" (§753). For it is at this point that we begin to create something which Jung describes as "the beginning of individuation," a process whose "immediate goal is the experience and production of *the symbol of totality* [*die Herstellung des ganzheitlichen Symbols*]" (§753).

At the same time as he is exploring the relation between light and dark, Jung is working through the problem of God as light and dark that we find in Wolfram's *Parzival*, and in Parzival's attempt to answer the question, *waz ist got*, "What is God?" (§119, l. 17; vol. 1, p. 68, and §332, l.1; vol. 1, p. 188). Both the lesson in basic theology given by Herzeloyde in Book 3 (§119, ll. 18-§120, l.1; p. 68) — which recapitulates some key ideas from the opening prologue, including the opposition of *lieht* and *swarz* (§1, ll. 1-14; vol. 1, p. 3) — and its expansion in his conversation with Trevrizent in Book 9 (§465, l. 19-28 and §466, ll. 1-4; vol. 1, pp. 268), define God as light, echoing the words found in the First Letter of John, "God is light, and in him there is no darkness" (*Deus lux est, et tenebrae in eo non sunt ullae*) (1 John 1:5).[60] This statement echoes the prologue to the Gospel of John, "In [God] was life, and the life was the light of men. And the light shineth in darkness, and the darkness did not comprehend it" (John 1:4-5), as well as Christ's

[60] DKV, vol. 2, pp. 519-520 and 676-677.

later declaration to the people, "I am the light of the world: he that followeth me, walketh not in darkness" (John 8:12). Similarly, Paul tells the Ephesians: "Therefore do not be partakers with them; for you were formerly darkness, but now you are light in the Lord; walk as children of light (for the fruit of the light consists in all goodness and righteousness and truth), trying to learn what is pleasing to the Lord. And do not participate in the unfruitful deeds of darkness, but instead even expose them; for it is disgraceful even to speak of the things which are done by them in secret. But all things become visible when they are exposed by the light, for everything that becomes visible is light. For this reason it says, 'Awake, sleeper, And arise from the dead, And Christ will shine on you'" (Ephesians 5:7-14).

Evidently this leaves open the problem of darkness; or, to put it another way, it leaves us with the problem of evil. It is a problem to which Jung returns on a number of occasions, including *Answer to Job* (1952), his correspondence with Victor White,[61] and indeed (as we shall see in Volume 4 in this series) in his *Red Book*. Now in theological terms, one of the responses to the problem of evil is the doctrine of *privatio boni*, which argues that evil is merely the absence or "privation" (i.e., lack) of good. This argument is an old one: In the *Timaeus* (43c), Plato argues that the physical world falls short of the ideal world, since it is merely a copy of the latter;[62] and, in the *Protagoras* (357d), Socrates claims that, "when people make a wrong choice of pleasures and pains — that, of good and evil — the cause of their mistake is lack of knowledge." Similarly, in his *Metaphysics* (Book Theta, Chapter 9) Aristotle suggests he

---

[61] See *The Jung-White Letters*, ed. Ann Conrad Lammers and Adrian Cunningham (London and New York: Routledge, 2007); and Ann Conrad Lammers, *In God's Shadow: The Collaboration of Victor White and C.G. Jung* (New York and Mahwah, NJ: Paulist Press, 1994).

[62] See Harold Cherniss, "The Sources of Evil According to Plato," *Proceedings of the American Philosophical Society*, vol. 98, no. 1 (February 1954), 23-30.

also thinks of evil as essentially a privation (or, rather, it has no essence at all): "Clearly, then, the bad does not exist apart from bad things; for the bad is in its nature posterior to the potency. And therefore we may also say that in the things which are from the beginning, i.e. in eternal things, there is nothing bad, nothing defective, nothing perverted (for perversion is something bad)." We find the clearest statement of the doctrine, however, in Plotinus and in his remarks in the eighth tractate of his First Ennead about evil as an absolute lack having no part whatsoever in the Good or the One:

> Evil is not in any and every lack; it is in absolute lack. What falls in some degree short of the Good is not Evil; considered in its own kind it might even be perfect, but where there is utter dearth, there we have Essential Evil, void of all share in Good; this is the case with Matter. Matter has not even existence whereby to have some part in Good: Being is attributed to it by an accident of words: the truth would be that it has Non-Being. Mere lack brings merely Not-Goodness: Evil demands the absolute lack [...]. In fine we are not to think of Evil as some particular bad thing — injustice, for example, or any other ugly trait — but as a principle distinct from any of the particular forms in which, by the addition of certain elements, it becomes manifest. [...] If all this be true, we cannot be, ourselves, the source of Evil, we are not evil in ourselves; Evil was before we came to be; the Evil which holds men down binds them against their will; and for those that have the strength — not found in all men, it is true — there is a deliverance from the evils that have found lodgement in the Soul. In a word since Matter belongs only to the sensible world, vice in men is not the Absolute Evil; not all men are vicious; some overcome vice, some, the better sort, are

> never attacked by it; and those who master it win by means of that in them which is not material."[63]

Via Neoplatonism, then, this doctrine reemerges in the Christian tradition in the thought of St. Augustine of Hippo who, in his *Enchiridion*, declared:

> For what is that which we call evil but the absence of good? In the bodies of animals, disease and wounds mean nothing but the absence of health; for when a cure is effected, that does not mean that the evils which were present —namely, the diseases and wounds — go away from the body and dwell elsewhere: they altogether cease to exist; for the wound or disease is not a substance, but a defect in the fleshly substance, — the flesh itself being a substance, and therefore something good, of which those evils — that is, privations of the good which we call health — are accidents. Just in the same way, what are called vices in the soul are nothing but privations of natural good. And when they are cured, they are not transferred elsewhere: when they cease to exist in the healthy soul, they cannot exist anywhere else.[64]

In Chapter 4 of his work *The Divine Names*, Pseudo-Dionysius the Areopagite declares that all being is good, on the basis that God or "this essential Good, by the very fact of its existence, extends goodness into all things."[65] And in Article 1 of Question 5 of the

[63] *Enneads*, Book 1, tractate 8, §5; in Plotinus, *The Six Enneads*, trans. Stephen MacKenna and B.S. Page (Chicago and London: Encyclopedia Britannica, 1955), p. 29.
[64] *Enchiridion*, §11; in *The Essential Augustine*, ed. Vernon J. Bourke (Indianapolis, IN: Hackett, 1974), p. 65.)
[65] Pseudo-Dionysius, *Complete Works*, p. 71.

First Part of his *Summa Theologiae*, St. Thomas Aquinas argues that "goodness and being are really the same, and differ only in idea,"[66] while elsewhere in his *Summa Theologiae* (First Part, Question 49), he suggests that even the theory of privation need not exclude positive factors: "It must be said that every evil in some way has a cause. For evil is the absence of the good, which is natural and due to a thing. But that anything fail from its natural and due disposition can come only from some cause drawing it out of its proper disposition. For a heavy thing is not moved upwards except by some impelling force; nor does an agent fail in its action except from some impediment. But only good can be a cause; because nothing can be a cause except inasmuch as it is a being, and every being, as such, is good."[67]

Yet all these arguments, however clever or sophisticated, might — for precisely this reason — be considered so many examples of what Jung described in 1926 as human beings "loving [their] own reason more than God's secret intentions"; instead, Jung placed an emphasis on God as an experienced reality rather than a matter of theological belief.[68] This is an important theme in the later interviews with Jung: in 1955, he told the *Daily Mail* that everything he had learned had led him step by step to "an unshakeable conviction of the existence of God," and he declared: "I only believe in what I know. And that eliminates believing. Therefore I do not take His existence on belief — I *know* that He exists."[69] And there was the famous moment in his interview in 1959 with John Freeman for

---

[66] Thomas Aquinas, *Summa Theologiae* [I, Q. 5, Art. 1]. Available online HTTP: <http://documentacatholicaomnia.eu/03d/1225-1274,_Thomas_Aquinas,_Summa_Theologiae-Prima_Pars_Edente,_EN.pdf>

[67] Thomas Aquinas, *Summa Theologiae* [I, Q. 49, Art. 1]. Available online HTTP: <http://documentacatholicaomnia.eu/03d/1225-1274,_Thomas_Aquinas,_Summa_Theologiae-Prima_Pars_Edente,_EN.pdf>

[68] See Kingsley, *Catafalque*, vol. 2, p. 475; citing William McGuire and R.F.C. Hull (eds),*C.G. Jung Speaking: Interviews and Encounters* (Princeton, NJ: Princeton University Press, 1977), pp. 251 and 427-428.

[69] McGuire and Hull (eds), *C.G. Jung Speaking*, p. 251.

the BBC TV program *Face to Faith* when the following exchange took place: "*And did you believe in God?* Oh, yes. *Do you now believe in God?* Now? [Pause.] Difficult to answer. I *know*. I don't need to believe. I know."[70] (Freeman never pressed Jung further on this point.) At the same time, we find in the account of Jung's school years in *Memories, Dreams, Reflections* various references to "these talks with the 'Other'" as his "profoundest experiences: on the one hand, a bloody struggle, on the other supreme ecstasy" (MDR, 65); to God as "annihilating fire and an indescribable grace" (MDR, 74) and as "one of the most certain and immediate of experiences" (MDR, 80); and to "God's world" as "everything superhuman — dazzling light, the darkness of the abyss [i.e., the abysmal darkness], the cold impassivity of infinite space and time, and the uncanny grotesqueness of the irrational world of chance," and as hence "anything but 'edifying'" (MDR, 91).

In particular, Jung drew a link between the insights arising from these experiences and Goethe's *Faust*, which he read at the instigation of his mother (MDR, 78). "The real problem," we are told, seemed to Jung to lie "with Mephistopheles, whose whole figure made the deepest impression on [him], and who" — or so Jung "vaguely sensed" — had "a relationship to the mystery of the Mothers" (MDR, 78). Indeed, in Goethe's *Faust*, Jung found confirmation that other people had seen that, far from being a *privatio boni*, evil had a "universal power" and played a "mysterious role [...] in delivering humankind from darkness and suffering" (MDR, 78-79). As we shall see (in Volume 2), the problem of evil plays an important role in the theological underpinning of Goethe's *Faust*.

Returning to Jung's letter of 1926, we find that Jung draws this conclusion: "Try to apply seriously what I have told you, not that you might escape suffering — nobody can escape it — but

[70] McGuire and Hull (eds), *C.G. Jung Speaking*, pp. 427-428.

that you may avoid the worst — *blind* suffering."[71] In *Catafalque*, Kingsley highlights this emphasis on the problem of suffering, arguing that "in today's world suffering has come to be treated as a highly individualized affair," into which "civilization rushes [...] with its fixes, all its sanitizing cures." Yet he goes on to suggest that "most people are far too frightened to ask [...] what kind of sanitization is possible in a world which itself is insane, is completely out of balance." The truth is, Kingsley says, that "beyond our personal sufferings lies another type of suffering," one that is "so horrific that anyone unfortunate, or fortunate, enough to encounter it would dearly love to be able to avoid it and be rid of it," and which he defines as "the suffering of experiencing how insanely and unsustainably selfish we have become as a culture, how unbearably forgetful." In such a world, Kingsley argues, there always have to be "a few people who through their conscious suffering are willing to balance the selfishness and foolishness and forgetfulness bearing down on the world we live in."[72]

Jung was one of these people. Or at least, this is what Kingsley claims, while adding that there is almost nobody who "cares to note the lengths Jung himself felt pulled to go so that he could suffer consciously for the sake of the sacred" — or, as Jung himself had written in 1926, he had "wanted God to be alive and free from the suffering man has put on him by loving his own reason more than God's secret intentions."[73] Although a single, unpublished

[71] Adler, "Aspects of Jung's Personality and Work," p. 12. In so writing, Jung is picking up a theme from Nietzsche's *On the Genealogy of Morals* (1887), where he writes: "What really arouses indignation against suffering is not suffering as such but the senselessness of suffering," an insight which he develops at some length: "So as to abolish hidden, undetected, unwitnessed suffering from the world and honestly to deny it, one was in the past virtually compelled to invent gods and genii of all the heights and depths [...]" (GM II §7; Friedrich Nietzsche, *Basic Writings of Nietzsche*, ed. and trans. Walter Kaufmann (New York: Modern Library, 1968), p. 504).

[72] Kingsley, *Catafalque*, vol. 1, p. 26.

[73] Kingsley, *Catafalque*, vol. 1, p. 27; Adler, "Aspects of Jung's Personality and Work," p. 12.

letter might seem a frail hook onto which to hang such a heavy argument, Kingsley can point to other published works by Jung which make a similar argument. For instance, in his introductory address to a discussion at the Conference for Psychology held in Zurich in 1942 that was later published as "Psychotherapy and a Philosophy of Life" (*Psychotherapie und Weltanschauung*) (1943), Jung had defined "the principal aim of psychotherapy" as being "not to transport the patient to an impossible state of happiness, but to help him acquire steadfastness and philosophic patience in face of suffering" (CW 16 §185). In its profound modesty, this statement makes Jung sound almost like a Stoic, while his formulation also reminds one of Freud's description of the task of analysis as being to transform "hysterical misery into common unhappiness."[74] And when Jung goes on to say that "life demands for its completion and fulfilment a balance between joy and sorrow," one recalls that Faust's ambition is not simply to obtain happiness but rather: "Full-steeled to tread the world I feel my mettle, / Earth's woe, Earth's bliss, my soul can not unsettle, / I would not blench with storms to battle, / Nor quail amidst the shipwreck's crash and rattle! —" (ll. 464-467); and, in his wager with Mephisto, he insists:

> You hear! No dreams of joy am I caressing!
> The giddy whirl be mine, with agonized delight,
> With loving hatred, quickening despite.
> My bosom, healed now from the lust of learning,
> Henceforth unto no pain shall close its portals;
> And in myself I'll gratify each yearning,
> Assigned in sum to the whole race of mortals.
> All heights and depths my mind shall compass single;

[74] Freud, "The Psychotherapy of Hysteria," in Josef Breuer and Sigmund Freud, *Studies in Hysteria* [*Standard Edition of the Complete Psychological Works*, vol. 2], ed. James Strachey (London: Hogarth Press; Institute of Psycho-Analysis, 1955), pp. 253-305 (p. 305).

All weal and woe within my breast shall mingle;
Till mine own self to mankind's self expanded,
Like it at last upon Time's reef be stranded.
(ll. 1765-1775)

Elsewhere in "Psychotherapy and a Philosophy of Life" Jung defends such doctrines as original sin, the meaning of suffering, and immortality precisely not as "doctrines," i.e., "logical arguments," but as "emotional facts [...] felt and experienced" (CW 16 §186). To experience them as such, he adds, is "a charism" — a charism that "no human arts can compel" but which only "unreserved surrender" can achieve (§186). Such surrender does not lie within the grasp of everyone, and he describes "the most healing, and psychologically the most necessary, experiences" as "the treasure hard to attain,"[75] a treasure that Kingsley equates with the Grail itself.[76] Like the Grail, to acquire this "treasure" requires "something out of the common" (§187). From clinical experience, Jung argues, this "something-out-of-the-common" proves to be "an invasion by archetypal contents," the assimilation of which cannot be achieved by "current philosophical or religious ideas," but which demands rather "pre-Christian and non-Christian conceptions," which are more compatible with "the archaic symbolism of the material" (§188).

Lumen naturae and the Grail Dream

Medieval physicians, Jung claims in "Psychotherapy and a Philosophy of Life," seem to have practiced a philosophy "whose roots can be traced back to pre-Christian times and whose nature exactly corresponds to our experiences with patients today" (§189):

[75] See Jung, *Psychology and Alchemy* (CW 12 §155, §205, §222, §438, §442-§446 and §448); cf. *Symbols of Transformation* (CW 5 §393, §450, §510, §569 and §659).
[76] Kingsley, *Catafalque*, vol. 1, p. 184.

> These physicians recognized, besides the light of divine revelation, a *lumen naturae* as a second, independent source of illumination, to which the doctor could turn if the truth as handed down by the Church should for any reason prove ineffective either for himself or for the patient. (CW 16 §189)

What is the *lumen naturae*? In her recent study — an attempt to rehabilitate this notion of a purely immanent, non-supernatural form of enlightenment and to apply both to modern art (Paul Cezanne, Mark Rothko, Sol LeWitt, Lee Krasner) and to modern science (the concept of space, the notion of randomness, the shape of the cosmos, and other puzzles of the universe) — Matilde Marcolli describes *lumen naturae* as "a form of Enlightenment that proceeds not from supernatural causes, like divine intervention, but fully from an immanent investigation of nature and matter":

> This nonsupernatural Enlightenment is what one may envision as a form of higher insight and awareness that emanates from poetry and art, or from the contemplation of the beauty of abstract concepts. It is the elegance of the natural universe described by physical laws, and the poetic imagination of abstract mathematics. It is a purely immanent Enlightenment, which does not involve any religion or any transcendental form of spirituality.[77]

[77] Matilde Marcolli, *Lumen Naturae: Visions of the Abstract in Art and Mathematics* (Cambridge, MA, and London: MIT Press, 2020), p. 2. In Chapter 11 of her study, Marcolli discusses the relation between graphical illustration and scientific text, from ancient forms of manuscript illumination to Jung's *Red Book* and the work of such contemporary artists as the German Dadaist and Surrealist Max Ernst (1891-1976) and the American conceptual artist Sonya Rapoport (1923-2015) (see pp. 317-322).

For a definition contemporary to the medieval period, however, we can turn to the treatise *Caput de morbis somnii* (*On Diseases of Dreams*) where Paracelsus (c. 1493-1641) declares the following:

> Look at Adam and Moses and others. They sought in themselves what was in man and have revealed it and all kabbalistic arts and they knew nothing alien to man neither from the Devil nor from the spirits, but derived their knowledge from the Light of Nature. This they nurtured in themselves [...] it comes from nature which contains its manner of activity within itself. It is active during sleep and hence things must be used when dormant and not awake — sleep is waking for such arts — for things have a spirit which is active for them in sleep. Now it is true that Satan in his wisdom is a Kabbalist and a powerful one. So, too, are these innate spirits in man [...] for it is the Light of Nature which is at work during sleep and is the invisible body and was nevertheless born like the visible and natural body. But there is more to be known than the mere flesh, for from this very innate spirit comes that which is visible [...] the Light of Nature which is man's mentor dwells in this innate spirit.[78]

Jung himself quotes this passage in a footnote to "Paracelsus as Spiritual Phenomenon," a lecture delivered to the Swiss Society for the History of Medicine and the Natural Sciences at the annual meeting of the Society for Nature Research in 1941, held on the

[78] Paracelsus, "Caput de morbis somnii," in *Sämtliche Werke*, ed. Karl Sudhoff and Wilhelm Matthiessen, section 1, *Medizinische, naturwissenschaftliche und philosophische Schriften*, 14 vols (Munich and Berlin: Oldenbourg, 1922-1933), vol. 9, pp. 359-362 (p. 360); cited in Jung, "Paracelsus as a Spiritual Phenomenon" (CW 13 §148, fn. 6).

occasion of the 400th anniversary of the death of Paracelsus (and subsequently published in a small volume called *Paracelsica* in 1942).[79] This lecture opens with a section that is programmatically titled "The Two Sources of Knowledge: The Light of Nature and the Light of Revelation" (CW 13 §145-§168) and here Jung glosses the term *lumen naturae* with reference to Paracelsus as follows:

> The light of nature [*lumen naturae*] is the *quinta essentia*, extracted by God himself from the four elements, and dwelling "in our hearts." It is enkindled by the Holy Spirit. The light of nature is an intuitive apprehension of the facts, a kind of illumination. It has two sources: a mortal and an immortal, which Paracelsus calls "angels." "Man," he says, "is also an angel and has all the latter's qualities." He has a natural light, but also a light outside the light of nature by which he can search out supernatural things. The relationship of this supernatural light to the light of revelation remains, however, obscure. Paracelsus seems to have held a peculiar trichotomous view in this respect. (CW 13 §148)[80]

[79] With good reason, one survey of the significance of Paracelsus describes him as "elusive"; see Owsei Temkin, "The Elusiveness of Paracelsus," *Bulletin of the History of Medicine*, vol. 26, no. 3 (May-June 1952), 201-217. For further discussion, see Paracelsus, *Selected Writings*, ed. Jolande Jacobi (Princeton, NJ: Princeton University Press, 1979); Walter Pagel, *Paracelsus: An Introduction to Philosophical Medicine in the Era of the Renaissance*, 2nd edn (Basel: Karger, 1982); Paracelsus, *Essential Readings*, ed. Nicholas Goodrick-Clarke (Berkeley, CA: North Atlantic Books, 1999); Philip Ball, *The Devil's Doctor: Paracelsus and the World of Renaissance Magic and Science* (London: Heinemann, 2006); and Paracelsus, *Essential Theoretical Writings*, ed. and trans. Andrew Weeks (Leiden and Boston: Brill, 2008).

[80] See Paracelsus, *Astronomia magna*, in *Sämtliche Werke*, ed. Sudhoff, vol. 12, pp. 1-444 (pp. 36 and 304); *Das Buch Paragranum*, ed. Franz Strunz (Leipzig: Diederichs, 1903), p. 36 (*auß dem Liecht der Natur / das angezuendet wirdt durch den heiligen Geist*); *Labyrinthus medicorum errantium* [*On the Going-Astray of Doctors*, 1537/1538], in *Sämtliche Werke*, ed. Sudhoff, vol. 11, pp. 161-221 (chapter 8 = pp. 199-204); and *De nymphis*, in *Sämtliche Werke*, ed. Sudhoff, vol. 14, pp. 115-151 (p. 115).

In this lecture, Jung pays close attention to the notion of the *lumen naturae* or the light of nature, pointing out that it is "indeed of great importance in alchemy," for "just as, according to Paracelsus, it enlightens the individual as to the workings of nature and gives them an understanding of natural things 'by cagastric magic' (*per magiam cagastricam*), so it is the aim of alchemy to beget this light in the shape of the *filius philosophorum*" (CW 13 §161),[81] that is, the "philosophers' child," often (but not always) the philosopher's stone (*lapis philosophorum*). (By the *cagastrum*, Paraclesus means a negative kind of *iliaster*, his term for the prime matter of body and soul (i.e., *hyle* [matter] + *astrum* [star]). In order to explicate what this light actually involves, Jung cites a number of ancient treatises and their definitions (CW 13 §161):

- "See therefore that the light which is in thee be not darkness" (*Tractatus Aristotelis*)
- "My light excels all other lights, and my goods are higher than all other goods. I beget the light, but the darkness too is of my nature. Nothing better or more worthy of veneration can come to pass in the world than the union of myself with my son" (*Tractatus aureus*, where Mercury is speaking)
- "I enlighten all that is mine, and I make the light manifest on the journey from my father Saturn. […] I make the days of the world eternal, and I illumine all lights with my light" (*Dicta Belini*; again, it is Mercury speaking)
- "They embrace and the new light is begotten of them, which is like no other light in the whole world" (Mylius, *Philosophia reformata*; said with reference to the "chymical marriage" from which the *filius philosophorum* arises)

[81] See Paracelsus, *Liber Azoth*, in *Philosophi et Medici Opera Bücher und Schrifften*, ed. Johannes Huser, 2 vols (Strasbourg: Zetzner, 1603-1616), vol. 2, pp. 519-543 (p. 522).

With Paracelsus as with other alchemists, Jung argues, "this idea of the light [...] coincides with the concept of Sapientia and Scientia," so that we could safely call the light "the central mystery of philosophical alchemy" (CW 13 §162).

We should also note that there is an important link between this doctrine of *lumen naturae* and Jung's Grail dream of 1938. "The 'natural light of man' or the 'star in man' sounds harmless enough, so none of the authors had any notion of the possibilities of conflict that lurked within it," Jung explains, adding: "Yet that light or *filius philosophorum* was openly named the greatest and most victorious of all lights, and set alongside Christ as the Saviour and Preserver of the world!", i.e., the *servator* or *salvator mundi* (CW 13 §163):

> Whereas in Christ God himself became man, the *filius philosophorum* was extracted from matter by human art and, by means of the opus, made into a new light-bringer. In the former case the miracle of man's salvation is accomplished by God; in the latter, the salvation or transfiguration of the universe is brought about by the mind of man — "Deo concedente," as the authors never fail to add. In the one case man confesses "I under God," in the other he asserts "God under me." (CW 13 §163)

And so, fatefully, "Man takes the place of the Creator" (§163) — a development that informs the entire philosophical outlook of Nietzsche, as we shall see. As a result, medieval alchemy prepared the way for "the greatest intervention in the divine world order that man has ever attempted," and an epochal shift takes place:

> Alchemy was the dawn of the scientific age, when the daimon of the scientific spirit compelled the forces of nature to serve man to an extent that had never been

> known before. It was from the spirit of alchemy that Goethe wrought the figure of the "superman" Faust,[[82]] and this superman led Nietzsche's Zarathustra to declare that God was dead and to proclaim the will to give birth to the superman, to "create a god for yourself out of your seven devils."[[83]] Here we find the true roots, the preparatory forces deep in the psyche, which unleashed the forces at work in the world today. (CW 13 §163)

In relation to what has arisen as a result of these "true roots [...] which unleashed the forces at work in the world today," Jung sounds a note of immense urgency, commenting that "science and technology have indeed conquered the world, but whether the psyche has gained anything is another matter" (CW 13 §163).

Aside from the specific links drawn here to Goethe's *Faust* and Nietzsche's *Zarathustra*, there is another important connection to be made. As Tatsuhiro Nakajima has pointed out, the figure of the wounded king in Wolfram's *Parzival* can be read as prophesying in a symbolic way the paradigm shift that Edward Grant describes as "something important occurr[ing] between approximately 1200 and 1600 that proved conducive for the emergence of the Scientific Revolution."[84] In mythology in general and, in particular, in

[82] See *Faust*, Part One, l. 490: *Welch erbärmlich Grauen / Faßt Übermenschen dich!* ("What mortal dread, thou man of more than mortal essence, / Gets hold on thee?"), the Earth Spirit exclaims.

[83] See *Thus Spoke Zarathustra*, Part One, "Of the Way of the Creator" (Z I 17). In his seminar on *Zarathustra*, Jung glossed this passage as follows: "Here Nietzsche is going to create a god out of his conflict, out of his seven devils. He cannot help seeing what he is doing, but he cannot draw the necessary conclusion. It is not he who is creating a god, not the man Nietzsche who declared that God was dead, but the god is creating himself" (SNZ, vol. 1, p. 723).

[84] Tatsuhiro Nakajima, "Psychology of the 12th Century Renaissance in Wolfram von Eschenbach's *Parzival*," *Studia Hermetica Journal*, vol. 8, no. 1 ("Hermetism and the Underworld") (2018), 23-40 (p. 37); citing Edward Grant, *A History of Natural Philosophy: From the Ancient World to the Nineteenth Century* (Cambridge: Cambridge University Press, 2007), p. 329.

alchemy, the goal of healing the sick king does not so much signify the restoration of the older order as rather point to the renewal of the old world *through transformation* (37).[85] In the second volume of *Mysterium coniunctionis*, Jung offers the following analysis of the symbolic representation of the figure of the king in medieval alchemy:

> The fact that the king played a large role in medieval alchemy for several hundred years proves that, from about the thirteenth century onwards, the traces of the king's renewal surviving from Egyptian and Hellenistic times began to gain in importance because they had acquired a new meaning. For as the West started to investigate nature, till then completely unknown, the doctrine of the *lumen naturae* began to germinate too. Ecclesiastical doctrine and scholastic philosophy had both proved incapable of shedding any light on the nature of the physical world. The conjecture thereupon arose that just as the mind revealed its nature in the light of divine revelation, so nature herself must possess a "certain luminosity" which could become a source of enlightenment. (CW 14 §425).

Many years earlier, in 1921, Jung was already arguing that such early forms of knowledge as astrology and alchemy were essentially "projected psychology," whereas astronomy and modern chemistry had arisen from a process of withdrawal of projection, or (in Jung's

[85] For further discussion of the links between the Age of the Discovery of the Americas and the Age of Discovery in science, and between the works of such late medieval alchemists as Roger Bacon, Arnaldus de Villa Nova, and Ramon Llull and the early modern literature of the conquest of America, see Ralph Bauer, *The Alchemy of Conquest: Science, Religion, and the Secrets of the New World* (Charlottesville: University of Virginia Press, 2019).

own words) "the de-psychologizing work of objective science" (CW 6 §12).[86]

As Nakajima argues, Wolfram's *Parzival* stands exactly at the turning point between the projection by astrologers and alchemists of the natural philosophy of the Hermetic and Aristotelian traditions onto celestial movements and chemical substances, and the withdrawal of those projections that initiated the rise of modern science — a shift which, in *Mysterium coniunctionis*, Jung describes as follows:

> It is therefore understandable that for those individuals whose particular interest lay in the investigation of natural things the dogmatic view of the world should lose its force as the *lumen naturae* gained in attraction, even though the dogma itself was not directly doubted. The more serious alchemists, if we are to believe their statements, were religious people who had no thought of criticizing revealed truth. There is in the literature of alchemy, so far as I can judge, no attack on dogma. The only thing of this kind is a depreciation of the Aristotelian philosophy sponsored by the Church in favour of Hermetic Neoplatonism.[[87]] Not only were the

[86] Nakajima, "Psychology of the 12th Century Renaissance in Wolfram von Eschenbach's *Parzival*," p. 37.

[87] At this point, Jung refers in a footnote to the following passage from Gerhard Dorn's *Speculativae philosophiae, gradus septem vel decem continens* [*Speculative Philosophy, containing the seven or ten steps*]: "Whoever wishes to learn the Chemical Art ought to study philosophy — not the Aristotelian variety of course, but that which teaches the truth. A disciple of Aristotle might say, 'Are you calling Aristotle a liar?' I am not, but he himself does, for his entire doctrine consists of ambiguity, which is the most effective cloak of liars. Since he himself rebuked Plato and the rest merely to seek fame, no instrument could be found more fitting than that which he used in those rebukes, namely ambiguity, by which he protects his writings against attack from one quarter by creating a subterfuge in another quarter, and vice versa. This kind of sophistry can be seen in all his writings [...]" (*Theatrum chemicum*, vol. 1, Ursel 1602, pp. 255-310 [p. 271]; translated in *The Speculative*

> old Masters not critical of ecclesiastical doctrine, they were, on the contrary, convinced that their discoveries, real or imaginary, would enrich the doctrine of the correspondence of heavenly and earthly things, since they endeavoured to prove that the "mystery of faith" was reflected in the world of nature. They could not guess that their passion for investigating nature would detract as much as it did from revealed truth, and that their scientific interests could be aroused only as the fascination of dogma began to pall. And so, as in dreams, there grew up in their unconscious the compensating image of the king's renewal. (CW 14 §425).

Now this shift is reflected in Wolfram's conception of the Grail: on the one hand, self-evidently religious and transcendent; on the other, less mystical in its conception than Chrétien's and, as tangible stone, more immanent. *Daz was ein dinc, daz hiez der Grâl* ("that thing which men call 'The Grail'"), so Wolfram's narrator tells us, and rather than a dish or a cup or a ciborium, it is a stone.[88] In Chrétien's *Perceval*, the hero witnesses a procession in which a young man carries a bleeding lance, two boys carry candelabras, and finally a beautiful young girl emerges, bearing an elaborately decorated *graal,* or "grail." (For Chrétien, this object is not necessarily unique: It is "*a* grail" (*un graal*),[89] and it seems to have resembled a dish or a bowl, containing a single Communion wafer that keeps alive the

Philosophy of Gerhard Dorn [Magnum Opus Hermetic Sourceworks, no. 34], trans. Paul Ferguson (Kilbirnie: Alchemy Website and Bookshop, 2008).

[88] DKV, vol. 2, pp. 580-581.

[89] In his commentary in the Pléiade edition, Daniel Poirion notes that "un graal" was used in medieval times and in a monastic context to indicate a bowl or a platter (*scutellum*), pointing out that the fact it has to be held in two hands suggests it is something large, less like goblet and more like a plate or a basket; in the Morvan dialect of the Burgundian language, *grô* signified "basket," and in the ancient mystery cults a basket is said to have played a central rôle (Chrétien de Troyes, *Œuvres complètes*, p. 1349).

Grail King — the Fisher King's father and Perceval's uncle — as it has done for the last 15 years [ll. 6413-6431], although it is unclear how often — once a year? — he eats the wafer.)[90] In Robert de Boron's verse romance *Joseph of Arimathea* (composed between 1191 and 1202), the grail becomes *the* Holy Grail, i.e., the chalice used by Christ at the Last Supper and subsequently used by Joseph of Arimathea to collect Christ's blood when he was removed from the cross.[91] Later (c. 1220-1225) in *The Quest of the Holy Grail* (*Queste del Saint Graal*), part of the prose *Lancelot* (which is in turn the longest part of the *Lancelot-Grail* Cycle), the search for the Grail has become more or less allegorical, and the Grail itself a symbol of divine grace — and transformation.

In this respect, the Grail emerges from a long conceptual lineage. In the *Timaeus*, Plato uses the image of the *kratēr*, a mixing bowl for wine and water, as a metaphor for the creation of the universe — in which the Demiurge creates the World Soul, the human soul, and living creatures — through mixing different elements (Being, the Same, and the Different) in this transformative

[90] In Chrétien's *Perceval*, the Grail King is the brother of Perceval's mother and the Fisher King is his mother's nephew, meaning that the Grail King is Perceval's uncle and the Fisher King is his cousin. However, because (a) Perceval's mother has told him that his father, who died of grief after his two older sons were killed on the same day, had been wounded between the legs — a medieval circumlocution for castration or sterility — and, as a consequence, his land has gone into decline; and (b) Perceval's cousin explains that the Fisher King is wounded and his land has become a barren wasteland, is it possible that the Fisher King is Perceval's own dead father and the Grail King his grandfather? (See Joseph J. Duggan, "Afterword," in Chrétien de Troyes, *Perceval: The Story of the Grail*, trans. Burton Raffel (New Haven and London: Yale University Press, 1999), pp. 293-307 [pp. 297 and 299].) Whatever, it is clear that Chrétien's *Perceval* is, like Wolfram's *Parzival*, permeated by the theme of lineage or, to put it another way, **the theme of the ancestors.** For further discussion from an analytical psychological perspective in relation to Jung himself, see Andreas Jung, "The Grandfather," *Journal of Analytical Psychology*, 56 (2011), 653-673.

[91] Likewise, in the *Estoire del Saint Graal* the Grail is the vessel ("*escuele*," a bowl) used by Christ at the Last Supper, which Joseph of Arimathea takes from the Upper Room where that meal was shared with the disciples and uses to collect Christ's blood at the Entombment (not at the Crucifixion).

vessel.[92] Likewise, in a discourse in the *Corpus Hermeticum* called "The Mixing Bowl or the Monad," Hermes gives an account of how the craftsman (or the Demiurge) "made the whole cosmos by reasoned speech, not by hand." Wishing to "make this offering and to adorn the earth," he "sent the man below, an adornment of the divine body, mortal life from life immortal."[93] Thus humankind "became a spectator of god's work," and "looked at it in astonishment" (15). But although God shared reason among all people, he did not share mind (*nous* or Νους); not because he begrudged it or out of envy, but because he wanted to put it "between souls [...] as a prize for them to contest" (15), and in order to do so, he did the following:

> "He filled a great mixing bowl with it and sent it below, appointing a herald whom he commanded to make the following proclamation to human hearts: 'Immerse yourself in the mixing bowl if your heart has the strength, if it believes you will rise up again to the one who sent the mixing bowl below, if it recognizes the purpose of your coming to be.'
>
> "All those who heeded the proclamation and immersed themselves in mind participated in knowledge and became perfect people because they received mind. But those who missed the point of the proclamation are people of reason because they did not receive <the gift of> mind as well and do not know the purpose or

[92] See Plato, *Timaeus*, 35a-b, 37a-c, and 41d-e. For further discussion, see Renate Schlesier, "KRATĒR. The Mixing-Vessel as Metaphorical Space in Ancient Greek Tradition," in Fabian Horn and Cilliers Breytenbach (eds.), *Spatial Metaphors. Ancient Texts and Transformations* (Berlin: Edition Topoi, 2016), pp. 69-84; and Luc Brisson, "How to Make a Soul in the *Timaeus*," in Chad Jorgenson, Filip Karfík, and Štěpán Špinka (eds), *Plato's "Timaeus": Proceedings of the Tenth Symposium Platonicum Pragense* (Leiden and Boston: Brill, 2021), pp. 70-91.

[93] Brian P. Copenhaver, *Hermetica: The Greek "Corpus Hermeticum" and the Latin "Asclepius" in a new English translation* (Cambridge: Cambridge University Press, 1992), pp. 15-16.

> the agents of their coming to be. These people have sensations much like those of unreasoning animals, and, since their temperament is willful and angry, they feel no awe of things that deserve to be admired; they divert their attention to the pleasures and appetites of their bodies; and they believe that mankind came to be for such purposes. But those who participate in the gift that comes from god, O Tat, are immortal rather than mortal if one compares their deeds, for in a mind of their own they have comprehended all — things on earth, things in heaven and even what lies beyond heaven. Having raised themselves so far, they have seen the good and, having seen it, they have come to regard the wasting of time here below as a calamity. They have scorned every corporeal and incorporeal thing, and they hasten toward the one and only. This, Tat, is the way to learn about mind, to {resolve perplexities} in divinity and to understand god. For the mixing bowl is divine."[94]

In his commentary on this passage, Brian Copenhaver notes that a *kratēr* is a "vessel for mixing wine" and that *kratērizō* can mean the "mixing or pouring of wine to be used in an initiation or sacrifice" (134). In the Septuagint version of Scripture, the figure of Wisdom in the Book of Proverbs is said to have "mingled her wine in a bowl [*kratēra*]," while commending those who "leave folly [...] seek wisdom, and improve understanding by knowledge [*en gnōsei*]" (see Proverbs 9:1-6); and in a work of alchemical and spiritual advice called the *Final Accounting*, Zosimus urges Theosebeia to "rush to Poimandres and, having been baptized in the krater, rise up to your race" (cited 134).

[94] Copenhaver, *Hermetica*, pp. 15-16.

Here, then, the overtones of *gnosis* and baptism are unmistakable; and, in his seminar on dream symbolism held in 1937 in New York, Jung drew a link between one of Wolfgang Pauli's pictures, showing a lake in a crater surrounded by four mountains, and the use of the word *krater* in the alchemical writings of Zosimos and in this discourse from the *Corpus Hermeticum*.[95] He highlighted this account's emphasis on how human beings are created "in a state of *anoia*," interpreted as a state "of not knowing, of mindlessness, unconsciousness" (275-276). And this is why the Demiurge created a "wonderful vessel, a krater, and filled it with *nous*, with mind" — that is, with *pneuma* or spirit: "So God filled the vessel with *nous* and sent it to earth for those who were not satisfied with their state of *anoia*, and they could then dip themselves in the krater in order to be transformed and to attain a new state of *ennoia*, that is, [a] state of consciousness, of being conscious or [aware] of, which would mean mindful of, or, filled with mind, by means of which they really became spiritual beings" (276).[96]

As a result, Jung concluded in his lecture, this discourse in the *Corpus Hermeticum* can help us understand why, in the *Final Accounting*, Zosimos gave Theosebeia — whose name means "the one that worships God" — advice, not just in the form of "alchemistic prescriptions" about "how to produce changes in metals" and "how to melt the ores," but also to "seek the aid of the krater": "to go right away down to the krater, to dip herself or to get baptized," since to be dipped in the krater means to "transform into

[95] C.G. Jung, *Dream Symbols of the Individuation Process: Notes of C.G. Jung's Seminars on Wolfgang Pauli's Dreams*, ed. Suzanne Gieser (Princeton, NJ, and Oxford: Princeton University Press, 2019), p. 275. For further discussion, see M.J. Edwards, "The Vessel of Zosimus the Alchemist," *Zeitschrift für Papyrologie und Epigraphik*, 90 (1992), 55-64; and H.S. El Khadem, "A Translation of a Zosimos' Text in an Arabic Alchemy Book," *Journal of the Washington Academy of Sciences*, vol. 84, no. 3 (September 1996), 168-178.

[96] For Jung's discussion of this discourse in the previous year (i.e., 1936), see SNZ, vol. 2, p. 936.

a new kind of human being, a pneumatic being" (276 and 275).[97] (In addition, as a receptacle for the divine food, be it a wafer or blood, the Grail recalls the function of the *cista mystica,* or "holy box" or "basket," of the ancient Greek mystery cults, from which typically a snake or serpent would arise.)[98]

Returning to Wolfram's *Parzival*: Here, the Grail is explicitly associated with light, thanks to the six glass vials carried before it: "And lights both rare and costly before the Grail they bore / Six glasses tall, transparent — and wondrous balsam's flame / Burnt within with a strange sweet perfume" (§236, ll. 1-4; vol. 1, p. 135). In Book 9, Trevrizent relates how, each year on Good Friday, a brilliant white dove descends, bringing to the Grail an equally white Communion wafer with life-sustaining powers:

> For ever upon Good Friday a messenger takes her way.
> From the height of the highest Heaven a Dove on her flight doth wing,
> And a Host, so white and holy, she unto the stone doth bring.
> And she layeth It down upon It; and white as the Host the Dove
> That, her errand done, swift wingeth her way to the Heaven above.
> Thus ever upon Good Friday doth it chance as I tell to thee:
> And the stone from the Host receiveth all good that on earth may be

[97] By a "pneumatic" being, Jung is using the Hermetic and Gnostic distinction between the higher "spiritual" (*pneumatikos*) as opposed to the lower "psychic" life (*psuchikos*) (see Copenhaver, *Corpus Hermeticum*, p. 135).

[98] William A. Nitze, "The Fisher King in the Grail Romances," *Publications of the Modern Language Association*, vol. 24, no. 3 (1909), 365-418 (p. 400). See also his "Who was the Fisher King: A Note on Halieutics," *Romanic Review*, vol. 33, no. 2 (April 1947), 97-104.

> Of food or of drink, the earth beareth as the fulness of
> Paradise.
> (§470, ll. 1-15; vol. 1, p. 271)

And in Book 16, it is Repanse de Schoye who brings forth the Grail because of her radiant beauty, "And the Grail, so men have told me, might be borne by her hands alone; / Pure was her heart, and radiant as sunlight her fair face shone," *ir vel des blickes flôrî* (or as Hatto translates these lines, "the flesh without was a blossoming of all brightness") (§809, ll. 10-14; vol. 2, p. 176).

The world of the Grail is thus symbolically associated with a universe of light, as well as — through Parzival's failure to ask the question — with immense suffering on the part of Anfortas. Suffering is, too, a central theme in Jung's letter of 1926 — "the secret meaning of Christian symbolism," he writes, is "a path of blood and suffering" — and what this letter demonstrates, on Kingsley's account, is just how far Jung took the practice of conscious suffering.[99] In this way, it also forms an important point of connection back to Wolfram's *Parzival*, and its question "What ails thee?" variously formulated as "*hêrre, wie stêt iuwer nôt?*" (i.e., "Sire, what ails you?") or as "*oeheim, waz wirret dir?*", (i.e., "Uncle, what ails you?") (§484, l. 27, cf. §795, l. 29).

At the beginning of Book 16, Wolfram's narrator underscores the horrific nature of Anfortas's suffering, the cosmic dimension of which is signaled by means of an astrological reference:

> And the time was near when the planet, its course in
> high heaven run,
> Mars or Jupiter, glowing wrathful, its station had
> well-nigh won,
> And the spot whence it took its journey — Ah! then
> was an evil day

[99] Kingsley, *Catafalque*, vol. 1, p. 475.

That wrought ill to the wound of Anfortas, and the torment would have its way;
And maiden and knight must hearken as the palace rang with his cries,
And the help that no man might give him he besought with despairing eyes,
For past all aid was he wounded, and his knights could but share his grief—
Yet the tale saith he drew ever nearer who should bring him alone relief.

Then oft as the bitter anguish in its bondage the hero held,
The taint of the wound to banish, the hall was with sweetness filled,
For before him they spread on the carpet Terebinth, and odours fair
Of aromatic spices and sweet woods filled the scented air.

(§789, ll. 4-24; vol. 2, p. 166)

This astrological reference recalls the link drawn by Flegetanis between the Grail and astrology (§444, ll. 24-30; vol. 1, p. 262) and the reference made in Book 15 by Cundrie at the end of her speech, using Arabic names for the planets in a way that is comprehensible to Feirefiz, to the favorable astrological constellation observable in the skies (§782, ll. 6-12; vol. 2, p. 160), even if the specific detail of whether Mars or Jupiter was in the ascendent does not really make sense.[100]

[100] DKV, vol. 2, pp. 772-773. For the suggestion that the descriptions of astrological constellations in *Parzival* refer to the idea of *großes Planetenjahr*, see Wilhelm Deinert, *Ritter und Kosmos im "Parzival": Eine Untersuchung der Sternkunde Wolframs von Eschenbach* (Munich: Beck, 1960), pp. 23-29. By contrast, Paul

The subsequent list of perfumes used to sweeten the air and to mask the stench of Anfortas's wound (§789, l. 21-§790, l. 13) is but a prelude to the impressive list of no fewer than 58 precious stones, all with beneficial medicinal properties, that adorn Anfortas's bed (§790, l. 18-§792, ll. 1-30). (The list corresponds almost exactly to the 60 stones listed by Marbod of Rennes (c. 1035-1123) in his treatise *De lapidibus* of c. 1090.)[101] Within the overall narrative economy of Wolfram's epic, Parzival's quest to rediscover the Grail forms the necessary counterpart to Anfortas's waiting for his release from suffering: "And once more would they wait his coming whose joy [*sîn vreude*] there had waxen weak, / And the hour that should bring them healing from the question his lips should speak" (§788, ll. 17-20; vol. 2, 166). That release from suffering can only be achieved through Parzival's own painful journey as he discovers his identity — or, in other words, as he discovers his true identity as the lord of the Grail. To the Grail, as to Anfortas's release from suffering, there are no shortcuts. In the terms of Jung's letter of 1926, no one, not even Parzival, can "escape suffering" — and Anfortas in particular cannot escape it — but Parzival is able to "avoid the worst — *blind* suffering."

In Wolfram's *Parzival*, the hero rediscovers the "healing vessel," the *servator mundi*, which Anfortas so urgently needs (cf. MDR, 313); in his dream of the Grail Castle of 1938 as retold in

---

Kunitzsch and Arthur B. Groos suggest that the order in which the list of planet names in Arabic is given by Cundrie is a purely cataloglike presentation of the usual geocentric order (Kunitzsch, "Die Planetennamen im 'Parzival,'" *Zeitschrift für deutsche Sprache*, 25 (1969), 169-174), and hence without any deeper astrological significance (Arthur B. Groos, "Cundrie's Announcement (*Parzival*, 781-782)," *Beiträge zur Geschichte der deutschen Sprache und Literatur*, 113 (1991), 384-414); cited in DKV, vol. 2, pp. 768-769. For the significance of astrological references in *The Red Book*, see Liz Greene, *The Astrological World of Jung's "Liber Novus": Daimons, Gods, and the Planetary Journey* (London and New York: Routledge, 2018); and for discussion of Jung's interest in astrology more generally, see Liz Greene, *Jung's Studies in Astrology: Prophecy, Magic, and the Qualities of Time* (London and New York: Routledge, 2018).

[101] DKV, vol. 2, p. 774.

Memories, Dreams, Reflections, Jung implicitly presents himself (and, according to Kingsley, in the Jaffé Protocols, he more or less explicitly presents himself) as the healing vessel itself, as a Christlike preserver and savior of the world.[102] And he does so in a way that ties up, so Kingsley argues, with Jung's claim in his letter of 1926 to have adopted for himself the practice of conscious suffering by "consciously and intentionally" making his life miserable, because he wanted God to be "alive and free from the suffering man has put on him," and his description in his introductory address of 1942 of psychotherapy as a way to help the individual "acquire steadfastness and philosophic patience in face of suffering" (CW 16 §185).

As Kingsley puts it when concluding his account of the version in the Jaffé Protocols of Jung's 1938 Grail Castle dream, this is the point at which "all these interesting details become really fascinating — because it's as if suddenly a back door has sprung open into Jung's own scientific writings."[103] Now if this is so, then all this has important implications for Jung's identity or rather his status as not just an intellectual, but a prophetic figure:

> His extended use of the Grail mythology here, just a few years before he died, in explaining the real meaning of individuation gives the lie to the very rational and unfortunately very fashionable idea nowadays that Jung saw his evolutionary task as being to leave the antiquated world of mythology behind so he could introduce people instead to a scientific or "post-mythic" world of psychology. On the contrary: his psychological work was aimed specifically at renewing forgotten myths and mysteries by restoring them, as a true scientist, to life.[104]

[102] Kingsley, *Catafalque*, vol. 1, p. 134.
[103] Kingsley, *Catafalque*, vol. 1, p. 134.
[104] Kingsley, *Catafalque*, vol. 2, p. 533.

In other words, Jung saw his own task and the project of analytical psychology as something essentially transformative. But it also has implications for what we could call Jung's communicative strategy.

In an unpublished letter to J.B. Lang of 9 March 1918, Jung highlighted the importance of Gnosticism and Neoplatonism as "the systems that contain the materials which are suited to form the basis of a theory of the unconscious spirit," adding that he had "already been working on this [him]self for a long time" — surely, a reference to the genesis of *The Red Book* — and had had "ample opportunity to compare [his] experiences at least partially with those of others."[105] Then again, in his letter of 1926 that Gerhard Adler published in 1975, Jung declared: "There is a mystical fool in me that proved to be stronger than all my science,"[106] an expression that Kingsley glosses as Jung's "own, shorthand way of using standard prophetic language to describe the prophet who goes unrecognized, unacknowledged; unheard."[107] Kingsley points out that that origin of this phrase is in the book of Hosea, where the prophet declares, "Know ye, Israel, that the prophet was foolish, the spiritual man was mad, for the multitude of thy iniquity, and the multitude of thy madness" (Hosea 9:7),[108] and one might add that there is a parallel pagan tradition here, which looked on those who were inspired by Apollo in the same light (see H, 471). For instance, there is Virgil's account in Book 5 of the *Æneid* of when Aeneas consults the Cumaean Sibyl, the priestess presiding over the Apollonian oracle at Cumae:

> Thus, from the dark recess, the Sibyl spoke,
> And the resisting air the thunder broke;
> The cave rebellow'd, and the temple shook.

[105] Jung, letter to J.B. Lang of March 1918; cited in RB, 47.
[106] Adler, "Aspects of Jung's Personality and Work," p. 12; cited in *Catafalque*, vol. 1, p. 71.
[107] Kingsley, *Catafalque*, vol. 1, p. 343.
[108] See also 4 Kings 9:11; Ezekiel 3:25; Ezekiel 33:30; and Jeremiah 29:26.

> Th' ambiguous god, who rul'd her lab'ring breast,
> In these mysterious words his mind express'd;
> Some truths reveal'd, in terms involv'd the rest.
> At length her fury fell, her foaming ceas'd,
> [*Ut primum cessit furor et rabida ora quierunt*]
> And, ebbing in her soul, the god decreas'd.
> (Book 6, translated Dryden)

and Cicero, in discussion with Quintus in *On Divination*, challenges the view of Cratippus thus: "But what weight is to be given to that frenzy of yours, which you term 'divine' and which enables the crazy man to see what the wise man does not see, and invests the man who has lost human intelligence with the intelligence of the gods [*ea videat insanus, et is qui humanos sensus amiserit divinos adsecutus sit*]?" (Book 2, §54).[109]

In his essay "The Concept of the Unconscious" (1936; 1954), Jung remarked that "if, thirty years ago, anyone had dared to predict that our psychological development was tending towards a revival of the medieval persecutions of the Jews, that Europe would again tremble before the Roman fasces and the tramp of legions, that people would once more give the Roman salute, as two thousand years ago, and that instead of the Christian Cross an archaic swastika would lure onward millions of warriors ready for death — why, that man would have been hooted at as a mystical fool," adding: "And today? Surprising as it may seem, all this absurdity is a horrible reality" (CW 9/i §98). And in *Memories, Dreams, Reflections*, Jung firmly rejects the label of being "wise" (*weise*) or being "a sage" (*ein »Wissender«*), and he attributes to those occasions when he was (presumably, like Socrates) "overpowered" (*überflügelt*) or "gripped" (*gedrängt*) by his inner daimon (*ein Dämon in mir*) the

[109] Cicero, *De Senectute; De Amicitia; De Divinatione*, trans. William Armistead Falconer (Cambridge, MA; London: Harvard University Press, 1923), p. 495.

fact that at times he had "to hasten on, to catch up with my vision," with the result that "my contemporaries, understandably, could not perceive my vision, they saw only a fool rushing ahead [*einen sinnlos Davonlaufenden*]" (MDR, 389).

And in his exchanges with Eugen Rolfe in November and December 1960 (or, in other words, shortly before his death in 1961), not only is Jung's sense of isolation highly reminiscent of his Grail dream of 1938, when he realizes that there is no one else but him who can search for the Grail, but he tells Rolfe that "to live an archetypic life is no reason for an inflation as it is the ordinary life of Man,"[110] a phrase which Kingsley glosses as follows: "Where [Jung] ends up is a place of such simplicity that it's hard for anyone to understand. For him the totally extraordinary has become the utterly ordinary which, what's more, was the normal state of humanity right from the start."[111]

After drawing attention to a passage in Jung's *Zarathustra* seminar explaining how religious systems are "not inventions, but are revelations" (SNZ, vol. 2, p. 971), Kingsley introduces the notion of *Uroffenbarung* (328, 331), in relation to which Jung's scientific pretensions were a *Bekleidungsstoff* or "cloak" (329). From this perspective, Jung's most important works are *Aion* (1951), a work arising from Jung's experience of ecstatic mystical union in 1944 and which stands in a special relation to the figure of Joachim of Fiore (c. 1135-1202); and *Answer to Job* (1952), a work whose true significance, it is said, that few have grasped, with the exception of Erich Neumann (356). And if it is true that "it takes a prophet to understand a prophet" (632), Kingsley does little to hide the prophetic dimension of his own book in two volumes, *Catafalque*. So whereas Jung's task was "to translate his mission and message to the world out from the language of prophecy into

[110] Eugene Rolfe, *Encounter with Jung* (Boston: Sigo Press, 1989), p. 178.
[111] Kingsley, *Catafalque*, vol. 1, p. 142.

the language of science" (696), Kingsley reverses this process. Thus, psychology and religion are said to be fundamentally the same (662, n. 53), inasmuch as prophets "speak on behalf of" the divine reality inside them (647, n. 36).

In turn, this argument should prompt us to consider how Wolfram von Eschenbach presents his epic work, for he explicitly foregrounds questions about communication and structure in his famous "bowstring parable," to which we shall now turn.

The Bowstring Parable

In a significant excursus that is inserted in Book 5, Wolfram uses the famous "bowstring parable" to describe his narrative technique:[112]

> Methinks that I then shall show ye the bowstring without the bow.
> 'Tis a symbol good, the bowstring, for swift as ye deem the bow,
> Yet the shaft that the bowstring speedeth findeth swifter its aim, I trow!
> And not without thought I said it, for the string, it seemeth me,
> Is like to the simple story wherewith men well-pleased shall be;
> For it goeth straight to its ending, while he who aside shall stray,
> Tho' his goal at last he reacheth findeth all too long his way.
> When unbent the bow thou sawest, then straight was, I ween, the string,

[112] For further discussion, see DKV, vol. 2, pp. 586-588; and Arthur B. Groos, Jr., "Wolfram von Eschenbach's 'Bow Metaphor' and the Narrative Technique of *Parzival*," *Modern Language Notes*, vol. 87, no. 3 (April 1972), 391-408.

From the straight line thou erst must draw it, ere the
shaft to its goal may wing.
But he who his story aimeth at the ear of a fool shall
find
His shaft go astray, for no dwelling it findeth within
his mind.
Too wide is the road, I think me, and that which he
chance to hear
Ere yet he may know the meaning flies out at the other
ear.
Far rather at home I'ld bide me than in such ears my
story tell,
A beast, or a stock, I think me, as a hearer would serve
as well.

(§241, ll. 8-30; vol. 1, p. 138)

Later, in Book 16, Wolfram returns to this metaphor in a brief reprise, when the narrator interjects: "Nor my tale like the bow shall be bended, but straight as an arrow flies" (§805, ll. 14-15; vol. 2, p. 174). On both occasions, the bow metaphor occurs in a context that is significant: on the first occasion, at the moment of Parzival's lapse and the beginning of his hardships when, following his failure ask Anfortas about his affliction, the entourage leaves the banquet hall (and later the Grail Castle itself, thus depriving him of the opportunity to make good his lapse and to fulfill his destiny); and, on the second, at the pinnacle of Parzival's success after he has been called back to the Grail Castle.[113] What, however, does the parable mean?

To begin with, the metaphor needs to be seen in the context of the classical and medieval distinction, based on Horace's *Ars poetica* and the *Rhetorica ad Herennium* (formerly attributed to Cicero or Cornificius, but in fact of unknown authorship), between stylistic

[113] Groos, "Wolfram von Eschenbach's 'Bow Metaphor' and the Narrative Technique of *Parzival*," pp. 400-401, cf. pp. 391-392.

adornment, i.e., the *ornatus*, and narrative structure, i.e., the *ordo* or *dispositio*. In turn, the *ordo* can be divided into two kinds: the order of discourse chosen by the narrator, i.e., the *ordo artificialis* (or *artificiosus*); and the succession of events in a story, i.e., the *ordo naturalis*. (This distinction recurs in more recent literary theory: in Formalist theory, for instance, in the distinction between *fabula* and *syzuhet*, i.e., between events and narrative construction, or in other words between the "story" or the chronological sequence of events and the "plot" or the manner in which the narrative presents them;[114] in structuralist literary theory, in the distinction between *langue* and *parole*;[115] and in psychoanalytic approaches to literature, where the task of psychoanalysis is to read the past in order to be able to make sense of the present.)[116]

For medieval rhetors and commentators, both sacred and pagan literature (that is, both the Bible and, say, Virgil's *Aeneid*) served as examples of an "artistic" disposition, demonstrating what

[114] Ann Jefferson and David Robey, *Modern Literary Theory: A Comparative Introduction* (London: Batsford, 1986), p. 39. A classic example of this approach to narrative is Viktor Shklovsky's famous essay on *Tristram Shandy*, first published in Russian in 1921 (see Viktor Shklovsky, "Stern's *Tristram Shandy*: Stylistic Commentary," in Lee T. Lemon and Marion J. Reis (eds), *Russian Formalist Criticism: Four Essays* (Lincoln, NB: University of Nebraska Press, 1965), pp. 25-57.

[115] Jefferson and Robey, *Modern Literary Theory*, p. 99. Two examples of the narratological approach would be Tzvetan Todorov's analysis of the 14th-century collection of novellas by the Renaissance humanist Giovanni Boccaccio (Tzvetan Todorov, *Grammaire du Décameron* (The Hague: Mouton, 1969); and Gérard Genette's "Le discours du récit" of 1972, in which he defines the subject of his study as "narrative discourse" (Gérard Genette, *Narrative Discourse: An Essay in Method*, trans. Jane E. Lewin (Ithaca, NY: Cornell University Press, 1980), p. 29).

[116] Jefferson and Robey, *Modern Literary Theory*, p. 150. In this respect, Freud's case histories have been compared to detective stories (see E.A. Loewenstein, "The Freudian Case History: A Detective Story or a Dialectical Progression? Reflections on Psychoanalytic Narratives from a Lacanian Perspective," *Psychoanalytic Psychology*, vol. 9, no. 1 (1992), 49-59). And such theorists as Peter Brooks and Jonathan Culler have discovered an analogy between the Russian Formalist distinction (see above) of *fabula* and *syuzhet* and the narrative that arises in the psychoanalytic situation (Peter Brooks, "Fictions of the Wolfman," *Diacritics*, vol. 9, no. 1 (1979), 72-83; and Jonathan Culler, "*Fabula* and *syuzhet* in the Analysis of Narrative," *Poetics Today*, vol. 1, no. 3 (1980), 27-37).

Remegius of Auxerre (c. 841-908) in his commentary on Martianus Capella's *De Nuptiis Philologiae et Mercurii et de septem Artibus liberalibus libri novem* (or *On the Wedding Day of Philology and Mercury and of the Seven Liberal Arts, in Nine Books*), called a narrative scheme that was *voluntate et ingenio*, i.e., by choice and ingenious.[117] These distinctions between adornment and arrangement, and in turn between artistic and natural arrangement, form the background to Wolfram's parable.

Similarly, the bow metaphor itself has both biblical[118] and pagan analogs. To begin with, there are two principal biblical sources of the metaphor, in the Book of Psalms, "Except you will be converted, he will brandish his sword; he hath bent his bow, and made it ready. And in it he hath prepared the instruments of death, he hath made ready his arrows for them that burn" (Psalm 7:13-14), and the Book of Job, "My glory shall be always renewed, and my bow in my hand shall be repaired" (Job 29:20). In his *Expositions on the Book of Psalms*, St. Augustine allegorically interprets the relationship between the Old and New Testaments in terms of the bending of the bow by the bowstring, in order to dispatch sacred truths like shot arrows: "That bow then I would readily take to be the Holy Scripture, in which by the strength of the New Testament, as by a sort of string, the hardness of the Old has been bent and subdued. From thence the Apostles are sent forth like arrows, or divine preachings are shot."[119] And in his *Moralia in Job*, St. Gregory the Great explores the interaction between the bow and

---

[117] D.H. Green, *The Beginnings of Medieval Romance: Fact and Fiction, 1150-1220* (Cambridge: Cambridge University Press, 2004), Chapter 5, "Fiction and structure" (pp. 93-133).

[118] For further discussion, see David Finnemore Hill, *An Archer Looks at the Bible: A Study of the Literal and Figurative Allusions to the Bow and Arrow* (Durham: Pentland Press, 1994).

[119] On Psalm 7, §14 (on v. 13), in *Expositions on the Book of Psalms*, vol. 1, *Psalms I-XXXVI* Library of the Fathers, vol. 24] (Oxford; London: Parker; Rivington, 1847), p. 56.

the bowstring as a metaphor for the rigidity of the Old Testament law being bent by the spiritual interpretation of the New Testament.

Commenting on Job 29:20, but also referring to Psalm 7:13-14 and to a passage in Isaiah, "With arrows and with bows they shall go in thither" (Isaiah 7:24), Gregory writes:

> What then in this place is to be understood by the name of the bow but sacred Revelation? For by the string the New Testament, while by the bow the Old Testament, is understood. Now in a bow, when the string is drawn, the horn is bended: so in this same sacred Revelation, when the New Testament is read, the hardness of the Old is rendered pliant. For to the spiritual and mild precepts of this, the rigidness of the letter of the other bends itself; because whilst the New Testament as it were by a kind of arm of good practice is drawn, in the Old Testament the claims of severity are relaxed. Nor do we improperly say that the string accords with the New Testament, which it is certain came out by the Incarnation of the Lord. And so as it were the string is drawn and the horns bent; because when in the New Testament the Incarnation of our Mediator is seen, the rigidness of the Old Testament is made to bend to a spiritual signification. (Book 19, §55)[120]

Consequently, Gregory equates a true understanding of scripture with a life lived in accordance with scriptural principles:

> "A bow in the hand" is Holy Writ in the practising. For he holds "a bow in his hand," who performs by the practising

[120] Gregory the Great, *Morals on the Book of Job* [*Library of the Fathers*, vol. 38], vol. 2 (Parts 3 and 4) (Oxford; London: Parker; Rivington, 1845), p. 443.

> the divine revelations which he learns by apprehension. Thus the "bow is renewed in the hand," in that whatever is learnt belonging to Holy Revelation by studying is fulfilled by living accordingly. (Book 19, §56)[121]

The quotation from Psalm 7 also forms the starting point of Hugh of St. Victor's discussion of allegory in the *Didascalicon* (book 6, chapter 4),[122] and Arthur B. Groos, Jr., concludes that "in the light of this extensive tradition, Wolfram von Eschenbach's bow metaphor could be viewed as an analogy to the commonplace bow exegesis of medieval Biblical commentaries which he employs to defend and elucidate the artistic disposition of his narrative" (397).

At the same time, there are significant links to the nonbiblical context of pagan literature, such as Virgil's *Aeneid* where, in the account in Book 19 of Turnus's siege of the Trojan camp, we read that "Jove bow'd the heav'ns, and lent a gracious ear, / And thunder'd on the left, amidst the clear. / Sounded at once the bow; and swiftly flies / The feather'd death, and hisses thro' the skies" (Book 19, ll. 704-705),[123] or even the *Histories* of Herodotus where, in the account in Book 8 of Xerxes's taking of the Acropolis after the defeat of the Greek fleet at Thermopylae in the Greco-Persian wars, we learn how "the Persians took up their position upon a hill which the Athenians call the Areiopagos and which faces the Acropolis, and then began their siege of the place in this way": "They wrapped their arrows with hemp fiber and, after setting them on fire, shot them at the barricade" (Book 8, §52).[124] Ultimately,

---

[121] Gregory the Great, *Morals on the Book of Job*, p. 443.

[122] *The Didascalicon of Hugh of St. Victor: A Medieval Guide to the Arts*, trans. Jerome Taylor (New York and London: Columbia University Press, 1961), pp. 139-144.

[123] Translated by John Dryden, in Virgil, *Works*, vol. 4 (London: Bathurst, 1782), p. 39. The passage is discussed in Montaigne, *Essays*, book 1, no. 48, "On War-Horses" (Michel de Montaigne, *The Complete Essays*, ed. and trans. M.A. Screech (Harmondsworth: Penguin, 2003), p. 325).

[124] Robert B. Strassler (ed.), *The Landmark Herodotus: The Histories* (London: Quercus, 2008), p. 621.

however, the bow metaphor can be traced back to the image of the bow and the lyre in Heraclitus:

> Listening not to me but to the account [*logos*], it is wise to agree that all things are one. [...] They do not comprehend how, in differing, it agrees with itself — a backward-turning connection, like that of a bow and a lyre. (DK 22 B 50, 51)[125]

As is so often the case in Heraclitus, the reading and meaning of almost every key word is in dispute. Is the word for "agreement" *homologeei* or (as in the manuscripts of Hippolytus) *homologeein*? Is the word for "back-turning" *palintropos* or *palintonos* ("back-stretched," "back-bending")? And what does the word *harmoniē* actually mean — "joining" or "fitting together" (in the sense of carpentry or shipbuilding), "agreement" or "compact" (as between hostile parties), "fitting together" (in the sense of tuning a musical instrument or using different strings to produce a desired scale or key), or even "adjustment" or "reconciliation" (in the Pythagorean sense in which opposing powers of the cosmos are held together)?[126]

Leaving these specific questions on one side, however, the logic of Heraclitus's simile seems to be that when the arrow leaves the string, the archer's hands are pulling in opposite ways to each other and to the different parts of the bow (cf. Plato,

[125] Jonathan Barnes, *Early Greek Philosophy* (Harmondsworth: Penguin, 1987), p. 102.

[126] See Charles H. Kahn, *The Art and Thought of Heraclitus* (Cambridge: Cambridge University Press, 1979), pp. 195-196. For further discussion, see Seth Bernadete, *The Bow and the Lyre: A Platonic Reading of the "Odyssey"* (Lanham, MD: Rowman & Littlefield, 1997), although the central allusion here is not to the *Symposium* or even to Heraclitus but to the use of the lyre as a simile for Odyesseus's bow in *Odyssey*, Book 21, ll. 406-411. For discussion of how the "bow composition" is a narrative technique developed by Heraclitus to reveal his conception of the world, see Celso Vieira, "Heraclitus' Bow Composition," *Classical Quarterly*, vol. 63, no. 2 (2013), 473-490.

Republic, 439b); that a similar combination of tension and retention allows the lyre to make sweet musical sounds; and that the entire universe itself is maintained and sustained by the equilibrium that results from opposing tensions.[127] In fact, this fragment is cited in Plato's *Symposium* at a significant juncture in the dialogue where Erixymachus uses Heraclitus's example of the bow and the lyre as an illustration of how harmony may be brought into being between the two opposites of the high-pitched and the low:

> And so not merely is all medicine governed, as I propound it, through the influence of this god, but likewise athletics and agriculture. Music also, as is plain to any the least curious observer, is in the same sort of case: perhaps Heracleitus intends as much by those perplexing words, "The One at variance with itself is drawn together, like harmony of bow or lyre." Now it is perfectly absurd to speak of a harmony at variance, or as formed from things still varying. Perhaps he meant, however, that from the grave and acute which were varying before, but which afterwards came to agreement, the harmony was by musical art created. For surely there can be no harmony of acute and grave while still at variance: harmony is consonance, and consonance is a kind of agreement; and agreement of things varying, so long as they are at variance, is impossible. On the other hand, when a thing varies with no disability of agreement, then it may be harmonized; just as rhythm is produced by fast and slow, which in the beginning were at variance but later came to agree. In all these cases the agreement is brought about by music

[127] Lewis Campbell (ed.), *The Theaetetus of Plato* (Oxford: Oxford University Press, 1861), p. xl; cited in R.G. Bury (ed.), *The Symposium of Plato* (Cambridge: Heffer, 1932), p. 49.

> which, like medicine in the former instance, introduces a mutual love and unanimity. Hence in its turn music is found to be a knowledge of love-matters relating to harmony and rhythm. (186e-187c)[128]

By communicating lowness to the high and highness to the low, the stretched cord of the bow or the lyre brings contrary, and even contradictory, aspects into harmonious union, thereby creating harmony out of these two extremes.[129] Tellingly, for the ancient Greeks the principal attributes of Apollo, the god of archery and the god of music and dance (among other things), were the bow (in fact, a golden bow and a quiver of silver arrows) and the lyre.[130]

What, however, is the purpose of the bow metaphor in Wolfram's *Parzival*? If we follow Arthur Groos in his reading, it has at least three functions. First, both Wolfram and biblical exegetes interpret the bow "as a figure of speech, presented as a 'bîspel' or a 'similitudine,' which characterizes the adaptation or exposition of a text to render it intelligible to an audience," and hence the bow and bowstring are "associated in an analogous manner with two parts or aspects of each work" — i.e., the natural order of a story and its artificial arrangement, or the Old and New Testaments — "which are ultimately made coherent by the adaptor or commentator" (Groos, 398). (In the case of Wolfram, the metaphor fits with the theme of his deviation from Chrétien and his adherence to the problematic

[128] Plato, vol. 5, *Lysis; Symposium; Gorgias*, trans. W.R.M. Lamb (London; New York: Heinemann; Putnam, 1925), pp. 127-129. For further discussion, see John E. Ziolkowski, "The Bow and the Lyre: Harmonizing Duos in Plato's *Symposium*," *The Classical Journal*, vol. 95, no. 1 (October-November 1999), 19-35; and Kenneth Dorter, "The Significance of the Speeches in Plato's *Symposium*," *Philosophy & Rhetoric*, vol. 2, no. 4 (Fall, 1969), 215-234.

[129] Ziolkowski, "The Bow and the Lyre," pp. 31-32.

[130] According to Diodorus Siculus, Hermes had discovered the three-stringed lyre (cf. book 1.16.1), while Apollo had presumably added an additional four strings, which were subsequently rediscovered by the Muses, Linus, Orpheus, and Thamyas (*Library of History*, book 3, §59).

figures of Kyot and, in turn, Flegetanis.) Second, both Wolfram and the biblical exegetes "state that the resultant action of bending the bow by the string propels the 'arrow' or message rapidly to its goal" (Groos, 399). Or as Wolfram puts it, "now you think a bow is swift: yet what it lets fly is swifter" (*nu dunket iuch der boge snel: / doch ist sneller daz diu senewe jaget*) (§24, ll. 10-11; trans. Hatto).

Third, there is a parallel between the attempts Wolfram makes to differentiate the symbolical significance of his own narrative bow from a bow that is twisted or *krump*, and the exegetical tradition of preferring a variant reading of Psalm 77:57, where *pravum* is read as *perversum*, thereby suggesting an association between the crooked bow and the deceitful intentions of false exegetes. In the bowstring parable, Wolfram equates crookedness with deceit and attributes this intention to his opponents: "But when a storyteller takes you round about, he is out to delude you" (*swer iu sager von der krümbe, / der wil iuch leiten ümbe*) (§24, ll. 15-16). In his *Enarrationes*, Augustine comments on the biblical passage in question as follows: "'They were turned,' he saith, 'into a crooked,' or, as some copies have it, 'into a perverse bow.' But what this is doth better appear in that which followeth, where he saith (v. 58), 'And unto wrath they provoked Him with their hills' (v. 59). It doth signify that they leaped into idolatry. The bow then was perverted, not for the name of the Lord, but against the name of the Lord: who said to the same people, 'Thou shalt have none other Gods but Me' [Exodus 20:3]. But by the bow He doth signify the mind's intention."[131]

The narrative context in which Wolfram introduces the bowstring parable is, as mentioned above, as follows: Parzival has failed to ask the question of Anfortas, and as the Grail entourage leaves the banquet hall, it passes a chamber in which Parzival sees "thro' the open door / Within an outer chamber, on a folding couch

[131] *Expositions on the Book of Psalms*, vol. 4, *Psalms LXXVI-CI* [Library of the Fathers, vol. 32] (Oxford; London: Parker; Rivington, 1850), p. 76.

[…] / The fairest of old men ancient whom ever his eyes had seen, / Grey was he as mists of morning" — this is, of course, Titurel (Anfortas's grandfather and hence Parzival's great-grandfather), but this is information that, at this point, Wolfram strategically withholds with the following justification:

> — Nor o'er rash is the tale, I ween,
> Who he was shalt thou know hereafter, when a fitting time shall be,
> The host, his Burg, and his kingdom, yea, all will I name to ye,
> And all shall be clear and in order, no halting my tale shall know;
> Methinks that I then shall show ye the bowstring without the bow.
>
> (§241, ll. 1-8; vol. 1, p. 137)

The final line in this quotation, *ich sage die senewen âne bogen* ("I give you the bowstring, not the bow"; trans. Hatto, p. 128), has a variant reading (in some G-class manuscripts), *ich sage diu senewe ungelogen* ("I tell you the story truthfully" or "I tell you the story straight"). (Or, as Edwin H. Zeydel and Bayard Quincy Morgan translate this couplet, "And no digression will I show: / Straight string and not the bow" [p. 128].)[132] This promise equally anticipates Wolfram's later claim in Book 16 that "this story goes straight and truthfully, not curved like a bow" (*ez ist niht krump alsô der boge, / diz mære ist wâr unde sleht*) (§805, ll. 14-15; trans. Hatto, p. 400).

[132] Groos, "Wolfram von Eschenbach's 'Bow Metaphor' and the Narrative Technique of *Parzival*," p. 399. In the variant reading in some G-class manuscripts of the previous line, i.e., *unde allez rehte vur gezogen* instead of *unde ân allez für zogen* (§241, l. 7), Groos detects an echo of the doctrine of the *ordo artificialis*, the rearrangement of events according to an order of discourse deemed "*voluntate et ingenio*" by the narrator (p. 394).

Now the proximity to a phrase found in Chrétien, namely *la droite voie aler* (*Erec*, ll. 55777 and 5583; *Lancelot*, l. 6271) points to a link that is more than simply philological or imagistic; it is also existential.

After all, in the "Prologue in Heaven" in *Faust*, Part One, the Lord tells Mephistopheles, "That a good man, by his dim impulse driven, / Of the right way hath ever consciousness [*Ist sich des rechten Weges wohl bewußt*]" (ll. 328-329). And the search for the right path and an extensive use of the image of the arrow are hallmarks of Nietzsche's thought, especially in *Thus Spoke Zarathustra*. In the Prologue, Zarathustra declares: "I love the great despisers, because they are the great adorers, and arrows of longing for the other shore. [...] I love him who loveth his virtue: for virtue is the will to down-going, and an arrow of longing. [...] Alas! there cometh the time when man will no longer launch the arrow of his longing beyond man — and the string of his bow will have unlearned to whizz!" (Z Prologue §4 and §5). In "On War and Warriors," Zarathustra advises: "One can only be silent and sit peacefully when one hath arrow and bow; otherwise one prateth and quarrelleth. Let your peace be a victory!" (Z I 10). In "On the Friend" he declares: "Thou canst not adorn thyself fine enough for thy friend; for thou shalt be unto him an arrow and a longing for the Superman" (Z I 14), while asking in "On Child and Marriage": 'Thirst in the creating one, arrow and longing for the Superman: tell me, my brother, is this thy will to marriage?" (Z I 20). And in "On the Thousand and One Goals" he extends this image, declaring that "'To speak truth, and be skilful with bow and arrow' — so seemed it alike pleasing and hard to the people from whom cometh my name — the name which is alike pleasing and hard to me" (Z I 15).

In Part Two, in the chapter called "The Grave-Song" that proved in his seminar on *Zarathustra* to be of almost endless fascination to Jung, Zarathustra cries out in agony:

> To kill ME, did they strangle you, ye singing birds of my hopes! Yea, at you, ye dearest ones, did malice ever shoot its arrows — to hit my heart!
>
> And they hit it! Because ye were always my dearest, my possession and my possessedness: ON THAT ACCOUNT had ye to die young, and far too early!
>
> At my most vulnerable point did they shoot the arrow—namely, at you, whose skin is like down — or more like the smile that dieth at a glance!
>
> (Z II 11)

In "Of Old and New Law Tablets," Zarathustra cries out in ecstasy:

> Thus did my wise longing, born in the mountains, cry and laugh in me; a wild wisdom, verily! — my great pinion-rustling longing.
>
> And oft did it carry me off and up and away and in the midst of laughter; then flew I quivering like an arrow with sun-intoxicated rapture:
>
> — Out into distant futures, which no dream hath yet seen, into warmer souths than ever sculptor conceived, — where gods in their dancing are ashamed of all clothes:
>
> (That I may speak in parables and halt and stammer like the poets: and verily I am ashamed that I have still to be a poet!)
>
> (Z III 12 §1)

and at the end of this discourse Zarathustra solemnly declares:

> — That I may one day be ready and ripe in the great noontide: ready and ripe like the glowing ore, the

> lightning-bearing cloud, and the swelling milk-udder:—
> — Ready for myself and for my most hidden Will: a bow eager for its arrow, an arrow eager for its star:—
> — A star, ready and ripe in its noontide, glowing, pierced, blessed, by annihilating sun-arrows:—
> — A sun itself, and an inexorable sun-will, ready for annihilation in victory!
> O Will, thou change of every need, MY needfulness! Spare me for one great victory! —
>
> (Z III 12 §30)

Finally, in the concluding chapter of Part Four, "The Sign," we read: "And verily, there came down upon him as it were a cloud, like a cloud of arrows which poureth upon a new enemy. But behold, here it was a cloud of love, and showered upon a new friend" (Z IV 20).

In his seminar on *Zarathustra*, Jung discusses the inter-connectedness of such images as the star, the wheel, and the golden ball (SNZ, vol. 1, pp. 52-53), and he might well have added that the image of the arrow is cognate with the images of the bolt of lightning and "the heavy drop out of the cloud" as symbols of the *Übermensch*. In *Twilight of the Idols*, Nietzsche presents this Zarathustrian conception of the arrow — in a chapter itself titled "Maxims and Arrows" (!) — in the following aphorism: "Formula of my happiness: a Yes, a No, a straight line, a *goal* ..." (TI Maxims §44). And he returns to it in *Ecce Homo* where, looking back on his life, Nietzsche freely admits: "As the outcome of this 'Idealism' I regard all the blunders, the great aberrations of instinct, and the 'modest specializations' which drew me aside from the task of my life; as, for instance, the fact that I became a philologist — why not at least a medical man or anything else which might have opened my eyes?" (EH Why I am So Clever §2).

Indeed, in *Ecce Homo* Nietzsche enunciates the general principle: "The fact that one becomes what one is, presupposes that one has not the remotest suspicion of what one is. From this standpoint even the blunders of one's life have their own meaning and value, the temporary deviations and aberrations, the moments of hesitation and of modesty, the earnestness wasted upon duties which lie outside the actual life-task. In these matters great wisdom, perhaps even the highest wisdom, comes into activity [...]" (EH Why I am So Clever §9). Like Parzival, Nietzsche realizes that there *is* a path; and, like Parzival, he discovers that it is not always easy to follow it; but as Zarathustra also puts it, "A thousand paths are there which have never yet been trodden" (Z I 22 §2), and as he adds in "Of the Spirit of Gravity," "'This — is now MY way, — where is yours?' Thus did I answer those who asked me 'the way.' For THE way — it doth not exist!" (Z III 11 §2).

In *Ecce Homo*, Nietzsche discusses *Zarathustra* on several occasions, on one of which he notes: "People have never asked me as they should have done, what the name of Zarathustra [i.e., Zoroaster] precisely meant in my mouth, in the mouth of the first immoralist; for that which distinguishes this Persian from all others in the past is the very fact that he was the exact reverse of an immoralist." He goes on to explain that, in historical terms, "Zarathustra was the first to see in the struggle between good and evil the essential wheel in the working of things. The translation of morality into the realm of metaphysics, as force, cause, end-in-itself, is his work," and he adds: "But the very question suggests its own answer. Zarathustra created this most portentous of all errors, — morality; therefore he must be the first to expose it." Finally, Nietzsche offers the following encomium of the historical Zoroaster: "[...] Zarathustra was the most truthful of thinkers. In his teaching alone is truthfulness upheld as the highest virtue — that is to say, as the reverse of the cowardice of the 'idealist' who takes to his heels at the sight of reality. Zarathustra has more pluck in his body than all other thinkers put together. To tell the truth and to aim straight: that is the first Persian virtue. Have I made myself clear? ...” (EH Why I am a Destiny §2). Or as Wolfram puts it, “Nor my tale like the bow shall be bended, but straight as an arrow flies” (*ez ist niht krump alsô der boge, / diz mære ist wâr unde sleht*) (§805, ll. 14-15; vol. 2, p. 174).

Thus it is not so much a question of whether “the right path” (or, in Old French, *la droite voie*) is a narrative or an existential principle, it is that narration *is* an existential act. Hence the notion of straightness underling the bow metaphor applies *both* to how we tell stories *and* to how we live our life. In book 5, Parzival encounters the tattered and scantily clad Lady Jeschute of Karnant, sister of King Erec (see Chapter 2 above) and the wife of Duke Orilus. By jousting with Orilus, Parzival returns her to her jealous husband; and, in the battle between Parzival and Orilus, Wolfram’s narrator observes:

> And both they were right, I think me — He who ruleth the ways of life.
> Or straight they may be or crooked, ’twas His so to rule their strife
> [*der beidiu krump unde sleht / geschuof, künner scheiden*]
> That never to one nor the other the joust death for guerdon brought,
> Harm enow had they done to each other the while they so fiercely fought.
>
> (§264, ll. 25-29; vol. 1, p. 149)

In book 14, Gawan mistakes Parzival for Gramoflanz, and the two begin a terrible battle, until some of Arthur’s pages, who happen to be passing by, call out Parzival’s name, and Parzival reveals his identity. In response, Gawan exclaims,

"So, 'tis fitting, here Folly her goal hath found.
And her ways full straight hath she wroughten which aforetime but crooked wound.
[*sô was ez reht: / hiest krumbiu tumpheit worden sleht*]
Here have two hearts, leal and faithful, their hate 'gainst each other shown,
And thy hand which hath won the victory hath the twain of us overthrown. [...]"
(§689, ll. 25-29; vol. 2, p. 108)

These words about reconciling the *krump* ("crooked") with the *sleht* ("straight") might well also be applied to Parzival's striving for the Grail and the necessity of his being called to it, and in this sense how Wolfram directs Parzival's destiny as the hero is analogous to the way in which all human individuals are directed or guided by God. Or, Groos puts it, "as the manipulator of a narrative bow whose operation imitates the mediation between the Old and New Laws of justice and grace associated with the bow of the Divine Author, Wolfram guides Parzival" — just as, one might add, he guides his narrative — "between the *krump* and the *sleht*" (Groos, 401).

In other words, Wolfram's bow parable (in §241, ll. 8-30) which describes his narrative technique as comparable to the string without the bow — like the claim made by Wolfram in his apology to his audience at the end of Book 2 that his story proceeds without the guidance of books *because he cannot read* (cf. §115, ll. 21-30) — is, if taken at face value, implausible; but, if it is read (as Hans Eggers and Friedrich Ohly have argued it should be) as a secular adaptation of a commonplace in medieval biblical exegesis that associates the bow and the string (or learning and lack of learning) *in an analogous way* to the letter of the Old Testament and the spirit of the New, both these and other passages become intelligible (Groos, 405). Furthermore, this "implied antithesis between the letter and the spirit" underscores (at least, in *Parzival*, §241 and

§815; and §115) the relationship between "the natural order of narrative materials" and its "artistic arrangement" (Groos, 405) — or, more broadly, between what Jung in *The Red Book* calls "the spirit of this time" and "the spirit of the depths" (RB, 119). That is to say, what are the structural techniques involved in creating a narrative that originates in a "book" (*buoch*) or a "bow" (*bogen*) but then proceeds independently of it, "without the guidance of books" (*âne der buoche stiure*) or "without a bow" (*âne bogen*)? How do we transform ourselves into authentic beings, given that authenticity is something granted, not acquired; or, in Nietzsche's terms, how does one become what one is?

In his prooemium to *Ecce Homo*, Nietzsche undertakes to embark — "And so I tell myself my life" — on an exercise in self-narration that is equally an exercise in self-construction. Or as Jung puts it in *The Red Book*, "you should live your life" (RB, 319). This injunction from the chapter in *Liber Secundus* titled "Hell" offers a succinct summary of this theme that one finds elsewhere in *The Red Book*. In "The Way of What Is to Come" with which *The Red Book* opens, Jung offers the following advice: "Woe betide those who live by way of examples! Life is not with them. If you live according to an example, you thus live the life of that example, but who should live your own life if not yourself? So live yourselves" (RB, 125). In Chapter 2 of *Liber Primus* titled "Soul and God," Jung declares (at one point, echoing Pascal):

> The spirit of the depths even taught me to consider my action and my decision as dependent on dreams. Dreams pave the way for life, and they determine you without you understanding their language. One would like to learn this language, but who can teach and learn it? Scholarliness alone is not enough; there is a knowledge of the heart

> that gives deeper insight.[133] The knowledge of the heart is in no book and is not to be found in the mouth of any teacher, but grows out of you like the green seed from the dark earth. Scholarliness belongs to the spirit of this time, but this spirit in no way grasps the dream, since the soul is everywhere that scholarly knowledge is not. But how can I attain the knowledge of the heart? You can attain this knowledge only by living your life to the full. You live your life fully if you also live what you have never yet lived, but have left for others to live or to think. You will say: "But I cannot live or think everything that others live or think." But you should say: "The life that I could still live, I should live, and the thoughts that I could still think, I should think." (RB, 133)

Reflecting in the 10th chapter of *Liber Primus* titled 'Instruction' on his conversation with Elijah and Salome, Jung returns to this theme of existential authenticity:

> It is no small matter to acknowledge one's yearning. For this many need to make a particular effort at honesty. All too many do not want to know where their yearning is, because it would seem to them impossible or too distressing. And yet yearning is the way of life. If you do not acknowledge your yearning, then you do not follow yourself, but go on foreign ways that others have indicated to you. So you do not live your life but

[133] Compare with Pascal's dictum, *Le coeur a ses raisons que la raison ne connaît point* ("The heart has its reasons of which the reason knows nothing"), in Pascal, *Pensées*, trans A.J. Krailsheimer (Harmondsworth: Penguin, 1966), §423-*277* (p. 154), cf. *C'est le cœur qui sent Dieu et non la raison. Voilà ce que c'est la foi. Dieu sensible au cœur, non à la raison* ("It is the heart which perceives God and not the reason. That is what faith is: God perceived by the heart, not by the reason"), in *Pensées*, §424-*278* (p. 154).

> an alien one. But who should live your life if you do not live it? It is not only stupid to exchange your own life for an alien one, but also a hypocritical game, because you can never really live the life of others, you can only pretend to do it, deceiving the other and yourself, since you can only live your own life.
> [...]
> To live oneself means: to be one's own task. Never say that it is a pleasure to live oneself. It will be no joy [*keine Freude*] but a long suffering [*ein langes Leiden*], since you must become your own creator [*du musst dein eigener Schöpfer werden*].[134] If you want to create yourself, then you do not begin with the best and the highest, but with the worst and the deepest. Therefore say that you are reluctant to live yourself. The flowing together of the stream of life is not joy but pain, since it is power against power, guilt, and shatters the sanctified. (RB, 188-189)

In the third chapter of *Liber Secundus,* titled "One of the Lowly," Jung picks up this theme, as if echoing Zarathustra's injunction in the chapter of the third part of *Thus Spoke Zarathustra* titled "The Home-Coming," namely that "one should live on mountains" (Z III 9):

> Your heights are your own mountain, which belongs to you and you alone. There you are individual and

[134] In "On the Way of the Creator" (Z I 17), Zarathustra adumbrates the theme of creation and its relation to suffering to which he will, in "On the Blissful Islands," return as he declares:

> Creating — that is the great salvation from suffering, and life's alleviation. But for the creator to appear, suffering itself is needed, and much transformation.
> Yea, much bitter dying must there be in your life, ye creators! Thus are ye advocates and justifiers of all perishableness.
> For the creator himself to be the new-born child, he must also be willing to be the child-bearer, and endure the pangs of the child-bearer. (Z II 1)

> live your very own life. If you live your own life, you do not live the common life, which is always continuing and never-ending, the life of history and the inalienable and ever-present burdens and products of the human race. There you live the endlessness of being, but not the becoming. Becoming belongs to the heights and is full of torment. (RB, 237-238)

In "The Gift of Magic" in *Liber Secundus*, Jung castigates his readers for their "weakness," their "doubt," and their "fear" — "You will not bear going your way. [...] As if you were not yourself! Who should accomplish your deeds? Who should carry your virtues and your vices?" — and connects this theme to the figures of the dead: "You do not come to an end with your life, and the dead will besiege you terribly to live your unlived life" (RB, 384). Finally, in *Scrutinies* (*Prüfungen*), the role of the dead is more positively expressed by the shadow of the dead one who, raising its voice, tells Jung: "You see — or do you still not see, what the living do with your life. They fritter it away. But with me you live yourself, since I belong to you" (RB, 488). Yet — when Jung sees the sun swimming in a sea of blood and lamentation and asks the shadow of the dead one, "is this supposed to be the sacrifice of joy?" (*Soll es das Opfer der Freude sein?*), she tells him: "Joy [*Die Freude*] should neither be made nor sought; it should come, if it must come. [...] Joy can never be prepared, but it exists of itself or it does not exist" (RB, 491).

Wolfram's parable or allegory of the bowstring is thus *both* a point about literary composition and narrative construction, *and* about the narrative that we make of our own lives. It should prompt us to consider and appreciate the remarkable complexity of his *Parzival* epic, as a way of reflecting on the astonishing adventure of its hero's, Parzival's, threefold quest: for his identity, for *vröude* ("joy"), and for the Grail. In the course of this quest, Parzival himself is transformed from a fool to the lord of the Grail, and the power of the Grail brings about a collective transformation as well. Thus,

Wolfram's epic embodies the ambition, expressed in the words of the Jung-inspired tagline for the internet podcast *Aeon Byte Gnostic Radio*, to "write your own gospel and live your own myth."

Conclusion (A)

So what *is* the Grail? This is not the first time we have asked this question, nor can we pretend to have answered it fully. (As William Nitze observed, "the Grail symbolizes in its evasiveness the problem of its own origin.")[135] According to Chrétien, it is a "very holy thing" (*toute sainte chose est li Graax* [l. 6425]); according to Wolfram, it is the "wish of paradise" (*wunsch von pardîs*) (§235, l. 21, cf. §470, l. 14), it "outdoes all earthly wishes" (*erden wunsches überwal*) (§235, l. 24), it is the "fruit of holy bliss [*sælden*], the sweetness of the world [*der werlde süeze*]" (§238, ll. 21-22). And, in the case of Wolfram's *Parzival*, it is a stone and it resembles an emerald jewel. But what *is* it? Perhaps the clue lies in the reference to emerald; for in the so-called *Emerald Tablet of Hermes* (also known as the *Tabula Smaragdina* or the *Smaragdine Tablet*), and in other Hermetic works we find the celebrated maxim, "As above, so below," or (in its full form) "That which is above is like to that which is below, and that which is below is like to that which is above" (*Quod est superius est sicut quod inferius, et quod inferius est sicut quod est superius*).[136]

In his discussion of this Hermetic text as an alchemical tool for personal transformation, Dennis William Hauck draws a link between the *Emerald Tablet* and the seven operational stages of alchemy (i.e., calcination, dissolution, separation, conjunction, fermentation, distillation, and coagulation) as set out by a 15th-century writer known as Basilius Valentinus in his *Azoth, ou le moyen de faire l'or caché*

[135] Nitze, "The Fisher King in the Grail Romances," p. 365.

[136] For the entire text in translation, see Eric J. Holmyard, "The Emerald Table," *Nature*, 112 (6 October 1923), 525-526; and Robert Steele and Dorothea Waley Singer, "The Emerald Table," *Proceedings of the Royal Society of Medicine*, vol. 21, no. 3 (January 1928), 485-501 [41-57].

des philosophes (1624). In this work, Valentinus includes a series of illustrations, including one that is a kind of "meditative mandala" that illustrates and summarizes these seven alchemical steps in the following axion, "Visita interiora terræ rectificando invenies occultum lapidem" (i.e., "Visit the interior of the earth and [by] purifying [yourself] you will find the hidden stone").[137] (These seven alchemical steps are summarized in the alchemical phrase, *Solve et coagula* (i.e., "dissolve and coagulate") — or in Aniela Jaffé's paraphrase, "out of dissolution, unity!" —[138] cited by Jung in his foreword to *Mysterium coniunctionis* [CW 14 p. xiv].)

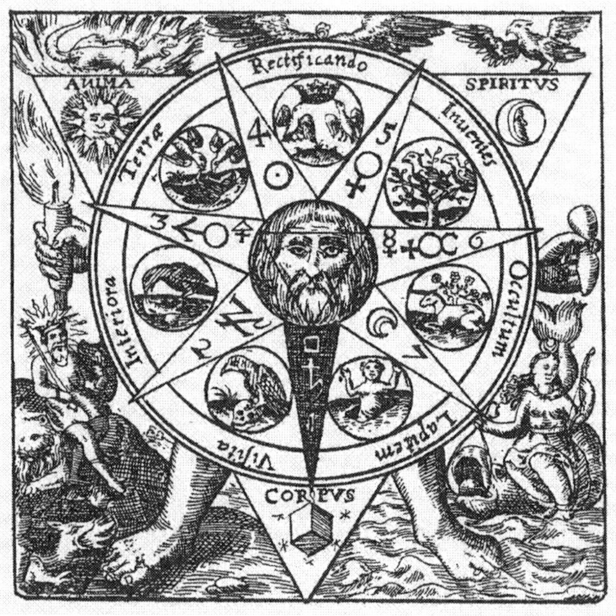

Figure 1: The Seven Operations of Alchemy or the Azoth Mandala.[139]

[137] Dennis William Hauck, *The Emerald Tablet: Alchemy for Personal Transformation* (New York: Penguin/Arkana, 1999), pp. 153-169 (p. 168), where the passage is translated, "Visit the innermost parts of the earth; by setting things right, you will find the hidden stone."

[138] See Aniela Jaffé, "Alchemy," in *From the Life and Work of C.G. Jung* [1968], trans. R.F.C. Hull and Murray Stein [1971] (Einsiedeln: Daimon Verlag, 1989), pp. 46-77 (p. 76).

[139] These images are available in the public realm HTTP: https://www.azothalchemy.org/azoth_ritual.htm and https://www.azothalchemy.org/downloads/Azoth%20Mandala.pdf.

According to Hauck, the letters "A" and "Z" in the name "Azoth" — "one of the more arcane names for the One Thing described in the tablet" — relate to "the Greek alpha and omega, the beginning and end of all things," and as a word is meant to "embrace the full meaning of the One Thing, which is both chaotic First Matter at the beginning of the Work and the perfected Stone at its conclusion."[140]

Now the notion of the hidden as well as the perfected stone naturally invites comparison with alchemical notions of the philosopher's stone; and, as we have seen, it is in the context of his writings on alchemy that Jung makes some of his most explicit references to Wolfram's *Parzival* (as we saw in Chapter 2 above). Yet alchemy itself becomes in the refining fire of Jung's intellect first and foremost a psychological (and, by the same token, an existential) endeavor — this is a transformation that does not just take place in the retort.

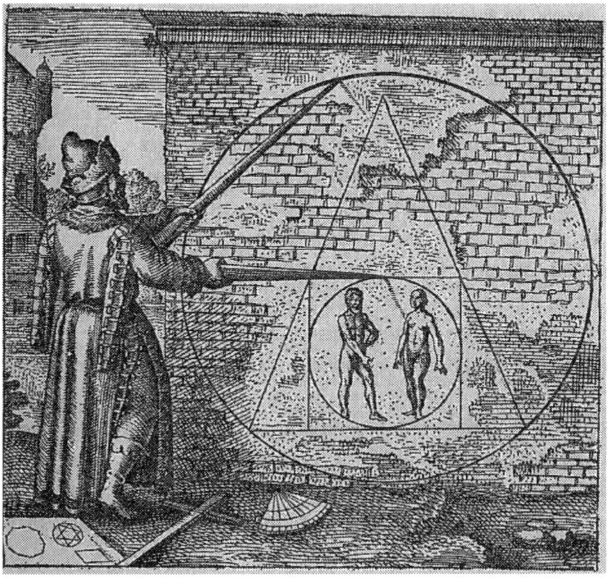

Figure 2: Michael Maier, *Atalanta Fugiens*, Emblem 21,
"The Philosophers' Stone."[141]

[140] Hauck, *The Emerald Tablet*, p. 153.
[141] Available in the public realm HTTP: https://en.wikipedia.org/wiki/Philosopher's_stone#/media/File:Michael_Maier_Atalanta_Fugiens_Emblem_21.jpeg

In the *Rosarium Philosophorum*, published as Part 2 of *De Alchimia Opuscula complura veterum philosophorum* (Frankfurt, 1550), a work to which in 1946 Jung dedicated an entire study (published as *The Psychology of the Transference*, and somewhat misleadingly hidden away toward the back of volume 16 of the *Collected Works*), the philosopher's stone is described in the following geometrical terms: "Make a round circle of the Man and Woman, and draw out of it a quadrangle, and out of the quadrangle a triangle, make a round circle, and thou shalt have the Stone of the Philosophers";[142] and in Michael Maier's *Atalanta Fugiens* (1617), this principle is reiterated: "Make of a man and woman a circle; then a quadrangle; out of this a triangle; make again a circle, and you will have the Stone of the Wise. Thus is made the stone, which thou canst not discover, unless you, through diligence, learn to understand this geometrical teaching."[143] The point here is not to make a series of esoteric moves (although, if one really wanted to, one could), by:

---

[142] *Rosarium philosophorum*, part 2; available online HTTP: http://www.levity.com/alchemy/rosary2.html; cf. Jung's Terry Lectures on "Psychology and Religion" given in 1937 (see CW 11 §92). Here Jung links the Philosopher's Stone to the *sphairos* of Empedocles (DK 31 B 27-29), to "the most blessed or fortunate god" (*eudaimonestatos theos*) (Aristotle, *Metaphysics*, Book 3, 1000b), and to the "all-round bisexual being" in Plato's *Symposium* (189d-190b) (CW 11 §93; cf. CW 12 §433; and SNZ, vol. 2, p. 95).

[143] Cited in J.B. Craven, *Count Michael Maier: Life and Writings, 1568-1622* [1910] (Lake Worth, FL: Ibis Press/Nicolas Hays, 1983), p. 90. For an alternative translation, see H.M.E. de Jong (ed.), *Michael Meier's Atalanta Fugiens: Sources of an Alchemical Book of Emblems* [1969] (York Beach, ME: Nicolas-Hays, 2002), p. 167:

> "Make a circle out of a man and a woman,
> From which a quadrangular body arises with equal sides,
> Derive from it a triangle, which is in contact on all sides with a round sphere:
> Then the Stone will have come into existence.
> If such a great things is not immediately clear in your mind
> Then know, that you will understand everything, if you understand the theory of Geometry."

For further discussion, see Hereward Tilton, *The Quest for the Phoenix: Spiritual Alchemy and Rosicrucianism in the Work of Count Michael Maier (1569-1622)* (Berlin and New York: de Gruyter, 2003), pp. 186-187 and 232.

- linking the etymology of the word "Grail" from the Celtic word *gar* (that is, "stone") and from *gar-al* (that is, "the cup of the stone");[144]
- making an association between a stone and greater works in stone, such as Chartres Cathedral, constructed by the Guild of Masons or the Children of Solomon;
- then looking back to Hiram Abiff, the architect of King Solomon's Temple, and a Hermetic alchemist;
- reminding the reader that, in Freemasonry, Hiram Abiff is identified as "the Son of the Widow," an epithet applied in Grail literature to Perceval (or Parzival);
- and finally identifying as the original Widow of the Grail bloodline Ruth the Moabite, who married Boaz to become the great-grandmother of David, thereby initiating the Davidic succession that issues in Jesus Christ — and, if some "alternative historians" are to be believed, in his descendants who came to Europe and intermarried, giving rise to the Merovingian dynasty, whose contemporary members are waiting in the shadows to seize political power.[145]

Yet elsewhere these sorts of historians come closer to what might be the real truth, namely, to the geometrical principle found in the *Rosarium philosophorum* — as well as in the fundamental axiom of Hermetic philosophy attributed to Hermes Trismegistus, that is, "As above, so below." At the heart of this axiom lies the principle that the universe is fundamentally harmonious, in the sense that there is a relation of proportion between the earth and the cosmos. Or, in other words, that there is something inherently *sacred* about

[144] Louis Charpentier, *The Mysteries of Chartres Cathedral*, trans. Ronald Fraser (Wellingborough: Thorsons [Research into Lost Knowledge Organisation], 1972), p. 113.

[145] Nearly all of these moves are made — on just one page! — by Laurence Gardner (see his *Bloodline of the Holy Grail: The Hidden Lineage of Jesus Revealed* [1996] (London: Element, 2002), p. 199).

geometry, and there is "a metaphysical pattern which determines the physical."[146] If it means anything (and it could, of course, mean a good number of things), the Grail is an expression and an embodiment (in its existence and in its transformative effect) of this cosmic significance of proportion.

To put it in linguistic structural terms, the Grail is a signifier; or, as Jacques Lacan (1901-1981) put it in his *Seminar III* (1955-1956), it is a "master-signifier," defined as follows: "Everything radiates out from and is organized around this signifier. It's the point of convergence that enables everything that happens in this discourse [to] be situated."[147] For a more expansive definition, we can turn to some of the work inspired by Slavoj Žižek:

> [B]ecause signifiers refer only to other signifiers, this produces a seemingly endless chain of reference [...]. For Žižek, this seemingly infinite sequence of referral can be fixed or anchored only "through the intervention of a certain 'nodal point' (the Lacanian *point de capiton*) which 'quilts' them, stops their sliding and fixes their meaning" [...]. And this nodal point or knot in the series of signifiers is the "master-signifier" — a signifier that, although essentially no different from any other signifier, is situated in such a way that it masters the entire sequence of referral by providing a kind of final reference or guarantee of meaning. It is able to do this, Žižek explains, not because it possesses some special significance — some positive content or fullness of meaning — but simply because it is able to halt the

[146] Nigel Pennick, *Sacred Geometry: Symbolism and Purpose in Religious Structures* (Wellingborough: Turnstone Press, 1980), p. 8.
[147] Jacques Lacan, *The Seminar of Jacques Lacan, Book III: The Psychoses, 1955-1956*, ed. Jacques-Alain Miller, trans. Russell Grigg (New York; London: Norton, 1993), p. 268.

> process of referral by the empty gesture of referring only to itself. This "reflective" signifier is nothing more than a kind of cul-de-sac in the chain of equivalences.[148]

Or as Kelsey Wood summarizes this concept as found in Lacan and Žižek, "the Master-Signifier is an empty signifier which has no signified content, and which unifies a field of meaning precisely through this very lack or inconsistency [...]. This means that 'beneath' the alleged unity of the field of meaning, there is only a tautological, self-referential, *performative* gesture. In other words, it is not some pre-existing, substantial fullness of meaning to which all of the particulars refer. The Master-Signifier is an empty signifier [...] the Master-Signifier is pure difference *misperceived* as pure identity."[149]

Here we find ourselves at the central point of confrontation between esoteric teachings and poststructuralist approaches: on the one hand, "the eternal," "purpose," "lost knowledge" — in short, the symbol; on the other, "emptiness," "self-referentiality," "pure difference *misperceived* as pure identity" — in short, the sign. (Analogously, as Kenneth Sylvan Guthrie [1871-1940] asked in *The Song of Mysticism* [1904], "Which is the Truth — the Symbol, or the Fact?").[150] This intellectual confrontation — but also this existential choice — was identified by Jung in *Psychological Types* (1921), where he defines the distinction between the symbolic and the semiotic as follows: Whereas the sign is "an analogue or an abbreviated designation for a *known* thing," a symbol is the "best

[148] David J. Gunkel, "Master-signifier," in Rex Butler (ed.), *The Žižek Dictionary* (Durham, NC: Acumen, 2014), pp. 190-193 (pp. 190-191). The quotation from Žižek comes from Slavoj Žižek, *The Sublime Object of Ideology* (London and New York: Verso, 1989), p. 87.

[149] Kelsey Wood, *Žižek: A Reader's Guide* (Malden, MA: Wiley-Blackwell, 2012), pp. 8-9.

[150] Kenneth Sylvan Guthrie, *The Song of Mysticism* (Medford, MA: Prophet Publishing House, 1904), section 1.

possible formulation of a relatively *unknown* thing" (CW 6 §815). As a result, the symbol is so much richer than the sign, for it is:

- "a product of an extremely complex nature"
- neither *rational* nor *irrational*, for it "has a side that accords with reason," but also "another side that does not"
- composed of rational data *and* irrational data "supplied by pure inner and outer perception [*Wahrnehmung*]"
- something that is rich in intuition and pregnant with significance [*das Ahnungsreiche und das Bedeutungs-schwangere*]
- something that appeals just as strongly to *thinking* [*das Denken*] as to *feeling* [*das Fühlen*]
- something whose "peculiar plastic imagery [*eigenartige Bildhaftigkeit*], when shaped into sensuous form [*zu sinnlicher Form gestaltet*], stimulates *sensation* [*die Empfindung*] as much as *intuition* [*die Intuition*]" (CW 6 §823)

This choice between the symbol and the sign — between presence and absence, between fullness and emptiness, between meaning and meaninglessness, between identity and difference — is aptly embodied in the symbolic legend of the Grail, which leaves both interpretations open (as an esoteric fullness of meaning and a poststructuralist absence of content), yet at the same time insists on the possibility of transformation. This transformativity takes place on different levels: most obviously, in the case of Anfortas, in the shift from suffering and sickness to healing; and, in the case of Parzival, in the shift from his despair at having failed to ask the question to his discovery of his true identity as the King of the Grail. Significantly, this is accompanied by a shift in Parzival's understanding of God, from his initial lack of understanding (as reflected in his question, *waz ist got?*) to the more nuanced theology of good and evil as expounded to him by Trevrizent. Given his emphasis on *Wandlung* in *Transformations and Symbols of the Libido* and in *The Red Book*, ultimately it is this *transformative* aspect that attracted Jung to the Grail. Is this transformation something essentially esoteric?

Not necessarily so. As Robert M. Price has put it, "the stuff that people have figured out about why we do what we do and what is going on in society" — that *is* the gnosis.[151] Yet Price was thinking less of the Nag Hammadi Library or the Dead Sea Scrolls (to say nothing of Hermeticism and alchemy), and more of Peter L. Berger and Thomas Luckman, authors of *The Social Construction of Reality: A Treatise in the Sociology of Knowledge* (1966); Erving Goffmann and his *The Presentation of Self in Everyday Life* (1956); Denis de Rougemont and his *Love in the Western World* (1939; 1956; 1972) and even Sigmund Freud. These and other thinkers, Price believes, offer "such an insight into why things happen and why people do [the] things [they do]," even if most people — in gnostic terms, the *psychikoi* (as opposed to the *pneumatikoi*) — do not have the occasion to learn this. To this list of thinkers, one could surely add Jung as well; and among the kinds of concepts that can not only theorize but actually bring about transformation, one might include the notion of proportion, the geometrical approach to the sacred, and the powerful maxim, "As above, so below."

Conclusion (B)

According to Aristotle, every tragedy has six constituent parts, namely (a) plot; (b) character; (c) diction; (d) thought; (e) spectacle; and (f) melody, and the most important of these is plot (or narrative), defined by Aristotle as "the arrangement of the incidents of the story" (*Poetics*, 1450a).[152] "In everything that is beautiful, whether it be a living creature or any organism composed of parts, these

[151]See the conclusion of AB Live 84, "The Sacred Scapegoat & Mimetic Violence," streamed live on 22 July 2022.

[152] Aristotle, *Complete Works*, ed. Jonathan Barnes, 2 vols (Princeton, NJ: Princeton University Press, 1984), vol. 2, p. 2320.

parts must not only be orderly arranged but must also have a certain magnitude of their own; for beauty consists in magnitude and ordered arrangement," Aristotle argues; accordingly, "as then creatures and other organic structures must have a certain magnitude and yet be easily taken in by the eye, so too with plots: they must have length but must be easily taken in by the memory" (1451b-1452a).[153] And then Aristotle goes on to make a point that is crucial in relation to the works discussed in this paper. "A plot does not have unity, as some people think, simply because it deals with a single hero," and "many and indeed innumerable things happen to an individual, some of which do not go to make up any unity" (1451a). Rather, "[a]s […] in the other arts of representation a single representation means a representation of a single object, so too the plot being a representation of a piece of action must represent a single piece of action and the whole of it; and the component incidents must be so arranged that if one of them be transposed or removed, the unity of the whole is dislocated and destroyed" (1451a).[154]

In other words, the unity must arise from the combination of various aspects of the narrative, much as the Self arises from the combination of the various components of consciousness and the unconscious, or as Jung puts it, "the self is not only the centre but it is the whole circumference which embraces both consciousness and unconscious; it is the centre of this totality, just as the ego is the centre of consciousness" (CW 12 §44). In this sense, "the self is our life's goal, for it is the complete expression of that fateful combination we call individuality" (CW 7 §404); the process of individuation might, then, be described as way of *narrating the Self into being*.

While Jung's works lend themselves to cherry-picking — a recent anthology calls itself *The Quotable Jung* (2016)! — it is

[153] Aristotle, *Complete Works*, vol. 2, pp. 2321-2322.
[154] Aristotle, *Complete Works*, vol. 2, p. 2320.

important not to overlook the structure of his argumentation (which often takes the form of a binary synthesis) or, in the case of *The Red Book*, its plot. The sequencing of the episodes that make up its storyline is as important as the textual (and visual) shape given to those episodes themselves. And there is a wider lesson here. That Jung-inspired tagline of *Aeon Byte Gnostic Radio*, "write your own gospel and live your own myth," thus has to be understood to mean that it is only if we *write* our own gospel that we shall be able to live our own myth. In this respect, what *The Red Book* enacts is a search for a style — albeit one that is "new and unaccustomed" to Jung (RB, 419) — which is also a search for a myth: a search for that moment when "the myth commences, the one that need only be lived, not sung, the one that sings itself" (RB, 453).

When discussing his dream of the knight and the customs official in *Memories, Dreams, Reflections*, Jung notes that "the world of the Knights of the Grail and their quest" was "in the deepest sense" *his* world; and thus a world which "had scarcely anything to do with Freud's" (MDR, 189). It is our task to make it *our* quest as well: As Jung put it, his "whole being was seeking for something still unknown" — *ein noch Unbekanntes* — "which might confer meaning upon the banality of life" (189). The quest for the Grail is thus the search for how to transform *die Banalität des Lebens* into a life replete with meaning (*Sinn*). This search for transformation continues in Goethe's *Faust*, itself set in the Middle Ages (and it is to this work that we shall turn in Volume 2 in this series). But can this quest for meaning itself have any meaning today, in our postmodern (or post-postmodern) world? One contemporary thinker who believes that it can is Bertrand Vergely.[155]

In his recent essay on the meaning of life, Vergely explicitly associates this meaning (*le sens de la vie*) with the Middle Ages (9). On his account, the Middle Ages saw life as a quest for meaning

[155] See Bertrand Vergely, *Notre vie a un sens!* (Paris: Albin Michel 2019).

— and in particular as a quest for a transcendent meaning of existence (14): "In the Middle Ages, culture was founded on the quest for meaning, and this journey of the soul was embodied in the pilrgimage, whether it was to the Holy Land or, across Europe, from one sacred place to another or from one monastery to the other" (19). In his essay, Vergely tries to reactivate this meaning of the quest, specifically linking it with the figure of the medieval knight. "One day, through an encounter, one is called by a word," he writes, and "called by this word, one begins to follow it," so that "living for it, in it, through it, life changes," and life "becomes a mission, a great mission" (215). (In the case of Parzival, these "words" takes the form of questions, namely: What is God? From what is Anfortas suffering? Whom does the Grail serve?) In the Middle Ages, Vergely argues, the knights lived *for* this quest:

> Their life became a great quest. Called by the chivalric ideal, they had no other aim than to become what this word *knight* involved, externally in the form of the strong and courageous warrior, internally in the form of the generous and spiritual nobleman. A knight was someone who, having passed from external nobility to interior and symbolic nobility, practised a kind of alchemical wedding with the spirit of life by transforming the lead of military violence into the gold of shining spiritual force. (215)

Vergely goes on to draw on the work of other commentators (albeit in a way that will undoubtedly be problematic for some, if not most, readers). In her recent study of masculinity, Jacqueline Kelen aligns the notion of spiritual chivalry with what she calls the "eternal masculine" (*éternal masculin*),[156] although this term

[156] Jacqueline Kelen, *L'Éternel masculin: Traité de chevalerie à l'usage des hommes d'aujourd'hui* (Paris: Robert Laffont, 1994). For a Jungian reading of the *Parzival*

draws, of course, on Goethe's (equally problematic) notion of the "Eternal Feminine." In his study of the anthropological structures of the imagination, Gilbert Durand (1921-2012) develops the gender symbolism latent in the tradition of the quest: in the symbolic imagination, he argues, the feminine is associated with the archetype of the cup or chalice, a symbol of infinite receptivity, while the masculine is associated with the sword, a symbol of infinite determination.[157] (As noted above, the gender stereotyping involved in such interpretations causes us immense difficulties today. For a moment, let us try to set those difficulties on one side, reading these distinctions as describing aspects of the individual psyche rather than as qualities of gendered individuals.) Picking up Durand's symbolic identification, Vergely agrees that much firmness is required to pass from the lead of violence to the gold of the spirit, adding that "to achieve such determination is a great adventure which demands the energy of an entire life" and "the spiritual knight is someone who suceeds in doing so" (215-216).

On this reading, the spiritual knight is a figure who existed "well before the age of chivalry" and who exists "beyond it as well" (216). Vergely equates the figure of the knight with the figure we found in Greek mythology in our introduction to the epic (Chapter 1) — namely, the hero as a symbol of valor and determination. According to the French psychologist Paul Diel (1893-1972), we can only understand these myths if we can see them as recounting how the human individual, as a true and living presence, must seek to be liberated from being a banal individual, without tipping over into tragedy — a false response to the nevertheless real danger

legend in terms of a quest for masculinity, see Robert A. Johnson, *He: Understanding Masculine Psychology: Based on the Legend of Parsifal and His Search for the Grail, Using Jungian Psychological Concepts* (New York: Harper & Row, 1974).

[157] Gilbert Durand, *Les Structures anthropologiques de l'imaginaire: Introduction à l'archétypologie générale* [1960; [2]1963] (Paris: Bordas, 1973), pp. 23-44.

of banality.[158] Following Diel, Vergely argues that it is precisely the existential danger of this banality that Hercules must strive ceaselessly to conquer, vanquishing one monster after another — slaying the Nemean Lion, slaying the nine-headed Lernaean Hydra, capturing the Golden Hind of Artemis, capturing the Erymanthian Boar, clearing the Augean stables (in a single day), slaying the Stymphalian Birds, capturing the Cretan Bull, stealing the Mares of Diomedes, obtaining the girdle of Hippolyta (the Queen of the Amazons), obtaining the cattle of the monster Geryon, stealing the apples of the Hesperides, and capturing Cerberus. The successful completion of these labors (representing symbolically an infinite number) displays the royal aspect of Hercules and his divinity, revealing him to be "an image of spiritual determination which, having received the light, reflects it, by being neither banal nor mad" (216). This "interior determination and, behind it, the shining light of the life one has received and which one reflects," exist for Vergely in a reciprocal relation, inasmuch as the light "brings this determination to life," and this determination "brings the light to life," in a way which "throws light on the heroism of the Ancients as well as the heroism of the moderns" (216).

Vergely transfers these labors from the mythological realm to the realm of philosophy (and, by extension, of psychoanalysis as well). In the first of his *Meditations on First Philosophy* (1641), Descartes recounts how he began to reflect on all the falsehoods he had believed in the course of his education and his life, and how he had built up an external knowledge of diverse and multiple facts, rather than a coherent, unified interior knowledge. On Vergely's reading, having various thoughts is not the same as being able to think; having various images is not the same as having a picture of the world — and, as a consequence, one must set out in search

[158] Paul Diel, *Le Symbolisme dans la mythologie grecque* [1966] (Paris: Payot, 1970), pp. 23-44.

of truth in order to know what is truly true or really real (217). This example is said to serve as an illustration of what a sense of mission, or a quest for meaning, or practicing spiritual chivalry really means: It is the search for an Archimedean point, a point so "firm and immovable" that it would enable one to move the entire globe from one place to another, or (in philosophical terms) to find absolute certainty (if only the certainty that there is nothing certain) (*Meditation II*, §1).

In other words, one has to follow Parzival's example and embark on an adventure (or *âventiure*), an aventure being something which first and foremost involves danger (218). And an adventure necessarily involves danger, because to get from *a* to *b* is always difficult because nothing ever happens as one expects and because there is a risk of defeat. Yet if one risks being distracted from one's goal and being led away from the true path under circumstances which are far more challenging than in normal life, there is always the prospect of success through overcoming this adversity.

Although the quest for meaning involves a focus on the individual, by no means does it entirely lack a social dimension. In the course of the adventure, one can have recourse to friends and allies; in the case of Parzival, for example, the advice that he receives from Herzeloyde, Gurnemanz, and, above all, the inestimable Trevrizent. Nor does the adventure simply involve trying to return everything to normality; rather, the overcoming of obstacles means leaving behind normal life in order to discover another, richer form of life (219).

In the introduction to the epic (Chapter 1) and elsewhere, we have drawn on the Homeric story of Odysseus as a paradigm of the Western epic tradition, symbolizing the overcoming of obstacles in order to return home — or in order to return to the self. In *En découvrant l'existence avec Husserl et Heidegger* (1949; ^{2}1967; ^{3}1974), Emmanuel Levinas (1906-1995) drew a contrast between this story, which he saw as exemplifying the primacy of thought that returns to itself, and the Judaic tradition with its biblical story of Abraham. Whereas Odysseus's trajectory illustrates the return of the self to the same inasmuch as he returns to the point of origin, Abraham becomes a model for a different kind of subjectivity which Levinas describes as "ethical," insofar as he leaves home only never to return. "To the myth of Ulysses returning to Ithaca," Levinas wrote, "I would like to oppose the history of Abraham leaving his country forever for an unknown land, and forbidding his servant to lead even his son back to this point of departure."[159] Yet are these two models really so different? After all, Jung defined the self as "a quantity that is superordinate to the conscious ego" and, because it "embraces not only the conscious but also the unconscious psyche," as being "therefore, so to speak, a personality which we *also* are" (CW 7 §274). As "our life's goal," the self is "the completest expression of that fateful combination we call individuality" — and we should note that Jung goes on to describe this "individuality" as "the full flowering not only of the single individual, but of the group, in which each adds their portion to the whole" (CW 7 §404); in this sense, then, the self *is* the Promised Land, *is* Paradise, and if in the quest for meaning and the quest for transformation we return to the starting point, we do so *at a higher level*.

As a result, Vergely is surely right when he argues that if the adventure involves obstacles and allies, it also involves something which surpasses obstacles and allies alike — something radically Other, something radically new (219). And he suggests that, surprisingly enough, Nietzsche had an intuition of this third element when he insisted on the need to go "beyond good and evil," declaring (in *Beyond Good and Evil*, §292) that "[a] philosopher —

[159] Emmanuel Levinas, "La trace de l'autre," in *En découvrant l'existence avec Husserl et Heidegger* (Paris: Vrin, 1974), p. 191; cf. Ann Katrin Jonsson, *Relations: Ethics and the Modernist Subject in James Joyce's "Ulysses," Virginia Woolf's "The Waves" and Djuna Barnes's "Nightwood"* (Oxford: Lang, 2006), p. 47.

is a human being who constantly experiences, sees, hears, suspects, hopes, and dreams extraordinary things."[160]

Vergely thus stakes himself on the quest for life, sense, freedom, and plenitude, embracing Bergson's notion of *élan vital* or the theological concept of spirit (*spiritus* in Latin, *pneuma* in Greek, *rouah* in Hebrew) (207), much as Jung himself will do in his seminar on Nietzsche's *Zarathustra* (as we shall see in Volume 3 in this series). Correspondingly, Pascal's belief that "all our dignity consists in thought" (§200-*347*),[161] and the Greek notion of the *kalos k'agathon* (i.e., the good and beautiful individual), both flow into the work of Micheline Sauvage, titled *L'Aventure philosophique* (1966). On her account, philosophy itself is an adventure, this time in the sense of discovering a buried treasure. For the act of thinking itself can make an extraordinary discovery which is capable of radically transforming our existence, just as in alchemy the discovery of the philosopher's stone enables the transformation of lead into gold (208). Sauvage suggests a significant parallel between philosophy and alchemy: Just as alchemy transforms the lead of our daily existence into spiritual gold,[162] so it is because we are alive that we sense that a more precious existence is possible — and seek to attain it (208). To the extent that we fail in our quest to do so, we suffer (and, in his letter of 1926, Jung is insistent on the inevitability of suffering); to the extent that we succeed, however, we experience that sense of joy which Spinoza (in his *Ethics*, part 5, prop. 42) calls *blessedness* or *beatitude* (*beatitudo*) —[163]

[160] Nietzsche, *Basic Writings*, ed. and trans. Kaufmann, p. 420.
[161] Pascal, *Pensées*, trans. Krailsheimer, p. 200. The context of this insight is the famous reflection that "Man is only a reed, the weakest in nature, but he is a thinking reed" (*L'homme n'est qu'un roseau, mais c'est un roseau pensant*).
[162] Micheline Sauvage, *L'Aventure philosophique* (Paris: Buchet-Chastel, 1966), pp. 226-247.
[163] Benedict de Spinoza, *On the Improvement of the Understanding; The Ethics; Correspondence* [*Works*, vol. 2], trans. R.H.M. Elwes (New York: Dover, 1955), p. 270.

or in Eschenbach's terms, joy (*vröude*). (Tellingly, one of Jung's contemporaries, the great French Catholic writer Patrice de la Tour du Pin (1911-1975) titled one his collections of poems *La Quête de joie* [1939].) It is this joy — the "true joy" (*die wahre Freude*) — which, in *The Red Book*, Jung will learn "is simple," because it "comes and exists from itself," and is the joy which "comes from fulfillment" (RB, 491-492), the joy which comes from fulfilling the quest for transformation and discovering the Grail of *vröude*.

Bibliography

Primary Texts and Editions

Jung, C.G. *Collected Works*, ed. Sir Herbert Read, Michael Fordham, Gerhard Adler, and William McGuire, 20 vols (London: Routledge & Kegan Paul, 1953-1983).

Jung, C.G. and Aniela Jaffé (ed.). *Erinnerungen, Träume, Gedanken von C.G. Jung*, ed. Aniela Jaffé (Olten und Freiburg im Breisgau: Walter-Verlag, 1990).

Jung, C.G. and Aniela Jaffé (ed.). *Memories, Dreams, Reflections of C.G. Jung*, ed. Aniela Jaffé, trans. Richard and Clara Winston (London: Routledge & Kegan Paul, 1963).

Jung, C.G. *Psychology of the Unconscious: A Study of the Transformations and Symbolisms of the Libido: A Contribution to the History of the Evolution of Thought*, trans. Beatrice M. Hinkle (London: Moffat, Yard, and Co., 1916; reprinted London: Routledge, 1991).

Jung, C.G. *Nietzsche's "Zarathustra": Notes of the Seminar given in 1935-1939*, ed. James L. Jarrett, 2 vols (London: Routledge, 1989).

Jung, C.G. *The Red Book: Liber Novus* [Reader's Edition], ed. Sonu Shamdasani, trans. Mark Kyburz, John Peck, and Sonu Shamdasani (New York and London: Norton, 2012).

Jung, C.G. *The Black Books, 1913-1932: Notebooks of Transformation*, ed. Sonu Shamdasani, trans. Martin Liebscher, John Peck, and

Sonu Shamdasani, 7 vols (New York and London: Norton, 2020).

Goethe, Johann Wolfgang. *Faust: Parts I and II*, trans. Albert G. Latham (London; New York: Dent; Dutton, 1908).

Nietzsche, Friedrich. *Thus Spake Zarathustra: A Book for All and None* [*Complete Works of Friedrich Nietzsche*, ed. Oskar Levy, vol. 4], trans. Thomas Common (Edinburgh and London: Foulis, 1909).

Wolfram von Eschenbach. *Parzival: A Knightly Epic*, trans. Jessie L. Weston [1894], 2 vols (New York: Stechert, 1912).

Wolfram von Eschenbach. *Parzival*, ed. Eberhard Nellmann, trans. Dieter Kühn, 2 vols (Frankfurt am Main: Deutscher Klassiker Verlag, 2006).

Other Works

[anon]. *Continuations of the Old French Perceval*, ed. William Roach (Philadelphia: University of Pennsylvania Press, 1949), vol. 1, *The first Continuation, Redaction of mss. TVD.*

[anon]. *La Queste del Saint Graal: Roman du XIII*[e] *siècle*, ed. Albert Pauphilet (Paris: Champion, 1923).

[anon]. *Le Haut Livre du Graal: Perlesvaus*, ed. William A. Nitze and T. Atkinson Jenkins, 2 vols (Chicago: University of Chicago Press, 1932-1937; reprinted New York: Phaeton Press, 1972).

[anon]. *Physiologus*, trans. Michael J. Curley [1979] (Chicago and London: University of Chicago Press, 2009).

[anon]. *Sir Gawain and the Lady of Lys*, trans. Jessie L. Weston [Arthurian Romances Unrepresented in Malory's "Morte d'Arthur," no. 7] (London: David Nutt, 1907).

[anon]. *The Death of King Arthur*, trans. James Cable (Harmondsworth: Penguin, 1971).

[anon]. *The High Book of the Grail: A Translation of the Thirteenth-Century Romance of Perlesvaus*, trans. Nigel Bryant (Cambridge: D.S. Brewer, 2007).

[anon]. *The Mabinogion*, trans. Gwyn Jones and Thomas Jones (London; New York: Dent; Dutton, 1974).

[anon]. *The Quest of the Holy Grail*, trans. Pauline Matarasso (Harmondsworth: Penguin, 1969).

[anon]. *The Turba Philosophorum or Assembly of the Sages*, trans. Arthur Edward Waite (London: Redway, 1896).

Adler, Gerhard. "Aspects of Jung's Personality and Work," *Psychological Perspectives*, vol. 6, no. 1 (1975), 11-21.

Andersen, Regine. *Governing Agrobiodiversity: Plant Genetics and Developing Countries* (London and New York: Routledge, 2016).

André, Hayen. "La théorie du lieu naturel d'après Aristote: Contribution à l'étude de l'hylémorphisme," *Revue néo-scolastique de philosophie*, 40, no. 53 (1937), 5-43.

Angelus Silesius. *The Cherubinic Wanderer*, trans. Maria Shrady, ed. Josef Schmidt (New York and Mahwah: Paulist Press, 1986).

Archibald, Elizabeth and A.S.G. Edwards (eds). *A Companion to Malory* (Cambridge: D.S. Brewer, 1996).

Aristotle. *Complete Works*, ed. Jonathan Barnes, 2 vols (Princeton, NJ: Princeton University Press, 1984).

Augustine of Hippo. *Expositions on the Book of Psalms*, vol. 1, *Psalms I-XXXVI* [Library of the Fathers, vol. 24] (Oxford; London: Parker; Rivington, 1847).

Augustine of Hippo. *Expositions on the Book of Psalms*, vol. 4, *Psalms LXXVI-CI* [Library of the Fathers, vol. 32] (Oxford; London: Parker; Rivington, 1850).

Augustine of Hippo. *The Essential Augustine*, ed. Vernon J. Bourke (Indianapolis, IN: Hackett, 1974).

Averbeck, Richard E. "Christian Interpretations of Isaiah 43," in Darrell L. Bock and Mitch Glaser (eds), *The Gospel According to Isaiah 53: Encountering the Suffering Servant in Jewish and Christian Theology* (Grand Rapids, MI: Kegel, 2012), pp. 33-60.

Ball, Philip. *The Devil's Doctor: Paracelsus and the World of Renaissance Magic and Science* (London: Heinemann, 2006).

Barber, Malcolm and Keith Bate (eds). *The Templars: Selected Sources* (Manchester: Manchester University Press, 2002).

Barber, Malcolm. *The New Knighthood: A History of the Order of the Temple* (Cambridge: Cambridge University Press, 1994).

Barber, Malcolm. *The Trial of the Templars*, 2nd edn (Cambridge: Cambridge University Press, 2006).

Barber, Richard. *The Holy Grail: Imagination and Belief* (London: Allen Lane, 2004).

Barnes, Jonathan. *Early Greek Philosophy* (Harmondsworth: Penguin, 1987).

Bärtges, Carol. "The Journey In, the Journey Out: The Waldorf Elementary and High School Curricula," *Renewal: A Journal for Waldorf Education*, vol. 20, no. 1 (Spring-Summer 2011), 28-32.

Bartsch, Karl. "Die Eigennamen in Wolframs *Parzival* und *Titurel*," *Germanistische Studien*, 2 (1875), 114-159.

Bauer, Ralph. *The Alchemy of Conquest: Science, Religion, and the Secrets of the New World* (Charlottesville: University of Virginia Press, 2019).

Beardsley, David A. *The Journey Back to Where You Are: Homer's "Odyssey" as Spiritual Quest* (Highland Park, NJ: Ideograph Media, 2014).

Beckingham, Charles F. and Bernard Hamilton (eds). *Prester John, the Mongols and the Ten Lost Tribes* (Aldershot: Variorum, 1996).

Bell, Clair Hayden. *The Sister's Son in the Medieval German Epic: A Study in the Survival of Matriliny* [*University of California Publications in Modern Philology*, vol. 10, no. 2, pp. 67-182] (Berkeley, CA: University of California Press, 1922).

Benz, Ernst. "Die heilige Höhle in der alten Christenheit und in der östlich-orthodoxen Kirche," *Eranos-Jahrbuch 1953*, vol. 22 (1954), 365-432.

Bernadete, Seth. *The Bow and the Lyre: A Platonic Reading of the "Odyssey"* (Lanham, MD: Rowman & Littlefield, 1997).

Berthelot, Marcellin (ed.). *Collection des anciens alchimistes grecs*, vols 2-3 (Paris: Steinheil, 1888).

Birch-Hirschfeld, Adolf. *Die Sage vom Graal: Ihre Entwicklung und dichterische Ausbildung in Frankreich und Deutschland, im 12. und 13. Jahrhundert: Eine literarhistorische Untersuchung* (Leipzig: F.C.W. Vogel, 1877).

Bishop, Paul (ed.). *The Archaic: The Past in the Present* (London and New York: Routledge, 2012).

Bishop, Paul. "On Reading Jung in German: Jung's Significance for *Germanistik*," in Jean Kirsch and Murray Stein (eds), *How and Why We Still Read Jung: Personal and Professional*

Reflections (London and New York: Routledge, 2013), pp. 66-85.

Bishop, Paul. "Telling Stories: Jung's *Red Book* as an Exercise in Narrative," in Raya A. Jones and Leslie Gardner (eds), *Narratives of Individuation* (New York and London: Routledge, 2019), pp. 111-131.

Bishop, Paul. *Analytical Psychology and German Classical Aesthetics: Goethe, Schiller, and Jung,* vol. 1, *The Development of the Personality*; vol. 2, *The Constellation of the Self* (London and New York: Routledge, 2008-2009).

Bishop, Paul. *The Dionysian Self: C.G. Jung's Reception of Friedrich Nietzsche* (Berlin and New York: de Gruyter, 1995).

Bishop, Paul. *Reading Plato through Jung: Why must the Third become the Fourth?* (Cham: Palgrave Macmillan, 2022).

Blamires, David. *Characterization and Individuality in Wolfram's "Parzival"* (Cambridge: Cambridge University Press, 1966).

Bloom, Harold. *The Western Canon: The Books and School of the* Ages (London: Macmillan, 1995).

Bonnechère, Pierre and Gabriela Cursaru. "Katábasis," *Cahiers des études anciennes*, 53 (2016), 7-14.

Brenner-Eglinger, Hans. "Briefe Jakob Burckhardts an Albert Brenner," *Basler Jahrbuch 1901*, 87-110.

Brewer, Derek and Jonathan Gibson (eds). *A Companion to the Gawain-Poet* (Cambridge: D.S. Brewer, 1997).

Brisson, Luc. "How to Make a Soul in the *Timaeus*," in Chad Jorgenson, Filip Karfík, and Štěpán Špinka (eds), *Plato's "Timaeus": Proceedings of the Tenth Symposium Platonicum Pragense* (Leiden and Boston: Brill, 2021), pp. 70-91.

Brock, Stephen L. *The Philosophy of Saint Thomas Aquinas: A Sketch* (Eugene, OR: Cascade, 2015).

Brooks, Peter. "Fictions of the Wolfman," *Diacritics*, vol. 9, no. 1 (1979), 72-83.

Brown, Arthur C.L. "Did Chrétien Identify the Grail with the Mass?", *Modern Language Notes*, vol. 41, no. 4 (April 1926), 226-233.

Büchler, Alfred. "Psalter und Zeitrechnung in Wolframs *Parzival*," *Amsterdamer Beiträge zur älteren Germanistik*, 50 (1998), 95-109.

Bumke, Joachim. *Courtly Culture: Literature and Society in the High Middle Ages* [*Höfische Kultur: Literatur und Gesellschaft im hohen Mittelalter*, 1986], trans. Thomas Dunlap [1991] (Woodstock, New York, London: Overlook Duckworth, 2000).

Bumke, Joachim. *Wolfram von Eschenbach*, 8th edn (Stuttgart: Metzler, 2004).

Burdach, Konrad. "Faust und die Sorge," *Deutsche Vierteljahrsschrift für Literaturwissenschaft und Geistesgeschichte*, 1 (1923), 1-60.

Burdach, Konrad. *Der Gral: Forschungen über seinen Ursprung und seinen Zusammenhang mit der Longinuslegende* [Forschungen zur Kirchen- und Geistesgeschichte, 14] (Stuttgart: Kohlhammer, 1938; reprinted Darmstadt: Wissenschaftliche Buchgesellschaft, 1974).

Burkert, Walter. *Greek Religion*, trans. John Raffan (Oxford: Blackwell, 1985).

Bury, R.G. (ed.). *The Symposium of Plato* (Cambridge: Heffer, 1932).

Busby, Keith and Roger Dalrymple (eds). *Arthurian Literature XII* (Cambridge: D.S. Brewer, 2005).

Campbell, Joseph. *The Hero with a Thousand Faces* (Princeton, NJ: Princeton University Press, 1968).

Campbell, Joseph. *The Masks of God*, vol. 4, *Creative Mythology* (New York: Viking Penguin, 1968).

Campbell, Lewis (ed.), *The Theaetetus of Plato* (Oxford: Oxford University Press, 1861).

Carey, John. "Henry Corbin and the Secret of the Grail," *Temenos Academy Review*, 14 (2011), 159-178.

Carey, John. *Ireland and the Grail* [Celtic Studies Publications, 11] (Aberystwyth: Celtic Studies Publications, 2007).

Charpentier, Louis. *The Mysteries of Chartres Cathedral*, trans. Ronald Fraser (Wellingborough: Thorsons [Research into Lost Knowledge Organisation], 1972).

Cherniss, Harold. "The Sources of Evil According to Plato," *Proceedings of the American Philosophical Society*, vol. 98, no. 1 (February 1954), 23-30.

Chrétien de Troyes. *Arthurian Romances*, trans. D.D.R. Owen (London: Dent, 1987).

Chrétien de Troyes. *Œuvres complètes*, ed. Daniel Poirion et al. (Paris: Gallimard, 1994).

Chrétien de Troyes et al. *The Complete Story of the Grail: Chrétien de Troyes' "Perceval" and its Continuations*, trans. Nigel Bryant (Cambridge: D.S. Brewer, 2015).

Christoph, Siegfried. "Conflict Resolution and the Concept of Honor in Wolfram's 'Parzival,'" *Colloquia Germanica*, vol. 15, no. 1/2 (1982), 32-45.

Cicero. *De Senectute; De Amicitia; De Divinatione*, trans. William Armistead Falconer (Cambridge, MA; London: Harvard University Press, 1923).

Cicora, Mary A. "Medievalism and Metaphysics: The Literary Background of *Parsifal*," in William Kinderman and Katherine R. Syer (eds), *A Companion to Wagner's "Parsifal"* (Rochester, NY, and Woodbridge: Camden House, 2005), pp. 8-53.

Clark, Raymond J. *Catabasis: Vergil and the Wisdom Tradition* (Amsterdam: Grüner, 1979).

Classen, Albrecht. "Jewish-Christian Relations in the Middle Ages — The Exploration of Alternative Voices? The Deconstruction of a Myth or Factual History? Literary-Historical Investigations," *Amsterdamer Beiträge zur Älteren Germanistik*, 58 (2003), 123-149.

Clement et al. *The Apostolic Fathers*, vol. 1, ed. and trans. Bart D. Ehrman (Cambridge, MA, and London : Harvard University Press, 2003).

Combes, Annie. "The Continuations of the *Conte du Graal*," in Norris J. Lancy and Joan Tasker Grimbert (eds), *A Companion to Chrétien de Troyes* (Cambridge: D.S. Brewer, 2005), pp. 191-201.

Copenhaver, Brian P. *Hermetica: The Greek "Corpus Hermeticum" and the Latin "Asclepius" in a new English translation* (Cambridge: Cambridge University Press, 1992).

Corbin, Henry. *En Islam iranien: Aspects spirituels et philosophiques*, vol. 2, *Sohrwardî et les Platoniciens de Perse* (Paris: Gallimard, 1971).

Corbin, Henry. *Jung, Buddhism, and the Incarnation of Sophia: Unpublished Writings from the Philosopher of the Soul*, ed. Michel Cazenave (Rochester, VT: Inner Traditions, 2019).

Cornford, Francis MacDonald. *Plato's Cosmology: The "Timaeus" of Plato* (Indianapolis, IN: Hackett, 1997).

Cory, Alexander Turner. *The Hieroglyphics of Horapollo Nilous* (London: Pickering, 1840).

Coyajee, J.C. *Studies in Shāhnāmeh* (Bombay: Taraporevala, 1939).

Craven, J.B. *Count Michael Maier: Life and Writings, 1568-1622* [1910] (Lake Worth, FL: Ibis Press/Nicolas Hays, 1983).

Culler, Jonathan. "*Fabula* and *syuzhet* in the Analysis of Narrative," *Poetics Today*, vol. 1, no. 3 (1980), 27-37).

Dahlstrom, Daniel. "Play and Irony: Schiller and Schlegel on the Liberating Prospects of Aesthetics," in Thomas Nenon (ed.), *Kant, Kantianism, and Idealism: The Origins of Continental Philosophy* [The History of Continental Philosophy, vol. 1] (Chicago: University of Chicago Press, 2010), pp. 107-129.

Deinert, Wilhelm. *Ritter und Kosmos im "Parzival": Eine Untersuchung der Sternkunde Wolframs von Eschenbach* (Munich: Beck, 1960).

Deinert, Wilhelm. *Ritter und Kosmos im Parzival: Eine Untersuchung der Sternkunde Wolframs von Eschenbach* (Munich: Beck, 1960).

Deleuze, Gilles. "A quoi reconnaît-on le structuralisme?" [1967], in François Châtelet (ed.), *Histoire de la philosophie*, vol. 8, *Le XXième siècle* (Paris: Hachette, 1972), pp. 299-335.

Deleuze, Gilles. "How do We Recognize Structuralism?", trans. Melissa McMahon and Charles Stivale, in Charles Stivale, *The Two-Fold Thought of Deleuze and Guattari* (New York: Guilford Press, 1998), pp. 258-282.

Dick, Ernst S. "*Katabasis* and the Grail Epic: Wolfram von Eschenbach's *Parzival*," *Res publica litterarum: Studies in the Classical Tradition*, vol. 1 (1978), 57-87.

Diel, Paul. *Le Symbolisme dans la mythologie grecque* [1966] (Paris: Payot, 1970).

Dieterich, Albrecht. *Nékyia: Beiträge zur Erklärung der neuentdeckten Petrusapokalypse* (Leipzig: Teubner, 1893; ²1913).

Diez, Friedrich. *Etymologisches Wörterbuch der romanischen Sprachen* (Bonn: A. Marcus, 1853).

Dilthey, Wilhelm. *The Formation of the Historical World in the Human Sciences* [*Selected Works*, vol. 3], ed. Rudolf A. Makkreel and Frithjof Rodi (Princeton, NJ, and Oxford: Princeton University Press, 2002).

Dorn, Gerhard. *Speculativae philosophiae, gradus septem vel decem continens*, in [anon], *Theatrum chemicum*, vol. 1 (Ursel: Zetzner, 1602), pp. 255-310.

Dorn, Gerhard. *The Speculative Philosophy of Gerhard Dorn* [Magnum Opus Hermetic Sourceworks, no. 34], trans. Paul Ferguson (Kilbirnie: Alchemy Website and Bookshop, 2008).

Dorter, Kenneth. "The Significance of the Speeches in Plato's *Symposium*," *Philosophy & Rhetoric*, vol. 2, no. 4 (Fall, 1969), 215-234.

Dover, Carol (ed.). *A Companion to the Lancelot-Grail Cycle* (Cambridge: D.S. Brewer, 2003).

Duggan, Joseph J. "Afterword," in Chrétien de Troyes, *Perceval: The Story of the Grail*, trans. Burton Raffel (New Haven and London: Yale University Press, 1999), pp. 293-307.

Durand, Gilbert. *Les Structures anthropologiques de l'imaginaire: Introduction à l'archétypologie générale* [1960; ²1963] (Paris: Bordas, 1973).

Edelstein, Ludwig. "The Function of the Myth in Plato's Philosophy," *Journal of the History of Ideas*, vol. 10, no. 4 (Oct. 1949), 463-481.

Edwards, M.J. "The Vessel of Zosimus the Alchemist," *Zeitschrift für Papyrologie und Epigraphik*, 90 (1992), 55-64.

El Khadem, H.S. "A Translation of a Zosimos' Text in an Arabic Alchemy Book," *Journal of the Washington Academy of Sciences*, vol. 84, no. 3 (September 1996), 168-178.

Ellis, Ralph. *The Grail Cypher: The Secrets of Arthurian Legends Revealed* (Chester: Edfu Books, 2015; expanded 2017).

Elsner, Tamara. "Text as thing. The dog lead in Albrecht's 'Jüngerer Titurel,'" in MEMO, 7 (2020) [Textual Thingness / Textuelle Dinghaftigkeit], 81-96.

Escudero, Jesús Adrián. "Heidegger on Discourse and Idle Talk: The Role of Aristotelian Rhetoric," *Gatherings: The Heidegger Circle Annual*, 3 (2013), 1-17.

Evola, Julius. *Revolt Against the Modern World* [*Rivolta contra il mondo moderno*, 1934], trans. Guido Stucco (Rochester, VT: Inner Traditions, 1995).

Evola, Julius. *The Mystery of the Grail: Initiation and Magic in the Quest of the Spirit*, trans. by Guido Stucco (Rochester, VT: Inner Traditions, 1997).

Fauch, Wolfgang. "Katabasis," in K. Ziegler and W. Sontheimer (eds), *Der kleine Pauly: Lexikon der Antike*, 5 vols (Stuttgart: Metzler, 1964-1975), vol. 3, pp. 152-153.

Ferry, Luc. *De Homère à Platon: La naissance de la philosophie* (Paris: Flammarion, 2012).

Ferry, Luc. *Sagesses d'hier et d'aujourd'hui* (Paris: Flammarion, 2014).

Fideler, David. "The Path Toward the Grail: The Hermetic Sources and Structure of Wolfram von Eschenbach's *Parzival*," *Alexandria:*

The Journal of the Western Cosmological Traditions, 1 (1991), 187-227.

Fischer, Steven R. *The Dream in the Middle High German Epic: Introduction to the Study of the Dream as a Literary Device to the Younger Contemporaries of Gottfried and Wolfram* (Bern, Frankfurt am Main, Las Vegas: Lang, 1978).

Franke, William. "On the Poetic Truth that Is Higher than History: Porphyry and the Philosophical Criticism of Literature," *International Philosophical Quarterly*, vol. 50, no. 44 (December 2010), 415-430.

Franz, Marie-Louise von (ed.). *"Aurora consurgens": Ein dem Thomas von Aquin zugeschriebenes Dokument der alchemistischen Gegensatzproblematik* [*Gesammelte Werke*, vol. 14/3] (Olten und Freiburg im Breisgau: Walter-Verlag, 1971).

Frensch, Michael (ed.). *Lust an der Erkenntnis: Esoterik: Von der Antike bis zur Gegenwart: Ein Lesebuch* (Munich and Zurich: Piper, 1991).

Freud, Sigmund. "Family Romances" [1909], in *Standard Edition of the Complete Works*, general eds James Strachey and Anna Freud, 24 vols (London: Hogarth Press; Institute of Psycho-Analysis, 1953-1974), vol. 9, pp. 237-241.

Freud, Sigmund. "The Psychotherapy of Hysteria" [1895], in Josef Breuer and Sigmund Freud, *Studies in Hysteria* [*Standard Edition of the Complete Psychological Works*, vol. 2], ed. James Strachey (London: Hogarth Press; Institute of Psycho-Analysis, 1955), pp. 253-305.

Gambero, Luigi. *Mary and the Fathers of the Church: The Blessed Virgin Mary in Patristic Thought* [1991], trans. Thomas Buffer (San Francisco: Ignatius, 1999).

Ganschinietz, Richard. "Katabasis," in Pauly-Wissowa, *Real-encyclopädie der classischen Altertumswissenschaft*, 85 vols (Stuttgart: Metzler, 1890-1980), vol. 10, cols 2359-2449.

Gardner, Laurence. *Bloodline of the Holy Grail: The Hidden Lineage of Jesus Revealed* [1996] (London: Element, 2002).

Garland, Henry and Mary. *The Oxford Companion to German Literature*, 2nd edn (Oxford and New York: Oxford University Press, 1986).

Gemelli Marciano, M. Laura et al. *Parmenide: suoni, immagini, esperienza* (Sankt Augustin: Academia Verlag, 2013).

Genette, Gérard. *Narrative Discourse: An Essay in Method*, trans. Jane E. Lewin (Ithaca, NY: Cornell University Press, 1980).

Giletti, Ann. "Early Witness: Thomas Aquinas, Albert the Great and Peter of Tarentaise in Ramon Martí's *Pugio fidei* (c. 1278)," in Görge K. Hasselhoff and Alexander Fidora (eds), *Ramon Martí's "Pugio fidei": Studies and Texts* (Santa Coloma de Queralt: Obrador Edèndum, 2017), pp. 121-156.

Goetz, Hermann. "Der Orient der Kreuzzüge in Wolframs Parzival," *Archiv für Kulturforschung*, vol. 2, no. 1 (1967), 1-42.

Goodrick-Clarke, Nicholas. *Black Sun: Aryan Cults, Esoteric Nazism, and the Politics of Identity* (New York and London: New York University Press, 2003).

Görres, Johann Joseph von (ed.). *Lohengrin, ein altteutsches Gedicht* (Heidelberg: Mohr & Zimmer, 1813).

Grant, Edward. *A History of Natural Philosophy: From the Ancient World to the Nineteenth Century* (Cambridge: Cambridge University Press, 2007).

Green, D.H. *The Art of Recognition in Wolfram's "Parzival"* (Cambridge: Cambridge University Press, 1982).

Green, D.H. *The Beginnings of Medieval Romance: Fact and Fiction, 1150-1220* (Cambridge: Cambridge University Press, 2004).

Greene, Liz. *Jung's Studies in Astrology: Prophecy, Magic, and the Qualities of Time* (London and New York: Routledge, 2018).

Greene, Liz. *The Astrological World of Jung's "Liber Novus": Daimons, Gods, and the Planetary Journey* (London and New York: Routledge, 2018).

Gregory of Nyssa. *The Life of Moses*, ed. and trans. Abraham J. Malherbe and Everett Ferguson (New York and Mahwah, NJ: Paulist Press, 1978).

Gregory the Great. *Morals on the Book of Job* [*Library of the Fathers*, vol. 38], vol. 2 (Parts 3 and 4) (Oxford; London: Parker; Rivington, 1845).

Groos, Arthur B. "Cundrie's Announcement (*Parzival*, 781-782)," *Beiträge zur Geschichte der deutschen Sprache und Literatur*, 113 (1991), 384-414.

Groos, Arthur B. "Time Reference and the Liturgical Calendar in Wolfram von Eschenbach's *Parzival*," *Deutsche Vierteljahrsschrift für Literaturwissenschaft und Geistesgeschichte*, 49 (1975), 43-65.

Groos, Arthur B., Jr. "Wolfram von Eschenbach's 'Bow Metaphor' and the Narrative Technique of *Parzival*," *Modern Language Notes*, vol. 87, no. 3 (April 1972), 391-408.

Guénon, René. *Le Roi du monde* (Paris: Charles Bosse, 1927).

Guénon, René. *The Lord of the World*, trans. Carolyn Shaffer and Olga de Nottbeck, rev. Anthony Cheke and Anthony Blake (Ellingstring: Coombe Springs Press, 1983).

Gunkel, David J. "Master-signifier," in Rex Butler (ed.), *The Žižek Dictionary* (Durham, NC: Acumen, 2014), pp. 190-193.

Guthrie, Kenneth Sylvan. *The Song of Mysticism* (Medford, MA: Prophet Publishing House, 1904).

Hadfield, Andrew (ed.). *The Cambridge Companion to Spenser* (Cambridge: Cambridge University Press, 2001).

Haferland, Harald. "Parzivals Pfingsten: Heilsgeschichte im *Parzival* Wolframs von Eschenbach," *Euphorion: Zeitschrift für Literaturgeschichte*, 88 (1994), 263-301.

Halbach, Kurt Herbert. "Epik des Mittelalters," in Wolfgang Stammler (ed.), *Deutsche Philologie im Aufriß*, second edn, vol. 2 (Berlin: Erich Schmidt, 1960), cols 397 and 683.

Hall, Manly P. *The Secret Teachings of All Ages* [Reader's Edition] (New York: Tarcher/Penguin, 2003).

Hall, Manly Palmer. *Neoplatonism: Theology for Wanderers in the New Millennium* (Los Angeles, CA: Philosophical Research Society, 2010).

Hall, Manly Palmer. *The Adepts in the Western Esoteric Tradition: Orders of the Quest* (Los Angeles, CA: Philosophical Research Society, 1949).

Harpur, Patrick. *The Philosophers' Secret Fire: A History of the Imagination* (Harmondsworth: Penguin, 2002).

Hasty, Will (ed.). *A Companion to Wolfram's "Parzival"* (Rochester, NY, and Woodbridge: Camden House, 1999).

Hasty, Will. "Introduction," in Will Hasty (ed.), *A Companion to Wolfram's "Parzival"* (Rochester, NY, and Woodbridge: Camden House, 1999), pp. ix-xxx.

Hathaway, Ronald F. *Hierarchy and the Definition of Order in the "Letters" of Pseudo-Dionysius: A Study in the Form and Meaning of the Pseudo-Dionysian Writings* (The Hague: Nijhoff, 1969).

Hatto, A.T. "An Introduction to a Second Reading," in Wolfram von Eschenbach, *Parzival* (Harmondsworth: Penguin, 1980), pp. 412-438.

Hatto, A.T. "Herzeloyde's Dragon-Dream," *German Life and Letters*, vol. 22, no. 1 (October 1968), 16-31.

Hauck, Dennis William. *The Emerald Tablet: Alchemy for Personal Transformation* (New York: Penguin/Arkana, 1999).

Haug, Walter. "Die Symbolstruktur des höfischen Epos und ihre Auflösung bei Wolfram von Eschenbach," *Deutsche Virteljahrsschrift für Literaturwissenschaft und Geistesgeschichte*, vol. 45 (1971), 668-705.

Hegel, G.W.F. *Aesthetics: Lectures on Fine Art*, trans. T.M. Knox, 2 vols (Oxford: Clarendon Press, 1975).

Hegel, G.W.F. *Lectures on the Philosophy of Religion: One-Volume Edition: The Lectures of 1827*, ed. Peter C. Hodgson, trans. Robert F. Brown, Peter C. Hodgson, and J. Michael Stewart (Oxford: Clarendon Press, 2006).

Hegel, G.W.F. *Philosophie der Kunst oder Ästhetik: Nach Hegel. Im Sommer 1826: Mitschrift. Friedrich Carl Hermann – Victor von Kehler*, ed. Annemarie Gethmann-Siefert et al. (Munich: Fink, 2004).

Hegel, G.W.F. *Preface and Introduction to the Phenomenology of Mind*, ed. Lawrence S. Stepelevich (New York and London: Macmillan, 1990).

Hegel, G.W.F. *Texts and Commentary: Hegel's Preface to His System in a New Translation*, ed. and trans. Walter Kaufmann (Notre Dame, IN: University of Notre Dame Press, 1977).

Heidegger, Martin. *Being and Time* [1929], trans. John Macquarrie and Edward Robinson (Oxford: Blackwell, 1962).

Heinzle, Joachim (ed.). *Wolfram von Eschenbach: Ein Handbuch*, 2 vols in 1 [vol. 1, *Autor Werk, Wirkung*; vol. 2, *Figuren-Lexikon, Beschreibendes Verzeichnis der Handschriften, Bibliographien, Register, Abbildungen*] (Berlin and Boston: de Gruyter, 2011).

Helmig, Christoph. "Plutarch of Chaeronea and Porphyry on Transmigration: Who Is the Author of Stobaeus I 445.14-448.3 (W.-H.)?", *The Classical Quarterly* [NS], vol. 58, no. 1 (May 2008), 250-255.

Hermias. *On Plato: Phaedrus 227A-245E*, trans. Dirk Baltzly and Michael Share (London: Bloomsbury, 2019).

Hicks, Stephen R.C. *Explaining Postmodernism: Skepticism and Socialism from Rousseau to Foucault* (Tempe, AZ and New Berlin/Milwaukee, WI: Scholargy Publishing, 2004).

Hill, David Finnemore. *An Archer Looks at the Bible: A Study of the Literal and Figurative Allusions to the Bow and Arrow* (Durham: Pentland Press, 1994).

Hollinrake, Roger. *Nietzsche, Wagner, and the Philosophy of Pessimism* (London: Allen & Unwin, 1982).

Holmyard, Eric J. "The Emerald Table," *Nature*, 112 (6 October 1923), 525-526.

Holznagel, Franz-Josef. "Die Lieder," in Joachim Heinzle (ed.), *Wolfram von Eschenbach: Ein Handbuch* (Berlin and Boston: de Gruyter, 2011), pp. 83-143.

Homans, Peter. *Jung in Context: Modernity and the Making of a Psychology* (Chicago and London: University of Chicago Press, 1979).

Homer. *The Odyssey*, ed. and trans. Albert Cook, 2nd edn (New York and London: Norton, 1993).

Horace. *Satires, Epistles, and Ars Poetica*, trans. H. Rushton Fairclough (London; Cambridge, MA: Heinemann; Harvard University Press, 1926).

Horapollo. *The Hieroglyphics of Horapollo*, trans. George Boas [1950] (Princeton, NJ: Princeton University Press, 1993).

Houlgate, Stephen. "Hegel's Aesthetics," in *Stanford Encyclopedia of Philosophy*, online https://plato.stanford.edu/entries/hegel-aesthetics/.

Hugh of St. Victor. *The Didascalicon of Hugh of St Victor: A Medieval Guide to the Arts*, trans. Jerome Taylor (New York and London: Columbia University Press, 1961).

Huxley, Aldous. *The Perennial Philosophy* (London: Chatto & Windus, 1947).

Introvigne, Massimo. "Grail Traditions in Western Esotericism," in Wouter J. Hanegraaff et al. (eds), *Dictionary of Gnosis & Western Esotericism* (Leiden and Boston: Brill, 2006), pp. 416-418.

Jaeger, Werner. *Paideia: The Ideals of Greek Culture*, vol. 1, *Archaic Greece: The Mind of Athens*, trans. Gilbert Highet, 2nd edn (New York and Oxford: Oxford University Press, 1965)

Jaffé, Aniela. "Alchemy," in *From the Life and Work of C.G. Jung* [1968], trans. R.F.C. Hull and Murray Stein [1971] (Einsiedeln: Daimon Verlag, 1989), pp. 46-77.

Jaffé, Aniela. *Streiflichter zu Leben und Denken C.G. Jungs* (Einsiedeln: Daimon Verlag, 2021).

Jefferson, Ann and David Robey. *Modern Literary Theory: A Comparative Introduction* (London: Batsford, 1986).

Johnson, Robert A. *He: Understanding Masculine Psychology: Based on the Legend of Parsifal and His Search for the Grail, Using*

Jungian Psychological Concepts (New York: Harper & Row, 1974).

Jones, Martin H. and Timothy McFarland (eds). *Wolfram's "Willehalm": Fifteen Essays* (Rochester, NY, and Woodbridge: Camden House, 2002).

Jong, H.M.E. de (ed.). *Michael Meier's Atalanta Fugiens: Sources of an Alchemical Book of Emblems* [1969] (York Beach, ME: Nicolas-Hays, 2002).

Jonsson, Ann Katrin. *Relations: Ethics and the Modernist Subject in James Joyce's "Ulysses," Virginia Woolf's "The Waves" and Djuna Barnes's "Nightwood"* (Oxford: Lang, 2006).

Jubber, Nicholas. *The Prester Quest* (London: Doubleday, 2005).

Jung, Andreas. "The Grandfather," *Journal of Analytical Psychology*, 56 (2011), 653-673.

Jung, C.G. and Victor White. *The Jung-White Letters*, ed. Ann Conrad Lammers and Adrian Cunningham (London and New York: Routledge, 2007).

Jung, C.G. and Wolfgang Pauli. *Atom and Archetype: The Pauli/ Jung Letters, 1932-1958*, ed. C.A. Meier, trans. David Roscoe (Princeton, NJ, and Oxford: Princeton University Press, 2001).

Jung, C.G. *Civilization in Transition* [*Collected Works of C.G. Jung*, vol. 10], trans. R.F.C. Hull, 2nd edn (London and New York: Routledge, 1970).

Jung, C.G. *Dream Analysis: Notes of the Seminar Given in 1928-1930*, ed. William McGuire (London: Routledge & Kegan Paul, 1984).

Jung, C.G. *Dream Symbols of the Individuation Process: Notes of C.G. Jung's Seminars on Wolfgang Pauli's Dreams*, ed. Suzanne

Gieser (Princeton, NJ, and Oxford: Princeton University Press, 2019).

Jung, C.G. *Mysterium Coniunctionis: An Inquiry into the Separation and Synthesis of Psychic Opposites in Alchemy* [*Collected Works of C.G. Jung*, vol. 14], trans. R.F.C. Hull, 2nd edn. Princeton, NJ: Princeton University Press, 1970).

Jung, C.G. *Psychological Types* [*Collected Works of C.G. Jung*, vol. 6], rev. R.F.C. Hull of trans. H.G. Baynes (Princeton, NJ: Princeton University Press, 1976).

Jung, C.G. *Psychology and Alchemy* [*Collected Works of C.G. Jung*, vol. 12], trans. R.F.C. Hull, 2nd edn (London: Routledge, 1968).

Jung, C.G. *The Spirit in Man, Art, and Literature* [*Collected Works of C.G. Jung*, vol. 15], trans. R.F.C. Hull (London: Routledge & Kegan Paul, 1966).

Jung, C.G. *Visions: Notes of the Seminar given in 1930-1934*, ed. Claire Douglas, 2 vols (London: Routledge, 1998).

Jung, Emma and Marie-Louise von Franz, *The Grail Legend* [1960], trans. Andrea Dykes (Boston: London: Sigo Press; Coventure, 1986).

Jung, Emma and Marie-Louise von Franz. *Die Graalslegende in psychologischer Sicht* (Zurich: Publications of the C.G. Jung Institute, 1960).

Kahane, Henry and Renée with Angelina Pietrangeli. *The Krater and the Grail: Hermetic Sources of the "Parzival"* (Urbana, IL: University of Illinois Press, 1965).

Kahane, Henry and Renée. "The Grail," in *Encyclopedia of Religion*, general ed. Mircea Eliade (New York and London: Macmillan, 1987), vol. 6, pp. 89-94.

Kahane, Henry and Renée. *Magic and Gnosticism in the "Chanson de Roland"* (Oakland, CA: University of California Press, 1959).

Kahane, Henry and Renée. "Wolframs Gral und Wolframs Kyot," *Zeitschrift für deutsches Altertum und deutsche Literatur*, 89 (1958-1959), 191-213.

Kahn, Charles H. *The Art and Thought of Heraclitus* (Cambridge: Cambridge University Press, 1979).

Kaltenbrunner, Gerd-Klaus. *Johannes ist sein Name: Priesterkönig, Gralshüter, Traumgestalt* (Zug/Schweiz: Die Graue Edition, 1993).

Katsen, Ingrid and Volker Mertens, "Aventure (âventiure)," in *Lexikon des Mittelalters* (LexMA), vol. 1 (Munich and Zurich: Artemis & Winkler, 1980), cols. 1289-1290.

Kelen, Jacqueline. *L'Éternel masculin: Traité de chevalerie à l'usage des hommes d'aujourd'hui* (Paris: Robert Laffont, 1994).

Kibler, William W. (ed.). *The Lancelot-Grail Cycle: Text and Transformations* (Austin: University of Texas Press, 1994).

Kinderman, William and Katherine R. Syer. *A Companion to Wagner's "Parsifal"* (Rochester, NY, and Woodbridge: Camden House, 2005).

Kingsley, Peter. *Catafalque: Carl Jung and the End of Humanity*, 2 vols (London: Catafalque Press, 2018).

Kirchweger, Franz (ed.). *Die Heilige Lanze in Wien: Insignie – Reliquie – Schicksalsspeer* (Vienna: Kunsthistorisches Museum, 2005).

Kirsch, Jean and Murray Stein (eds). *How and Why We Still Read Jung: Personal and Professional Reflections* (London and New York: Routledge, 2013).

Kittler, Friedrich A. *The Truth of the Technological World: Essays on the Genealogy of Presence* [2013], trans. Erik Butler (Stanford, CA: Stanford University Press, 2014).

Knight, Gareth. *Experience of the Inner Worlds: A Course in Christian Qabalistic Magic* (Cheltenham: Helios Book Service, 1975; Skylight Press, 2010).

Knight, Gareth. *The Secret Tradition in Arthurian Legend: The Archetypal Themes, Images and Characters of the Arthurian Cycle and the Place in the Western Magical Tradition* (Wellingborough: Aquarian Press, 1983).

Kranz, Margarita Kranz. "Sorge," in *Historisches Wörterbuch der Philosophie*, ed. Joachim Ritter and Karlfried Gründer, vol. 9 (Basel: Schwabe, 1995), cols. 1086-1090.

Kroll, Josef. *Beiträge zum Descensus ad Inferos* (Königsberg: Hartung, 1922).

Kroll, Josef. *Gott und Hölle: Der Mythos vom Descensuskampfe* (Leipzig and Berlin: Teubner, 1932; reprinted 1963).

Krueger, Roberta L. (ed.). *The Cambridge Companion to Medieval Romance* (Cambridge and New York: Cambridge University Press, 2000).

Kuhn, Hugo. *Tristan, Nibelungenlied, Artusstruktur* [*Bayerische Akademie der Wissenschaften, Philosophisch-historische Klasse, Sitzungsberichte*, vol. 5] (Munich: Verlag der Bayerischen Akademie der Wissenschaften, 1973).

Kunitzsch, Paul. "Die Planetennamen im 'Parzival,'" *Zeitschrift für deutsche Sprache*, 25 (1969), 169-174).

Lacan, Jacques. *The Seminar of Jacques Lacan, Book III: The Psychoses, 1955-1956*, ed. Jacques-Alain Miller, trans. Russell Grigg (New York; London: Norton, 1993).

Lamberton, Robert. *Homer the Theologian: Neoplatonist Allegorical Reading and the Growth of the Epic Tradition* (Berkeley, Los Angeles, and London: University of California Press, 1986).

Lammers, Ann Conrad. *In God's Shadow: The Collaboration of Victor White and C.G. Jung* (New York and Mahwah, NJ: Paulist Press, 1994).

Lancy, Norris J. and Joan Tasker Grimbert (eds). *A Companion to Chrétien de Troyes* (Cambridge: D.S. Brewer, 2005).

Lange, Hans-Jürgen. *Otto Rahn und die Suche nach dem Graal* (Engerda: Arun, 1999).

Layard, John. *A Celtic Quest: Sexuality and Soul in Individuation*, ed. by Anne S. Bosch (Dallas, TX: Spring Publications, 1985).

Le Saux, F.H.M. *A Companion to Wace* (Cambridge: D.S. Brewer, 2005).

Leisegang, Hans. "Das Mysterium der Schlange: Ein Beitrag zur Erforschung des griechischen Mysterienkultes und seines Fortlebens in der christlichen Welt (mit 14 Illustrationen)," *Eranos-Jahrbuch*, 9 (1939), 151-250.

Leisegang, Hans. "The Mystery of the Serpent," in *The Mysteries* [*Papers from the Eranos Yearbooks*, vol. 2], ed. Joseph Campbell (Princeton, NJ: Princeton University Press, 1955), pp. 194-260.

Levinas, Emmanuel. "La trace de l'autre," in *En découvrant l'existence avec Husserl et Heidegger* (Paris: Vrin, 1974), pp. 187-202.

Littleton, C. Scott and Linda A. Malcor. *From Scythia to Camelot: A Radical Reassessment of the Legends of King Arthur, the Knights of the Round Table, and the Holy Grail* [1994] (New York and Abingdon: Routledge, 2000).

Loeb, Paul S. and David F. Tinsley. "Translators' Afterword," in *Unpublished Fragments from the Period of "Thus Spoke Zarathustra" (Summer 1882 – Winter 1883/84)*, trans. Paul S. Loeb and David F. Tinsley [*Complete Works of Friedrich Nietzsche*, vol. 14] (Stanford, CA: Stanford University Press, 2019), pp. 717-797.

Loewenstein, E.A. "The Freudian Case History: A Detective Story or a Dialectical Progression? Reflections on Psychoanalytic Narratives from a Lacanian Perspective," *Psychoanalytic Psychology*, vol. 9, no. 1 (1992), 49-59.

Loomis, Roger Sherman. *The Grail: From Celtic Myth to Christian Symbol* (Princeton, NJ: Princeton University Press, 1991).

Lowell, James Russell. *The Vision of Sir Launfal* (Cambridge, MA: George Nichols, 1848).

Lucretius. *De rerum natura*, trans. W.H.D. Rouse, revised Martin Ferguson Smith (Cambridge, MA; London: Harvard University Press, 1992).

Lupack, Alan. *The Oxford Guide to Arthurian Literature and Legend* (Oxford and New York: Oxford University Press, 2005).

Maclellan, Alec. *The Secret of the Spear: The Mystery of the Spear of Longinus* (London: Souvenir Press, 2004).

Mann, Thomas. *Briefe, 1889-1955*, ed. Erika Mann, 3 vols (Frankfurt am Main: Fischer, 1961-1965).

Mann, Thomas. "The Making of *The Magic Mountain*," in *The Magic Mountain*, trans. H.T. Lowe-Porter (London: Secker and Warburg, 1971), pp. 719-729.

Marcel, Gabriel. *Homo Viator: Introduction to a Metaphysic of Hope* [1945], trans. Emma Craufurd (Chicago: Regnery, 1951).

Marcolli, Matilde. *Lumen Naturae: Visions of the Abstract in Art and Mathematics* (Cambridge, MA, and London: MIT Press, 2020).

Marino, John B. *The Grail Legend in Modern Literature* (Cambridge: D.S. Brewer, 2004).

Martensen, Hans Lassen. *Jacob Boehme: His Life and Teaching, or Studies in Theosophy*, trans. T. Rhys Evans (London: Hodder and Stoughton, 1885).

Matthews, Alastair. *The Medieval German "Lohengrin": Narrative Poetics in the Story of the Swan Knight* (Rochester, NY: Camden House, 2016).

Matthews, Caitlín and John Matthews. *Hallowquest: Tarot Magic and the Arthurian Mysteries* (Wellingborough: Aquarian, 1990).

Matthews, Caitlín and John Matthews. *The Arthurian Tarot* (Wellingborough: Aquarian Press, 1990).

Matthews, John. *Gawain: Knight of the Goddess: Restoring an Archetype* (Wellingborough: Aquarian Press, 1990).

Mazzeno, Laurence W. *Alfred Tennyson: A Companion* (Jefferson, NC: McFarland & Company, 2020).

McConnell, Winder. "Otherworlds, Alchemy, Pythagoras, and Jung: Symbols of Transformation in *Parzival*," in Will Hasty (ed.), *A Companion to Wolfram's "Parzival"* (Woodbridge and Rochester, NY: Camden House, 1999), pp. 203-222.

McConnell, Winder. "The Denial of the Anima in *Parzival*," *Quondam et Futurus*, vol. 2, no. 2 (Summer 1992), 28-40.

McDonald, William C. "Wolfram's Grail," *Arthuriana*, vol. 8, no. 1, *The Grail and The Quest* (Spring 1998), 22-34.

McGlathery, James M. "Erotic Love in Chrétien's *Perceval*, Wolfram's *Parzival*, and Wagner's *Parsifal*," in William Kinderman and Katherine R. Syer (eds), *A Companion to Wagner's "Parsifal"* (Rochester, NY, and Woodbridge: Camden House, 2005), pp. 55-79.

McGuire, William and R.F.C. Hull (eds). *C.G. Jung Speaking: Interviews and Encounters* (Princeton, NJ: Princeton University Press, 1977).

McGuire, William. "Firm Affinities: Jung's Relation with Britain and the United States," *Journal of Analytical Psychology*, 40 (1995), 301-326.

Mergell, Bodo. *Der Gral in Wolframs Parzival: Entstehung und Ausbildung der Gralsage im Hochmittelalter* (Halle (Saale): Niemeyer, 1952).

Michel de Montaigne. *The Complete Essays*, ed. and trans. M.A. Screech (Harmondsworth: Penguin, 2003).

Miller, Jeanine. "Holy Vessel, Holy Grail," *The Theosophist*, October 1989, 18-24.

Monier-Williams, Sir Monier. *A Sanskrit-English Dictionary: Etymologically and Philologically arranged with special reference to Cognate Indo-European Languages* (Oxford: Clarendon Press, 1899).

Morgan, Giles. *The Holy Grail* (Harpenden: Pocket Essentials, 2005).

Morgan, Peter. *The Critical Idyll: Traditional Values and the French Revolution in Goethe's "Hermann und Dorothea"* (Columbia, SC: Camden House, 1990).

Mosmann, Heinz. *Der "Parzival" Wolframs von Eschenbach: Erkenntnis und imaginative Gestaltung des Gralsmysteriums* (Stuttgart: Verlag Freies Geistesleben, 2020).

Murphy, G. Ronald, SJ. *Gemstone of Paradise: The Holy Grail in Wolfram's "Parzival"* (New York: Oxford University Press, 2006).

Murray, Gilbert. *Five Stages of Greek Religion* [[3]1955] (Mineola, NY: Dover, 2002).

Nagy, Gregory. *The Ancient Greek Hero in 24 Hours* (Cambridge, MA, and London: Belknap Press of Harvard University Press, 2013).

Nakajima, Tatsuhiro. "Psychology of the 12th Century Renaissance in Wolfram von Eschenbach's *Parzival*," *Studia Hermetica Journal*, vol. 8, no. 1 ("Hermetism and the Underworld") (2018), 23-40.

Nellmann, Eberhard. "Lapsit exillis? Jaspis exillix?: Die Lesarten der Handschriften," *Zeitschrift für deutsche Philologie*, vol. 119, no. 3 (2000), 416-420.

Nietzsche, Friedrich. *Basic Writings*, ed. and trans. Walter Kaufmann (New York: Modern Library, 1968).

Nietzsche, Friedrich. *The Gay Science*, ed. and trans. Walter Kaufmann (New York: Vintage Books, 1974).

Nitze, William A. "The Fisher King in the Grail Romances," *Publications of the Modern Language Association of America*, vol. 24, no. 3 (1909), 365-418.

Nitze, William A. "Who was the Fisher King: A Note on Halieutics," *Romanic Review*, vol. 33, no. 2 (April 1947), 97-104.

Noll, Richard. *The Aryan Christ: The Secret Life of Carl Jung* (New York: Random House, 1997).

Nordenhaug, Karin Elizabeth. *The symbolism of the Grail: A comparative analysis of the Grail in "Perceval ou Le Conte del Graal" by Chretien de Troyes and "Parzival" by Wolfram von*

Eschenbach. BA Thesis, Westhampton College, University of Richmond, 1962. Available HTTP: https://scholarship.richmond.edu/honors-theses/1077.

O'Sharkey, Eithne M. "The Maimed Kings in the Arthurian Romances," *Etudes Celtiques*, vol. 8, no. 2 (1959), 420-428.

Olympiodorus. *Commentary on Plato's "Gorgias": Translated with Full Notes*, trans. Robert Jackson, Kimon Lycos, and Harold Tarrant (Leiden: Brill, 1998).

Onfray, Michel. *La Résistance au nihilisme* [*Contre-histoire de la philosophie*, vol. 12] (Paris: Grasset, 2020).

Owen, D.D.R. "Introduction," in Chrétien de Troyes, *Arthurian Romances*, trans. D.D.R. Owen (London: Dent, 1987), pp. ix-xviii.

Pagel, Walter. *Paracelsus: An Introduction to Philosophical Medicine in the Era of the Renaissance*, 2nd edn (Basel: Karger, 1982).

Paracelsus. "Caput de morbis somnii," in *Sämtliche Werke*, ed. Karl Sudhoff and Wilhelm Matthiessen, section 1, *Medizinische, naturwissenschaftliche und philosophische Schriften*, 14 vols (Munich and Berlin: Oldenbourg, 1922-1933), vol. 9, pp. 359-362.

Paracelsus. *Essential Readings*, ed. Nicholas Goodrick-Clarke (Berkeley, CA: North Atlantic Books, 1999).

Paracelsus. *Essential Theoretical Writings*, ed. and trans. Andrew Weeks (Leiden and Boston: Brill, 2008).

Paracelsus. *Selected Writings*, ed. Jolande Jacobi (Princeton, NJ: Princeton University Press, 1979).

Paracelsus. *Astronomia magna*, in *Sämtliche Werke*, ed. Karl Sudhoff and Wilhelm Matthiessen, section 1, *Medizinische, naturwissenschaftliche und philosophische Schriften*, 14 vols

(Munich and Berlin: Oldenbourg, 1922-1933), vol. 12, pp. 1-444.

Paracelsus. *Das Buch Paragranum*, ed. Franz Strunz (Leipzig: Diederichs, 1903).

Paracelsus. *De nymphis*, in *Sämtliche Werke*, ed. Karl Sudhoff and Wilhelm Matthiessen, section 1, *Medizinische, naturwissenschaftliche und philosophische Schriften*, 14 vols (Munich and Berlin: Oldenbourg, 1922-1933), vol. 14, pp. 115-151.

Paracelsus. *Labyrinthus medicorum errantium* [1537/1538], in *Sämtliche Werke*, ed. Karl Sudhoff and Wilhelm Matthiessen, section 1, *Medizinische, naturwissenschaftliche und philosophische Schriften*, 14 vols (Munich and Berlin: Oldenbourg, 1922-1933), vol. 11, pp. 161-221.

Paracelsus. *Liber Azoth*, in *Philosophi et Medici Opera Bücher und Schrifften*, ed. Johannes Huser, 2 vols (Strasbourg: Zetzner, 1603-1616), vol. 2, pp. 519-543.

Pascal, Blaise. *Œuvres complètes*, ed. Louis Lafuma (Paris: Seuil, 1963).

Pascal, Blaise. *Pensées*, trans A.J. Krailsheimer (Harmondsworth: Penguin, 1966).

Peck, John. "Introduction," in C.G. Jung, *Dream Interpretation Ancient & Modern: Notes from the Seminar Given in 1936-1941*, ed. John Peck, Lorenz Jung, and Maria Meyer-Grass, trans. Ernst Falzeder with Tony Woolfson (Princeton, NJ, and Oxford: Princeton University Press, 2014), pp. xxi-lii.

Pennick, Nigel. *Sacred Geometry: Symbolism and Purpose in Religious Structures* (Wellingborough: Turnstone Press, 1980).

Pickens, Rupert T. "*Le Conte du Graal*: Chrétien's Unfinished Last Romance," in Norris J. Lacy and Joan Tasker Grimbert (eds), *A Companion to Chrétien de Troyes* (Cambridge: D.S. Brewer, 2005), pp. 169-187.

Pieper, Josef. *The Platonic Myths*, trans. Dan Farrelly (South Bend, IN: St Augustine's Press, 2011).

Pinion, F.B. *A Tennyson Companion: Life and Works* (Basingstoke: Macmillan Press, 1984).

Plato. *The Republic*, ed. and trans. Allan Bloom (New York: Basic Books, 1991).

Plato. *The Laws*, ed. and trans. Thomas L. Pangle (Chicago and London: University of Chicago Press, 1988).

Plato. *Works*, vol. 5, *Lysis; Symposium; Gorgias*, trans. W.R.M. Lamb (London; New York: Heinemann; Putnam, 1925).

Plotinus, *The Six Enneads*, trans. Stephen MacKenna and B.S. Page (Chicago and London: Encyclopedia Britannica, 1955).

Plotinus. *Porphyry on Plotinus; Ennead I*, trans. A.H. Armstrong (Cambridge, MA, and London: Harvard University Press, 1995).

Plotinus. *The Essential Plotinus: Representative Treatises from the Enneads*, ed. and trans. Elmer O'Brien, SJ (Indianapolis, IN: Hackett, 1964).

Porphyry, *On the Homeric Cave of the Nymphs*, in Porphyry, *Select Works*, ed. and trans. Thomas Taylor [TTS, vol. 2] (Westbury: Prometheus Trust, 1999), pp. 145-161.

Porphyry, *Select Works*, ed. and trans. Thomas Taylor [TTS, vol. 2] (Westbury: Prometheus Trust, 1999).

Proclus. *Commentary on Plato's "Parmenides,"* trans. Glenn R. Morrow and John M. Dillon, ed. John M. Dillon (Princeton, NJ: Princeton University Press, 1987).

Proclus. *Commentary on the First Book of Euclid's "Elements,"* trans. Thomas Taylor [TTS, vol. 19] (Sturminster Newton: Prometheus Trust, 2006).

Proclus. *On Plato Cratylus*, ed. and trans. Brian Duvick and Harold Tarrant (London and New York: Bloomsbury, 2007).

Proclus. *Commentary on Plato's "Republic,"* vol. 1, *Essays 1-6*, ed. and trans. Dirk Baltzly, John F. Finamore, and Graeme Miles (Cambridge and New York: Cambridge University Press, 2018).

Proclus. *Commentary on Plato's "Timaeus,"* vol 2, *Book 2: Proclus on the Causes of the Cosmos and its Creation*, trans. David T. Runia and Michael Share (New York: Cambridge University Press, 2008).

Proclus. *Proclus the Successor on Poetics and the Homeric Poems: Essays 5 and 6 of His "Commentary on the Republic of Plato,"* ed. and trans. Robert Lamberton (Atlanta, GA: Society of Biblical Literature, 2012).

Pseudo-Dionysius. *The Complete Works*, trans. Colm Luibheid, ed. Paul Rorem (New York and Mahwah, NJ: Paulist Press, 1987).

Rahn, Otto. *Kreuzzug gegen den Gral: Die Geschichte der Albigenser* [1933] (Engerda: Arun, 2000).

Ramm, Ben. "Locating Narrative Authority in *Perlesvaus: Le Haut Livre du Graal*," in *Arthurian Literature XII*, ed. Keith Busby and Roger Dalrymple (Cambridge: D.S. Brewer, 2005), pp. 1-19.

Rank, Otto. *The Myth of the Birth of the Hero and Other Writings*, ed. Philip Freund (New York: Knopf, 1959).

Ravenscroft, Trevor. *The Spear of Destiny: The Occult Power Behind the Spear which Pierced the Side of Christ* [1973] (Boston, MA; York Beach, ME: Weiser Books, 1982).

Reichert, Joachim. "'Slaying the Dragon': Der letzte Heilversuch an Anfortas im 'Parzival' Wolframs von Eschenbach (483, 6-18)," *Mediaevistik*, 14 (2001), 149-178.

Richey, Margaret F. "Ither von Gaheviez," *The Modern Language Review*, vol. 26, no. 3 (July 1931), 315-329.

Richey, Margaret F. "The 'Titurel' of Wolfram von Eschenbach: Structure and Character," *The Modern Language Review*, vol. 56, no. 2 (April 1961), 180-193.

Rieff, Philip. *The Triumph of the Therapeutic: Uses of Faith After Freud* (Harmondsworth: Penguin, 1973)

Robert de Boron. *Merlin and the Grail: Joseph of Arimathea, Merlin, Perceval*, trans. Nigel Bryant (Cambridge: D.S. Brewer, 2001).

Robertson, Ritchie. *Mock-Epic Poetry from Pope to Heine* (New York: Oxford University Press, 2009).

Rolfe, Eugene. *Encounter with Jung* (Boston: Sigo Press, 1989).

Rosenkranz, Karl [trans. D.J. Snider]. "Second Part of Goethe's Faust," *The Journal of Speculative Philosophy*, vol. 1, no. 2 (1867), 65-79.

Sanderson, Richard A. "Wounded Masculinity," available HTTP https://www.camilogallardo.com/index.php/resources/wounded-masculinity (accessed 19 February 2024).

Sauvage, Micheline. *L'Aventure philosophique* (Paris: Buchet-Chastel, 1966).

Schiller, Friedrich. *Essays*, ed. Walter Hinderer and Daniel O. Dahlstrom (New York: Continuum, 2005).

Schiller, Friedrich. *On the Aesthetic Education of Humankind* [1794], ed. and trans. Elizabeth M. Wilkinson and L.A. Willoughby (Oxford: Clarendon Press, 1982).

Schiller, Friedrich. *Über naïve und sentimentalische Dichtung* [1795-1796], ed. William F. Mainland (Oxford: Blackwell, 1957).

Schlesier, Renate. "KRATĒR. The Mixing-Vessel as Metaphorical Space in Ancient Greek Tradition," in Fabian Horn and Cilliers Breytenbach (eds.), *Spatial Metaphors. Ancient Texts and Transformations* (Berlin: Edition Topoi, 2016), pp. 69-84.

Schult, Arthur. *Die Weltsendung des Heiligen Gral im Parzival des Wolfram von Eschenbach* (Bietigheim-Bissingen: Turm-Verlag, 1975).

Schwietering, Julius. "Einwürkung der Antike auf die Entstehung des frühen deutschen Minnesangs" [1924], in *Philologische Schriften*, ed. Friedrich Ohly and Max Wehrli (Munich: Fink, 1969), pp. 237-253.

Shamdasani, Sonu. *C.G. Jung: A Biography in Books* (New York and London: Norton 2012).

Shamdasani, Sonu. *Cult Fictions: C.G. Jung and the Founding of Analytical Psychology* (London and New York: Routledge, 1998).

Shklovsky, Viktor. "Stern's *Tristram Shandy*: Stylistic Commentary," in Lee T. Lemon and Marion J. Reis (eds), *Russian Formalist Criticism: Four Essays* (Lincoln, NB: University of Nebraska Press, 1965), pp. 25-57.

Siebert, Johannes. "*Ecidemôn*," *Journal for German Philology*, 62 (1937), 248-264.

Sperber, Hans. "*lapsit exillis* und *sarapandratest*," *Zeitschrift für deutsches Altertum und deutsche Literatur*, vol. 87, no. 4 (1957), 270-275.

Spinoza, Benedict de. *On the Improvement of the Understanding; The Ethics; Correspondence* [*Works*, vol. 2], trans. R.H.M. Elwes (New York: Dover, 1955).

Steele, Robert and Dorothea Waley Singer. "The Emerald Table," *Proceedings of the Royal Society of Medicine*, vol. 21, no. 3 (January 1928), 485-501.

Stein, W.J. *The Ninth Century and the Holy Grail* [1928], trans. Irene Groves, revised John M. Wood (Forest Row: Temple Lodge Publishing, 2009).

Steiner, Rudolf. *The Mysteries of Initiation: From Isis to the Holy Grail* [*Collected Works*, vol. 144] (Forest Row: Rudolf Steiner Press, 2021).

Steiner, Rudolf. *The Holy Grail: The Quest for the Renewal of the Mysteries: Selections from the Work of Rudolf Steiner*, trans. revised by Christian von Arnim (Forest Row: Sophia Books, 2001).

Steiner, Rudolf. *The Mysteries of the Holy Grail: From Arthur and Parzival to Modern Initiation*, ed. and trans. Matthew Barton (Forest Row: Rudolf Steiner Press, 2010).

Stevens, Adrian. "Fiction, Plot and Discourse: Wolfram's *Parzival* and its Narrative Sources," in Will Hasty (ed.), *A Companion to Wolfram's "Parzival"* (Rochester, NY, and Woodbridge: Camden House, 1999), pp. 99-123.

Stewart, J.A. (trans.). *The Myths of Plato* (London: Macmillan, 1905).

Strassler, Robert B. (ed.). *The Landmark Herodotus: The Histories* (London: Quercus, 2008).

Stutley, Margaret and James. *A Dictionary of Hinduism: Its Mythology, Folklore and Development, 1500 B.C.-A.D. 1500* (London and Henley: Routledge & Kegan Paul, 1977).

Tatar, Maria. *The Heroine with a 1001 Faces* (New York: Liveright, 2022).

Taylor, Thomas. "Additional Notes on the *Gorgias*," in Plato, *Works*, vol. 4, trans. Thomas Taylor and Floyer Sydenham [TTS, vol. 12] (Westbury: Prometheus Trust, 1996), pp. 421-431.

Taylor, Thomas. "End Notes" to *On the Homeric Cave of the Nymphs*, in Porphyry, *Select Works*, ed. and trans. Thomas Taylor [TTS, vol. 2] (Westbury: Prometheus Trust, 1999), pp. 162-167.

Taylor, Thomas. "Extracts from the MS. Scholia of Proclus on the *Cratylus*," in Plato, *Works*, vol. 5, trans. Thomas Taylor and Floyer Sydenham [TTS, vol. 13] (Westbury: Prometheus Trust, 1996), pp. 542-614.

Taylor, Thomas. "The History of the Restoration of the Platonic Theology by the Later Platonists," in *Oracles and Mysteries* [TTS, vol. 7] (Frome: Prometheus Trust, 2001), pp. 129-244.

Taylor, Thomas. "The Wanderings of Ulysses," in Porphyry, *Select Works*, ed. and trans. Taylor [TTS, vol. 2] (Westbury: Prometheus Trust, 1999), pp. 201-224.

Temkin, Oswei. "The Elusiveness of Paracelsus," *Bulletin of the History of Medicine*, vol. 26, no. 3 (May-June 1952), 201-217.

Tennyson, Alfred Lord. *Tennyson: A Selected Edition*, ed. Christopher Ricks (Harlow: Longman, 1989).

Tether, Leah and Johnny McFadyen, with Keith Busby and Ad Putter (eds). *Handbook of Arthurian Romance: King Arthur's Court in Medieval European Literature* (Berlin and Boston: de Gruyter, 2017).

Thomas, Edward J. *The History of Buddhist Thought* (London: Routledge & Kegan Paul, 1833).

Thomas, Neil. "Wolfram von Eschenbach: Modes of Narrative Presentation," in Will Hasty (ed.), *A Companion to Wolfram's "Parzival"* (Woodbridge and Rochester, NY: Camden House, 1999), pp. 124-139.

Thompson, Stith. *Motif-Index of Folk-Literature*, revised edn, 6 vols (Bloomington, IN: Indiana University Press, 1955-1958).

Tilton, Hereward. *The Quest for the Phoenix: Spiritual Alchemy and Rosicrucianism in the Work of Count Michael Maier (1569-1622)* (Berlin and New York: de Gruyter, 2003).

Todorov, Tzvetan. *Grammaire du Décameron* (The Hague: Mouton, 1969).

Unger, Max. "The Persian Origins of 'Parsifal' and 'Tristan,'" *The Musical Times*, 73, no. 1074, (1 August 1932), 703-770.

Veltman, Willem Frederik. *The Temple and the Grail: The Mysteries of the Order of the Templars and the Grail and their Significance for Our Time* [^{2}1992], trans. Philip Mees (Forest Row: Temple Lodge Publishing, 2021).

Vergely, Bertrand. *Boulevard des philosophes: De la Renaissance à aujourd'hui* (Paris: Milan, 2005).

Vergely, Bertrand. *Notre vie a un sens!* (Paris: Albin Michel 2019).

Vergely, Bertrand. *Pascal ou l'expérience de l'infini* (Paris: Milan, 2007).

Vieira, Celso. "Heraclitus' Bow Composition," *Classical Quarterly*, vol. 63, no. 2 (2013), 473-490.

Virgil. *Works*, vol. 4, trans. John Dryden (London: Bathurst, 1782).

Wace and Layamon. *Arthurian Chronicles*, trans. Eugene Mason (London and Melbourne: Dent, 1962).

Wagner, Richard. *Das braune Buch: Tagebuchaufzeichnungen 1865 bis 1882*, ed. Joachim Bergfeld (Zurich and Freiburg im Breisgau: Atlantis, 1975).

Wagner, Richard. *Sämtliche Schriften und Dichtungen: Volks-Ausgabe*, 16 in 8 vols (Leipzig: Breitkopf & Härtel/Siegel, 1911).

Waite, Arthur Edward (ed.). *The Hermetic Museum*, trans. Arthur Edward Waite, 2 vols (London: Elliot, 1893).

Wansbrough, Henry (general ed.). *The New Jerusalem Bible* (London: Darton, Longman & Todd, 1985).

Warren, Henry Clarke (ed. and trans.). *A Buddhist Reader: Selections from the Sacred Books* [1896; [4]1906] (Mineola, NY: Dover, 2004).

Weber, Clifford. "The Allegory of the Golden Bough," *Vergilius*, vol. 41 (1995), 3-34.

Weber, Gottfried. *Der Gottesbegriff des Parzival* (Frankfurt am Main: Diesterweg, 1935).

Weber, Gottfried. *Parzival, Ringen und Vollendung: Eine dichtungs- und religionsgeschichtliche Untersuchung* (Oberursal: Kompaß-Verlag, 1948).

Weigand, Hermann J. "Die epischen Zeitverhältnisse in den Graldichtungen Chrestiens und Wolframs," *Publications of the Modern Language Association of America*, 54 (1938), 917-950.

Well, Benjamin van. "Sprache der Träume – Sprache der Kultur: Ein multiperspektivischer Blick auf den Traum der Herzeloyde in Wolframs von Eschenbach *Parzival*," in *Literaturstraße: Chinesisch-deutsche Zeitschrift für Sprach- und Literaturwissenschaft*, vol. 21, no. 2 (2020), 39-54.

Whitehead, Alfred North. *Process and Reality: An Essay in Cosmology*, ed. David Ray Griffin and Donald W. Sherburne (New York: The Free Press, 1979).

Willson, H.B. "The Grail King in Wolfram's 'Parzival,'" *The Modern Language Review* vol. 55, no. 4 (October, 1960), 553-563.

Wilson, Colin. *Religion and the Rebel* [1957] (Bath: Ashgrove Press, 1984).

Wilson, Simon. "René Guénon and the Heart of the Grail," *Temenos Academy Review*, 18 (2015), 146-167.

Wolf, Werner. "Der Vogel Phönix und der Gral," in Richard Kienast (ed.), *Studien zur deutschen Philologie des Mittelalters: Friedrich Panzer zum 80. Geburtstag* (Heidelberg: Winter, 1950), pp. 730-795.

Wolfram von Eschenbach. *"Parzival" and "Titurel,"* trans. Cyril Edwards (Oxford and New York: Oxford University Press, 2006).

Wolfram von Eschenbach. *Willehalm*, trans. Marion E. Gibbs and Sidney M. Johnson (Harmondsworth: Penguin, 1984).

Wood, Juliette. *Eternal Chalice: The Enduring Legend of the Holy Grail* (London and New York: Tauris, 2008).

Wood, Kelsey. *Žižek: A Reader's Guide* (Malden, MA: Wiley-Blackwell, 2012).

Wulsin, John. "Parzival — the journey of adolescence," *Renewal: A Journal for Waldorf Education*, vol. 15, no. 1 (Spring-Summer 2006), 3-5.

Wulsin, John. "Parzival — the journey of adolescence" [revised and expanded], *Journal for Waldorf/Rudolf Steiner Education*, 9 (2007), 9-13.

Ziolkowski, John E. "The Bow and the Lyre: Harmonizing Duos in Plato's *Symposium*," *The Classical Journal*, vol. 95, no. 1 (October-November 1999), 19-35.

Žižek, Slavoj. *The Sublime Object of Ideology* (London and New York: Verso, 1989).

Made in the USA
Coppell, TX
05 November 2026

11436091R00229